Praise for *Multiple Sclerosis: Coping With Complications*

"Few books provide advice on medical issues by physicians with extensive clinical and research experience who also suffer from the illness being discussed. This one was written by a compassionate medical expert with 24 years of MS. His advice is based on this unique blend of medical knowledge and personal experience. *Multiple Sclerosis: Coping With Complications* gives practical, tested solutions to common problems. Everybody with MS can benefit from its publication."

William R. Jarvis, MD

"As an epidemiologist, Dr. Farr conducted studies including many patients. After decades of MS, he became a master at studying his own illness to provide new answers (e.g., how to prevent pneumonia despite worsening nervous system damage). This book should help all patients with MS and many with similar problems due to other conditions (e.g., childbirth causes more cases of chronic rectal sphincter laxity than MS does)."

Robert J. Sherertz, MD

Multiple Sclerosis
Coping with Complications

Multiple Sclerosis
Coping with Complications

Barry Farr, MD

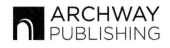

Archway Publishing books may be ordered through booksellers or by contacting:

Archway Publishing
1663 Liberty Drive
Bloomington, IN 47403
www.archwaypublishing.com
1 (888) 242-5904

Because of the dynamic nature of the Internet, any web addresses or
links contained in this book may have changed since publication and
may no longer be valid. The views expressed in this work are solely those
of the author and do not necessarily reflect the views of the publisher,
and the publisher hereby disclaims any responsibility for them.

ISBN: 978-1-4808-2922-0 (sc)
ISBN: 978-1-4808-2923-7 (hc)
ISBN: 978-1-4808-2924-4 (e)

Library of Congress Control Number: 2016941037

Print information available on the last page.

Archway Publishing rev. date: 6/6/2016

DISCLAIMER

A book about health-related issues NEVER takes the place of one's personal physician who will always have the advantage of knowing the patient's personal history, physical examination, laboratory values, etc. Ideas provided by such a book may be very useful, but should always be discussed with one's physician because there can be exceptions to any rule and one's physician is well positioned to know about exceptions applying to an individual patient (e.g., an MS patient who develops renal failure because of obstruction due to a high-pressure spastic bladder may have to do many things different from others).

MS patients are always at risk of something bad happening and must actively choose between a variety of options at every turn. As Robert Frost put it, "Two roads diverged in a yellow wood ... I took the one less traveled by, And that has made all the difference." For example, if an MS patient with hemiparesis rising from a toilet wishes to prevent urine leaking all over everything, she may have to use her only functional hand to do that. But doing that would make it impossible to keep that hand on a grab bar, which would increase the risk for falling. Each patient has to make a choice about which bad outcome she wants to prioritize. If the patient can't rise securely with her more functional leg braced against the toilet, then choosing to focus on preventing urine leakage would be a bad choice as compared with preventing falling. Urine leakage can cause a variety of problems that would have to be addressed as well, but the patient could choose to have a helper assist her with rising from the toilet every time, day and night. There are problems with that choice as well (e.g., expense, lack of privacy, etc). Active choices at every turn make "all the difference," and each patient must accept the consequences of her own choices. Discussing options with one's physician might help to make informed choices.

Dedication

To the millions who have suffered the frustration, indignity and pain of multiple sclerosis.

Contents

Foreword

Every person with multiple sclerosis should read this book. Professor Farr is in the unique position of having been a world renowned authority in epidemiology and infectious diseases before his career was cut short when he himself acquired the disease. In the 24 years of his illness he has used his training and experience as a clinician and investigator and his astute powers of observation to acquire perhaps the most intimate, personal knowledge of multiple sclerosis anyone has had. Accepting that there is yet no cure and that effectiveness of treatment is limited, Dr. Farr has addressed in penetrating detail the various clinical manifestations of this cruel and devastating process and the ways in which they can be mitigated. Multiple sclerosis has not made Dr. Farr a lesser man. Instead, he has discovered clever strategies of self-help and reserves of courage that empowered him through the arduous years of his illness. This knowledge will help readers who have multiple sclerosis or other neurological diseases or injuries causing similar morbidity.

Jack M. Gwaltney, Jr., M.D.
Professor Emeritus
Department of Medicine
University of Virginia

Preface

I NEVER intended to write a book about multiple sclerosis.

But then I never intended to have multiple sclerosis either. Like the way the family cat proudly deposits a dead mouse on your doorstep, life sometimes brings things you don't expect or want.

After many years of suffering with MS, it occurred to me that perhaps I should share some of the things I had learned about how to cope with the disease (for those coming along behind me who haven't had as much time to think about it yet).

Here are a few examples of my strategies for coping that I didn't find in other books about MS: 1) what is the best therapy for excruciatingly painful rib fractures for MS patients who can't tolerate narcotic analgesics (MS patients like me fall a lot and rib fractures are thus a common occurrence); 2) what is the best way to prevent recurrent, painful, pressure-related *Staphylococcus aureus* furuncles in the buttock of a leg being paralyzed by MS? 3) what is the best way to heal such furuncles when the MS patient can no longer tolerate antibiotic therapy because of gastrointestinal side effects and warm moist compresses don't seem to have enough oomph to quite get the job done despite eight weeks of application seven times per day? 4) what is the best way to control feculent odor after MS paralyzes the rectal sphincter making it incontinent for flatus? 5) once an MS patient starts choking on her own saliva, what's the best way to prevent aspiration pneumonia? 6) what is the best way to prevent shearing of the fragile skin on the buttock of a leg being paralyzed by MS? 7) what is the best thing to do after shearing the fragile skin on the buttock of a leg being paralyzed by MS? 8) what is the best way to keep from getting a high fever (and the profound weakness that can go with it – Uhthoff's phenomenon)? 9) most MS patients know about the hazards of heat, but what are its benefits to MS patients? 10) most books about MS recommend conventional medical wisdom for preventing urinary tract infections (e.g. drinking cranberry juice), but MS patients have a high risk of UTIs despite using those measures; is there an approach that works better? 11) why does a crisis of urinary urgency tend to reach maximal **just BEFORE** the MS patient reaches the toilet? 12) can an MS patient control such urgency and its embarrassing consequences without taking medications that make constipation worse? 13) why does taking a medication to control urinary urgency tend to be counterproductive if it makes constipation worse? 14) what is the best liquid to use for swallowing pills when getting up at night repeatedly for nocturia (waking at night to urinate) and why? 15) what is the best way to deal with the yucky taste of the methylprednisolone tablets used for treating MS relapses?

How did I manage to figure such things out?

More about this below, but necessity was an important ally. Necessity is said to be "the mother of invention," and it forced me to find an answer when medical science had no data or inadequate data regarding a problem. For example, recurrent, pressure-related, painful furuncles in the buttock of my increasingly paretic leg were DRIVING ME CRAZY. I kept asking my neurologist what could be done to stop them from happening. She kept saying, "we just don't have any data regarding that yet." So, I ended up thinking about this a lot and finally conducted a comparison between two different alternating air cushions from different companies that had a lot of positive testimonials on an independent website (there were not yet studies in the medical literature regarding the products of either company); my study showed that one worked very well and the other not well at all (more about this later).

I received neighborly help from another MS patient immediately after being hospitalized for my first attack of MS where I was given the diagnosis. I now want to return that favor and "pay it forward" [like in the movie by that name] by giving helpful information to other patients about coping with its complications.

Acknowledgment

It's always appropriate to be thankful at Thanksgiving and often at the beginning of a book, which usually is facilitated by others in one or more ways.

For a patient struggling with the paralytic effects of multiple sclerosis, the help of others becomes paramount. Writing a book is like running a marathon, and MS patients move more like a tortoise than a rabbit. Without the help of my wife and sons, I would not have been able to start writing this book, much less finish it. Without the help of nursing aides who assist me with activities of daily living, I also wouldn't have finished this book. Without the care of my neurologist, this book would not exist.

To help me illustrate how swallowed air can inflate the intestines and create problems in the pelvis of a patient with spastic, frequently unhappy excretory organs (bowel and bladder), Dr. Bruce Hillman, Dr. Alan Matsumoto and Dr. Eduard de Lange kindly provided me with a photograph of an abdominal x-ray. Dr. Robert Sherertz, Dr. William Jarvis, and Dr. Jack Gwaltney read and provided helpful comments on portions of the book. Frank Wood and Celia Wood also read and provided helpful comments on portions of the book.

Introduction

The Reason for This Book

The first question a thoughtful reader might ask will probably be, "why **YET ANOTHER** book about multiple sclerosis?"

Aren't there already many books about MS? Yes, but they're usually academic treatises written by physicians for other physicians.

Well aren't there already other books written by physicians for MS patients? Yes, but this one's different.

How? It's the advice of one MS patient (the author) to another MS patient (the reader) focusing upon common MS problems that go beyond what is usually addressed in an office visit with one's neurologist.

Do all MS patients get the same complications? No, there is a bewildering diversity of possible complications, and no MS patient gets them all. Virtually anything that the brain or spinal cord does can go haywire due to damage from MS (e.g., deafness, blindness, aphonia [inability to make sounds with vocal cords], inability to smell, inability to taste, inability to think, paralysis, numbness, ataxia, imbalance, tremor, dysarthria [difficulty talking], dysphagia [difficulty swallowing], vertigo, etc.). This is one of the reasons that the term "multiple" is so apt for multiple sclerosis. Just as every individual is unique, each MS patient's illness is unique, so what works for one won't necessarily be exactly what works for another. But there is sufficient commonality that MS patients reading about what worked for me will probably get ideas about what might work for them. Sometimes, it may be the same thing or the same thing except for a minor modification.

As stated above, MS is a disease capable of all sorts of disease manifestations, and I won't attempt encyclopedic coverage of all of them. In this book, I'll mainly address complications that I have faced and strategies I developed for dealing with them. An MS attack never made me blind or deaf, so I won't be able to talk about such things. But the problems I have had (e.g., weakness, constipation, spasticity, etc.) tend to be sufficiently common that most MS patients will probably be able to relate. My disease was worse than that of most MS patients (more relapses faster and quicker progression to requiring a cane [12.5 years] and wheelchair [16.4 years] than for the average patient [median 27.9 years among 2,319 patients until needing a cane]), so I've seen more complications than the average patient. [Tremlett H, Paty D, Devonshire V. Disability progression in multiple sclerosis is slower than previously reported. Neurology 2006; 66:172.]

As important as (or more important than) the specific strategies being described in this book is the process being used for devising new strategies as new complications develop. For example, my approach to controlling constipation is in many ways like that described in other books for MS patients (e.g., eating enough fiber, drinking enough fluids, using the proper amount of an osmotic laxative, etc.). But constipation has been a constant problem for me for over 24 years, and I had to modify the approach. Five of the most recent modifications weren't listed in the other books for MS patients and involved a rather different approach (e.g., other books for MS patients often counsel patience with constipation, emphasizing that a bowel movement every three days is adequate). Because constipation has caused multiple other intolerable complications for me, I was unable to view a bowel movement every three days as adequate.

I won't say, "don't try these things at home" because the point of the book is to help the MS patient struggling to cope. But before trying the strategies discussed in this book (or in any other book about MS), it would be best for the patient to discuss a plan with her physician.

Who Is This Book's Intended Audience?

It's primarily meant for MS patients, but those who care for (or care about) MS patients might be interested to read it as well to get a better idea about the "slings and arrows of outrageous fortune" that MS patients have to endure and some practical strategies for coping. Unlike some of the other books written for MS patients, this one's intended for patients who actually have to suffer through the illness because no panacea is actually yet available.

Physicians might find the observations in this book interesting and helpful – some of which I have published in the medical literature (e.g., using an alternating air cushion to prevent pressure-related furuncles in the buttock of a leg being paralyzed by MS) and others I have not (e.g., an "experiment of nature" that led me to conclude that there may be a better way to prevent aspiration pneumonia than the swallowing exercises often advocated).

Although I'm a man, it's important to note that most of the observations in this book are not gender specific (i.e., almost all of the strategies should be as useful to women as they are to men). For example, what I do for preventing aspiration pneumonia should work equally well for a woman.

As mentioned, this book is mostly about things that I figured out about coping with complications, but if my neurologist or someone else suggested an approach that worked well, I will share that as well since some of those approaches worked much better than others. For example, when I developed intolerable pain in a torn rotator cuff, I learned about the need to rest the shoulder from reading abstracts of some medical studies, but my wife suggested calming the inflammation with a brief course of methylprednisolone, which worked much faster than simple rest. When I first was embarrassed by loss of control of flatus, my neurologist recommended something that worked perfectly for the next 12 years despite progressive worsening of my MS-related bowel problems.

All progress in science is incremental, depending upon prior knowledge gathered by others. As Isaac Newton put it, "If I have seen further, it is by standing upon the shoulders of giants."

How This Book Fits in with Other Books about MS

As mentioned above, it's different. To give the reader an idea how it differs, I'll comment briefly on six other popular books written by physicians for MS patients: 1) *Multiple Sclerosis Diet Book* by Dr. Roy Laver Swank and Barbara Brewer Dugan; 2) *Overcoming Multiple Sclerosis* by Dr. George Jelinek; 3) *The Wahls Protocol* by Dr. Terry Wahls and Eve Adamson; 4) *MS for Dummies* by Rosalind Kalb, Dr. Barbara Giesser, and Kathleen Costello, 5) *Multiple Sclerosis Fact Book* by Dr. Richard Lechtenberg; and 6) *Navigating Life with Multiple Sclerosis* by Kathleen Costello, Dr. Ben W Thrower and Dr. Barbara S Giesser.

The focus of the first three books is completely different from this one. They focus not on dealing with complications of the disease but almost entirely on trying to prevent MS outright or cure it. The other three books focus on a wider range of topics related to the disease, so they deal with the same questions as the first three but also usually address the most frequent complications. This book thus overlaps with the latter three books but often disagrees with their recommendations. The six prior books often disagree with one another as well.

So, given all of this disagreement, why should an MS patient believe what I have to say?

As a physician, I know some things about MS that patients don't.

As a patient with MS for 24 years, I know some things about MS that neurologists don't. An example: on my way to a Pharmacy and Therapeutics Committee meeting, I stepped out of a building wearing only a physician's white coat on a cold winter day. A very intelligent and knowledgeable neurologist who knew that I had MS and was on his way to same meeting followed me out the door.

Noticing an immediate change in my gait, he said, "I thought heat was what affected MS patients." I said it did, but in a different way. If I stepped outside an air-conditioned building on a hot summer day, I became weaker within about 30 seconds, but on a cold day, my gait became more spastic within a few steps. This was obvious to me because I had been living with the problem for years.

As an epidemiologist, I may be more able to judge causal associations in epidemiologic studies than some other physicians authoring books for patients (e.g., what causes MS?).

And finally, I am an infectious diseases specialist, which makes prevention and therapy of infectious diseases more up my alley than it is for the other authors of books for patients (this is important because infectious diseases are important causes of suffering and death for MS patients).

Moreover, having had MS for decades, I may have suffered more than the authors of the other books written by physicians about MS for patients. This makes my point of view more like that of an MS patient and likely affects my opinions about treatment recommendations. For example, having had 23 different unpleasant side effects of 10 medications prescribed because of MS and its complications, I'm a whole lot less sanguine about the need for extra medications than Drs. Lechtenberg and Giesser for various MS complications. I'm probably more leery of a neurologist pulling out a prescription pad than of "Greeks bearing gifts." The use of DDAVP (desmopressin) for reducing nocturia is a good example to illustrate this effect. It doesn't eliminate nocturia, just makes it less frequent. It works. But it also has important side effects, and the most important of those is hyponatremia, which can result in other important, severe side effects. For that reason, fluid restriction by going NPO (i.e., taking nothing by mouth) from one hour before taking the dose until eight hours after taking the dose is recommended. Because of the potential, severe side effects and the requirement for going NPO through the night, I decided that I couldn't take this medication even though I was sorely tempted. I couldn't manage to go through the night without fluids because I have to take pills (e.g., zolpidem tartrate to get back to sleep and to quell the periodic limb movements that can prevent me going to sleep or wake me back up, analgesics for pain, and sometimes antibiotics).

The care of MS involves many judgment decisions. For this reason, Dr. Giesser says it is "as much an art as it is a science. It's more creative problem-solving than hard and fast rules." In other words, it's possible to approach the same problem multiple different ways. Among the various approaches that might work, mine is often influenced by the amount of suffering I've been through.

What Is This Book's Focus?

This book focuses on how I coped with complications of this disease. Unlike the books of Dr. Swank and Dr. Jelinek, this one won't promise MS patients a rose garden (i.e., that they can "overcome" MS).

MS reminds me of a line in the musical *Les Miserables*: "It's a struggle, it's a war..." That's how I think of my fellow patients with MS - *les miserables* ("the miserable ones"). This book will describe ways of trying to survive "the thousand natural shocks that flesh is heir to" with this disease. It will try to make their lives a little less miserable - partly by knowing someone else has suffered as much as they have and partly by knowing that someone else has not only endured the disease but sometimes managed to reestablish a modicum of control (using strategies described in this book). These strategies will usually not be ones that can be found in other books about dealing with MS because they are mostly strategies developed by the author. For example, most prior books on MS note that patients with MS often suffer fatigue and suggest a variety of drugs that might (or might not) help somewhat (and also might cause disturbing side effects). This book takes a different approach.

Some of the topics I address are unquestionably weightier than others. For example, counteracting the yucky taste of methylprednisolone tablets may seem trivial when compared with preventing aspiration pneumonia, but that taste was so repulsive to me that I gagged and snorted with disgust every time I had to swallow them, which was way too often. Finding ANYTHING that would mostly conceal that taste was a godsend. It greatly improved my quality of life.

Knowing what sort of problems occupied an MS patient's attention may interest neurologists who don't have the disease and aren't likely to take such a detailed history during an already overstuffed clinic visit.

Coping, Not Curing

It's important to understand that "coping" does not mean curing. At the end of the day, this disease will always win until a legitimate cure is found. ("I could not stop for Death. He kindly stopped for me." – Emily Dickinson)

But that is not specific to MS. It's true of many diseases. And every person's life ends with something bad happening – by means of a disease, an injury, etc.

I said "legitimate cure", because some books say that a cure for MS was found more than six decades ago, but most of the scientific community does not agree.

Is coping important? Yes. The average MS patient is reportedly diagnosed between 24 and 29 years of age, for women and men, respectively, and lives for about three decades. That's a long time to suffer. Coping can make things easier, even though it won't make the disease go away.

I have had some days and nights so bad that I didn't think I could go on if that was how it would stay from then on. But there is such a thing as natural variation – more at one time and less at another, with most days being in the middle. After an extreme day, there is usually a "regression to the mean" (i.e., a return to the middle or "the central tendency of the data."). For example, Roger Maris hit 61 home runs in 1961 but only 33 in 1962. He hit a mean of 23 home runs per year over 12 seasons of playing major league baseball, so the large number in 1961 was not typical of his usual batting performance. Knowing that one very bad day can be followed by a regression to the mean (and less severe problems) is one thing that helps me cope.

Some books say that MS is not a life limiting disease, but they're wrong. A recent national study lasting more than a decade and including more than 25,000 MS patients reported that the mean age of death of MS patients was 60.9 years – 14 to 19 years earlier than for American men and women in general, respectively. [Redelings MD, McCoy L, Sorvillo F. Multiple sclerosis mortality and patterns of co-morbidity in the United States from 1990 to 2001 *Neuroepidemiology.* 2006; 26:102-7.]

A Problem with This and Other Books about MS

MS complications can be highly associated (e.g., weakness and spasticity) and can influence one another (e.g., insomnia and daytime fatigue), which often makes it hard to talk about one problem without lapping over into another problem. For example, in the chapter on urinary urgency, it would be difficult for me to avoid discussing constipation. I will attempt to avoid unnecessary redundancy, but replication of some points will probably be unavoidable in a book trying to focus on different problems in different chapters.

A small amount of replication in different chapters may not be necessarily bad. When I joined the debate team in high school, our coach advised us, "to get a new point across, say it, say you said it, and say it again." She must have known her stuff; my debate colleague and I went undefeated at the state championship debate tournament that year, defeating the previous year's champion team who had also placed seventh in a national debate tournament.

See Chapter 25 for more discussion about the interrelatedness of MS complications.

Does This Book Have To Be Read in Order from the First Page to the Last to Be Understood?

Not really. Readers with a scientific background will probably prefer to start with Chapter 1 to see why epidemiologic studies are so important for understanding what causes what and what cures what.

But readers without a scientific background may prefer to jump straight to a chapter about a problem vexing them at the moment (e.g., regurgitation and aspiration of stomach contents). That's fine too. They can always come back later and digest the scientific information of Chapters 1 and 2 in smaller segments.

My sister said laymen don't care about scientific whys and wherefores – they just want the answers. But when an answer differs from one book to another, how does the reader know which to believe? Chapter 1 provides brief explanations of how such decisions are made scientifically. Chapter 2 provides specific examples of differences between this book and other books about MS often with explanations about points of disagreement or agreement.

Differences of opinion about science are not unique to the management of multiple sclerosis complications. History is full of examples: 1) When nuclear magnetic resonance imaging was first proposed, four Nobel laureates commented that it would never work. Now an MRI scan of the brain and spinal cord is a routine part of the initial battery of tests for patients diagnosed with multiple sclerosis. 2) When Copernicus published his conclusion that Earth orbited the sun, most astronomers disagreed. Galileo sided with Copernicus, made a telescope and produced data supporting the hypothesis. Galileo paid for advocating this "heretical" notion, however, by being sentenced to house arrest for the final decade of his life.

Supreme Court Justice Oliver Wendell Holmes Jr. wrote that, "The best test of truth is the power of the thought to get itself accepted in the competition of the market." Does that mean one can judge the accuracy of a book from the number of copies sold? No. Books falsely promising MS patients a rose garden sometimes sell like hotcakes. Desperate patients can want good news even if it eventually proves false. In our Judeo-Christian culture, the idea that a paralyzed patient can be told to "pick up your bed and walk" has been popular for millennia. Multiple best-selling authors have claimed that MS could be cured by something as simple as switching to a different diet; other books steadily insisted that such claims were false.

False or not, the more books wishful thinkers buy, the more additional copies will inevitably be sold because brisk sales stimulate further sales (i.e., bookstore shoppers prefer to buy "bestsellers," assuming that brisk sales imply scientific accuracy).

Chapter 1
Some Important Things to Understand before Considering My Strategies for Coping

1) **How to know what causes what**: Controlled comparisons are important for deciding anything about causation in epidemiology and in science in general. For example, a large English study confirmed that cigarette smoking was the principal cause of lung cancer in the 1940s, finding that lung cancer patients were 14-fold more likely to have been smokers than were healthy controls. [Doll R, Hill AB. Smoking and carcinoma of the lung: preliminary report. Br Med J. 1950 Sep 30;2(4682):739-48.] For such controlled comparisons to be valid, it's important that the control patients be as similar as possible to the lung cancer patients with respect to all variables except the one being studied (e.g., if the control patients happened to be 10-fold more likely to have exposure to other carcinogens such as asbestos or radon, this difference could have confounded the study results regarding the importance of smoking).

2) **One thing occurring before something else** doesn't mean that the first caused the second; in logic, this assumption is referred to as the "post hoc, ergo propter hoc" fallacy (i.e., "after this, therefore because of this"). But if it happens repeatedly, the interpretation can change.

3) **How to know that a difference isn't just due to chance:** Statistical tests can be used to estimate the probability that an observed difference could have occurred by chance alone. Before statistical tests are done, one can get an idea from the size of the observed difference: the larger the observed difference, the less likely this could have occurred by chance. For example, before trying streptomycin therapy for tuberculous meningitis, virtually "everybody" with the disease died. When the first patient treated with streptomycin for tuberculous meningitis survived at the Mayo Clinic, this large apparent difference suggested that streptomycin might be effective therapy. Likewise, when Josef Meister survived after being bitten by a rabid dog and receiving rabies vaccine from Louis Pasteur, many concluded that Pasteur's vaccine might be a breakthrough. When Conrad Roentgen published an x-ray photograph of his wife's hand showing the bones and her wedding ring, the scientific community was convinced that radiographs would be useful before studies could be done. When I was an epidemiology graduate student at the London School of Hygiene, the statistics faculty said that sometimes observed differences could be so large that calculating statistics becomes superfluous. This is a modern example of an ancient concept – *"res ipsa loquitur"* (i.e., "the thing speaks for itself").

4) **Is randomization necessary to determine causation?** No, there have never been randomized trials of smoking, but the data from other epidemiologic studies make it clear that smoking is the principal cause of lung cancer. Randomization can help assure the similarity of the two study groups that

was mentioned above, but it isn't absolutely necessary. Two recent meta-analyses (i.e., studies of other studies) compared the results of randomized trials with those of other types of epidemiologic studies of the same question and concluded that well-designed epidemiologic studies tend to give the same results whether randomized or not.[Concato J, Shah N, Horwitz RI. Randomized, controlled trials, observational studies, and the hierarchy of research designs. *New England Journal of Medicine.* 2000;342(25):1887-92.] [Benson K, Hartz AJ. A comparison of observational studies and randomized, controlled trials. *New England Journal of Medicine.* 2000;342(25):1878-86.]

5) **How does one decide that a new finding is representative of a particular population** (e.g., MS patients)? If the new finding is consistently found by different investigators in different sets of MS patients, this becomes clear. The larger the sample(s) showing this, the more confidence one has that the finding is representative.

6) In trying to figure out whether a treatment causes a difference or not from epidemiologic studies (i.e., studies involving human beings), **it's important to know what sample size was studied** (the larger the study groups, the easier it is to see the difference) **and what the postulated difference is** (the bigger the difference, the easier it is to detect). True differences in epidemiologic studies usually result in statistically significant results (i.e., calculated probability value <0.05) and a high strength of association between the putative cause and the observed result (i.e., a high relative risk or odds ratio, depending upon the type of epidemiologic study used). There also tends to be consistency of evidence across different studies of the same question evaluated by different investigators in different populations.

7) **Skepticism is good.** Most medical hypotheses throughout history have been wrong. So it's healthy to remain skeptical until data are convincing.

8) **Anecdote and testimonial have low value** for deciding an epidemiological association. It sometimes seems that the truth has to be obvious from reading a list of testimonials about the utility of a particular product, but suffice it to say that the plural of "testimonial" is "testimonials," not "data." Controlled medical studies with probability values so low that they are "unlikely to be due to chance" can still be wrong due to chance (random error) or to bias (systematic error).

If the reader can understand this, then it may be easy to comprehend why testimonials are more likely to be wrong. When trying to figure out what might prevent pressure-related furuncles in a leg being paralyzed by MS, I saw testimonials on an independent website that suggested that the alternating air cushions of two American companies might work equally well for preventing pressure-related ills. As I will elaborate in a subsequent chapter, this didn't pan out. Testimonials are an unreliable source of information. As bad as testimonials are, "science reports" in publications like *The National Enquirer*, which my mother would find in checkout aisles at the grocery and peruse for "cures" of MS, may be still more misleading. I told her that such articles claiming the efficacy of bee stings or of being hit by lightning bolts couldn't induce me to try them. Bee stings were later found ineffective in a randomized trial. [Wesselius T, Heersema DJ, Mostert JP, Heerings M, Admiraal-Behloul F, Talebian A, van Buchem MA, De Keyser J. A randomized crossover study of bee sting therapy for multiple sclerosis. Neurology. 2005 Dec 13;65(11):1764-8.]

For any therapy, there is a "therapeutic index," which compares the therapeutic dose with the toxic (or lethal) dose; because a single bolt of lightning can be lethal, there's no way lightning could be considered safe therapy.

9) **If something sounds too good to be true, it may well be false.** Some have claimed for 6 decades that eating particular

foods will cure MS. The vast majority of the scientific community remains unconvinced.

10) **"There's no such thing as a free lunch."** The idea in this adage is that changing one thing to make a problem better may make something else worse. For example, I stopped eating a particular food (MorningStar Farms Grillers) because they were causing unacceptable constipation. I avoided the constipation, but, to do that, I had to give up eating something that I liked that was helping me in other ways.

11) **Balancing risk and benefit:** This is something that physicians do for patients routinely using the "no free lunch" concept. It involves considering the pluses and minuses of everything in a patient's treatment plan before choosing an optimal regimen. As part of this process, the physician often tries to educate the patient that any medication can have adverse effects. MS patients may want their physicians to do all of this balancing, and the physicians will certainly try, but there are sometimes things that may have to be altered from day to day for best results. It's unlikely that physicians would be able to keep track of everything that is happening from one day to the next (e.g., if a patient needs to increase a laxative dose a bit because of increased constipation the day before). Before deciding to try to manage such day to day variation, the patient should discuss this with her physician.

When pain in my torn rotator cuff became intolerable, I decided to stop walking with my walker throughout the house and rely more on my motorized wheelchair. Doing this allowed me to rest the torn rotator cuff because my right shoulder served as a fulcrum when I walked with the walker and this seemed to be what was making my shoulder worse. But this solution caused my legs to get weaker because walking throughout the house with the walker had become my primary form of exercise as my disability increased.

A physical therapist evaluated the safety of my home environment when I retired due to physical disability and recommended not using a bedside floor mat because it could trip a patient with hemiparesis like me. After much thought, balancing risk and benefit, I decided that I had to use the mat and be careful because the mat provided multiple benefits (e.g., protecting my bare feet from the cold floor which could cause increased spasticity and increased urinary urgency. It also provided increased friction with the floor, which was important for a weak patient trying to stand up from the bed). The mat has helped me in such ways many times over years and hasn't caused me to fall. If a mat sliding is a problem, it could be taped to the floor with two-sided tape, but the mat I am using usually stays put because of a rubbery bottom. One thing that seems to move my bedside mat is my paretic left foot dragging the mat away from the bed when I am getting up after putting on my shoes. To prevent this, I found that positioning my walker with one or two wheels on the mat as I am maneuvering off of it will help keep the mat from moving.

Using extra MiraLAX can help a patient counter a bout of increased constipation but can cause fecal incontinence if used excessively. Balancing risk and benefit, I have used this approach successfully many times, but the risk of using too much is important to avoid because fecal incontinence can be a large problem that can result in still more problems (e.g., urinary tract infection requiring days of therapy, which can, of course, create still more problems).

12) **Cause is usually multifactorial,** meaning that there usually isn't just a single cause of a medical illness (e.g., MS) or a complication (e.g., MS related constipation); for example, a patient may have a certain amount of constipation due to MS, but it may get much worse after eating a particular food or swallowing a particular medication.

13) **How can a patient with MS figure out which foods are causing a problem?** Paying attention to one's body and taking notes are helpful. Without these, it's probably impossible.

Without paying careful attention, there are no observations at all, and without taking notes, all of the observations can merge into a blur over several weeks. The patient should also pay attention to "experiments of nature," where something happens that allows the patient to see what might be causing something else without designing an experiment. For example, when I tried to switch what I was eating for lunch from a plate of spaghetti to a couple of sandwiches using MorningStar Farms Grillers, I developed increased constipation the next day. Because I had just made this single change in diet, I suspected that that change could have been responsible, but not certain. So I stopped eating the Grillers and went back to the spaghetti. After trying to make the switch to Grillers five more times with identical results, a pattern was obvious: Grillers were associated with increased constipation.

14) **Trial and error:** It has been said that one definition of insanity is continuing to use the same measures while expecting different results. When things are not going well for a patient with MS, this can continue indefinitely. In order to get out of a rut, paying attention to one's body may be necessary, but there is often also a need for some judicious trial and error to see what works best for a particular problem (e.g., the right laxative in the right amount at a particular time). If you do this, change only one thing at a time. This makes it clearer what's going on when that change is followed by another. Doing that just one time won't be enough to make it totally clear that your change caused the other, but by doing this several times, you can establish a pattern.

15) **"There are truths that are neither for all men nor for all times."** This observation by Voltaire is an especially important concept for this book, because what works for a particular problem (e.g., constipation) in a particular MS patient can change continually, requiring frequent

modifications, fine tuning, etc. For example, I started having constipation with my first MS attack. What was required to treat it has changed over and over again. For this reason, this book won't tell the reader the exact dose of laxative she should be using at the moment for constipation, but no other book does that either. No book can provide such specific advice because all MS patients are relatively unique, and what's more, each patient can change over time, so a medication or a dosage that's appropriate for an individual patient can both change with time. As I became more physically disabled, everything physical got more difficult to do - walking, holding a glass, holding a book, holding the phone, wiping after a bowel movement, buttoning a button, tying a shoe, etc. This has continued throughout my worsening with MS for 24 years.

16) **Amounts can matter.** For example, exercise is good for MS patients, but overdoing it can cause problems. Aristotle advised "Moderation in all things," but many tend to sympathize with Mae West's contrary view that, "Too much of a good thing is wonderful." Ezra Pound said, "To know how much is enough, you have to know how much is more than enough." MS is "a long day's journey into night" and the further a patient goes down that road, the more important amounts can be (e.g., the amount of water the patient can and should drink to avoid terrible constipation from dehydration and avoid urinating all over his clothes from drinking too much; the amount of raisin bran she eats for breakfast to avoid getting increased constipation from eating too little and to avoid eating so much bulk that the colon becomes overloaded and occupies too much space in the pelvis, which can crowd the spastic bladder and result in urination all over her clothes from episodes of dire urinary urgency; etc.). Because amounts can matter, measuring can become important as the disease gets worse.

17) In ancient Chinese philosophy there were believed to be **two opposing causal principles – Yin and Yang**. As with Yin and Yang, things that increase MS-related constipation can be neutralized by those that relieve constipation. For example, MS-related constipation and constipating foods or medications can work together to increase constipation while polyethylene glycol 3350 (MiraLAX) and the antibiotic dicloxacillin (being used temporarily for a *Staphylococcus aureus* infection) can work together to cause diarrhea. If balanced together in the right combination, such opposing factors can result in regular bowel movements (in the same way that the correct amount of a strong acid during a titration can neutralize a strong base and result in an aqueous solution with a neutral pH of 7): more about this later.

18) **Murphy's Law** says that if anything bad can happen, it will, and the first corollary is that if anything worse can occur, it will as well. Murphy's Law wasn't created specifically for MS patients, but it sometimes seems that way because so many bad things happen routinely. Having MS is like playing chess against a chess master who is constantly maneuvering the patient into check and always seeking a final checkmate.

19) Alexander Pope mused that, "**A little learning is a dangerous thing**. Drink deep, or taste not the Pierian spring." ["Essay on Criticism" published in 1711]. In medicine, this seems correct; patients who get the wrong diagnosis or wrong therapy usually do worse. And Shakespeare said, "There are more things in heaven and earth than are dreamt of in your philosophy...." This is also true in medicine; new knowledge about the cause, diagnosis and optimal therapy of diseases is often discovered over time. Does eating saturated fat cause multiple sclerosis? Some books written for MS patients say that it does. Is this an example of a little learning being a dangerous thing? There will be more discussion of this question in the next chapter.

20) Another thing advised by Alexander Pope was, "**Be not the first by whom the new is tried,** nor yet the last to lay the old aside." Should MS patients avoid being the first to try something? It depends. I was apparently the first to compare two different alternating air cushions for preventing pressure-related furuncles in a leg being paralyzed by MS, but enough was known about such cushions that comparing them couldn't be considered dangerous. By contrast, being the first to expose oneself to something dangerous like a lightning bolt to see if it would cure MS would be foolhardy.

21) Yogi Berra said that 50% of baseball was **"90% mental."** Could this idea somehow relate to MS?

When I was training in medicine, fellow interns enjoyed contrasting patients' problems that were objective and "real" (e.g., an inflamed appendix) with those that were subjective and supratentorial (i.e., imagined or existing only in a patient's head). This was despite warnings from senior clinicians who insisted that a patient's problem is always a problem to the patient.

Because multiple sclerosis is due to damage to the central nervous system that is objective and easily documented by tests such as magnetic resonance imaging (MRI), an MS patient may feel that all of her MS related symptoms must be equally valid, but there are problems with a damaged central nervous system that can end up being supratentorial (i.e., "in the patient's head"). For example, most patients with MS develop problems with bladder control, but this problem can be made much worse by seeing or hearing something (i.e., something in the patient's head). How could this be?

Most readers are probably familiar with the conditioned reflexes made famous by Pavlov's experiment in which he rang a bell at supper for dogs. The dogs came to associate supper with the ringing bell and would salivate if Pavlov rang it without providing supper. Such conditioned reflexes have been shown to occur throughout much of the animal kingdom, including *Homo sapiens* (man). They occur in normal, healthy people but are more prominent in patients with MS (my neurologist speculated that this may be because damage to the central nervous system can keep it from exerting modulating influences). For example, healthy people hearing water running or seeing that they are approaching the bathroom might experience a mild increase in the urge to urinate, but a patient with MS can promptly wet her clothes. The fact that such reflexes occur and are recognized by the patient to be merely conditioned reflexes "in the head" doesn't lessen their spike in urinary urgency.

Chapter 2

More Details About How This Book Differs from Other Books about MS

Readers will probably want more details about this than were provided in the Introduction, but this chapter will not provide detailed critiques of everything said in the other books. The purpose of this chapter is not to debate everything the other authors say but merely to give readers a better understanding of how this book differs, using no more than two or three pages per book.

Dr. Swank's Book

Dr. Swank's book focuses almost entirely on his theory that the disease is caused by eating a diet high in saturated fat and can be controlled after diagnosis by switching to a diet low in saturated fat. Sounds easy, doesn't it? Just eat the right foods, and MS will disappear. H. L. Mencken said, "There is always an easy solution to every human problem—neat, plausible, and wrong."

Was Dr. Swank right? His theory was hatched in the 1940s and, try as he might, he never convinced the scientific community that his hypothesis was correct.

For example, here's what Dr. Lechtenberg's book had to say about this: "dietary approaches to modifying the frequency and severity of exacerbations have not been effective. Adherence to diets rich in specific nutritional factors, such as essential fatty acids (vegetable and fish oils), has been quite disappointing. Many of the failed therapies based on dietary manipulations grew out of nonmedical fads. The items involved required no special licensing for use, and so this approach to therapy has been more burdened than most by unjustified claims and unsafe regimens. Dietary adjustments are often valuable for individuals with MS, but they should never be misconstrued as treatment for demyelination or inflammation itself... No diet, sanitary precaution, or exercise routine protects an individual against the disease or ensures that the disease will not get worse once it appears. This has not deterred a virtual army of concerned physicians, articulate patients, and outrageous quacks from formulating and publicizing countless recommendations and routines that are alleged to relieve or eradicate this neurologic disease.... Various dietary regimens have failed to suppress flare-ups or improve re-myelination of damaged nerve pathways.... Claims for the potency of gamma linolenic acid and other polyunsaturated fatty acids in reducing the frequency and severity of acute exacerbations of the disease are grossly overstated in much of what has been written about multiple sclerosis. Their true value, if any, remains to be established."

Here is what Dr. Giesser's book has to say, "most scientists have concluded that no single thing in the environment or in a person's diet is directly responsible for the disease....Unfortunately, you can't eat your way around MS. Even though a variety of special diets have been promoted as MS cures, none have been shown in controlled trials to alter the course or severity of MS."

A different book written by physicians for other physicians [Handbook of Multiple Sclerosis edited by Dr. Stuart D Cook] dismissed

Dr. Swank's theory as follows: "Prior ecologic correlations suggesting that a higher intake of saturated fats and a lower intake of polyunsaturated fats might increase the risk of MS have been contradicted by the results of Zhang who found no relationship between intake of total fat or major specific types of fat and the risk of MS.[Zhang SM, Willett WC, Hernan MA, Olek MJ, Ascherio A. Dietary fat in relation to risk of multiple sclerosis among two large cohorts of women. *Am J Epidemiol* 2000;152(11):1056–1064.]"

Zhang et al also said, "no association between intake of animal fat or saturated fat and the risk of MS was found in most case-control studies," citing 9 retrospective case-control studies; 5 of the 9 found no association, and the other 4 reported some type of association, but there was inconsistency both within and between those 4 studies. Swank diet enthusiasts might view these 4 results as important confirmation, but Zhang termed the results of the four latter studies "inconsistent." For example, a Canadian study reported a doubling of the risk with ingestion of 33 extra grams of animal fat per day but reported the same doubling from eating 900 extra kilocalories per day; the same study reported that pork, hot dogs, sweets and candy were high-risk foods and that 11 different nutrients including bread and fruit juice were protective. None of the other three corroborated the finding of increased risk from eating any type of animal fat; instead, they each identified particular high-risk foods that differed from study to study. For example, an Italian study found that ingesting butter, lard and horseflesh were risk factors between infancy and adolescence as were bread, pasta, legume soup, coffee and tea; after adolescence none of those foods were risk factors, but eggs, wine and mineral water were. These results disagree with those of the Canadian study in multiple ways (e.g., one says bread is protective and the other says it promotes MS), and there is little reason to believe that bread, pasta, legume soup, coffee, tea, wine, or mineral water specifically predispose a patient to developing MS. A Croatian study reported increased risk with consumption of whole milk or potatoes with lard or meat but found the same level of risk with eating just "new potatoes." The latter finding is as dubious as the prior study's implication of legume soup, coffee, tea, wine and mineral water. A Russian study reported that children eating more meat than vegetables had significantly increased risk; this study partially corroborated the finding of the Italian study mentioned above that eating horsemeat before adolescence was a risk factor, but there was no corroboration of the Italian study's other results.

The most recent Cochrane meta-analysis of diet and MS reported no statistically significant benefit from dietary therapy of MS. [Farinotti M, Vacchi L, Simi S, Di Pietrantonj C, Brait L, Filippini G. Dietary interventions for multiple sclerosis. Cochrane Database Syst Rev. 2012 Dec 12;12:CD004192. doi: 10.1002/14651858.CD004192. pub3. Review]

If the reader is not already convinced, other reasons for doubting Dr. Swank's theory could be listed including the following:

1) Dr. Swank's study of 144 MS patients attempting to follow a diet containing less than 20 g of saturated fat per day was not set up as a controlled study. From reading Precept 1 in Chapter 1 of this book, the reader should know that that posed a serious problem.

Dr. Swank tried to circumvent this problem by conducting a post-hoc analysis in which patients with better compliance were compared with patients with poorer compliance. But doubt persisted despite the post-hoc analysis because it wasn't clear whether compliance was influenced by how patients were doing (i.e., which was the chicken and which the egg?). If patients destined to have the benign form of MS complied better because they thought the diet was working, this could have biased the study.

2) It's not clear how well Dr. Swank's study confirmed the diet of each participant because one of his principal supporters, Dr. Jelinek, has suggested in his own book that Dr. Swank's annual patient interviews underestimated the patients' consumption of saturated fat.

3) There have been no controlled, follow-up studies of patients eating Dr. Swank's diet.

4) Dr. Swank claimed huge differences in relapse rates (i.e.,

relapses declined by 95% in those with good compliance) and in survival (66% to 75% higher over 36 years in those with poor compliance vs. those with good compliance). From reading Precept 6 of Chapter 1 of this book, the reader knows that huge differences are easy to detect. This means that much smaller and briefer follow-up studies could have confirmed a huge difference in relapse rate. Despite this, there were no controlled follow-up studies documenting this finding. Dr. Swank claimed in his book that he cared for 3,500 patients with MS. In his study, he reported on only 4% of those patients. How did the other 96% do? Why were follow-up studies of the vast majority of his patients never published by Dr. Swank or by his colleagues working at the same university? If their outcomes were more like those usually expected with MS, that would have blunted enthusiasm for his diet. Did he fail to report on their outcomes for that reason?

5) According to Dr. Jelinek's book, the first publication of a randomized controlled trial of using a low-fat diet for treating MS was published in 2005. [Weinstock-Guttman B, Baier M, Park Y, Feichter J, Lee-Kwen P, Gallagher E, Venkatraman J, Meksawan K, Deinehert S, Pendergast D, Awad AB, Ramanathan M, Munschauer F, Rudick R. Low fat dietary intervention with omega-3 fatty acid supplementation in multiple sclerosis patients. Prostaglandins Leukot Essent Fatty Acids. 2005 Nov;73(5):397-404.] It compared patients consuming a diet in which fat constituted 15% of all calories [supplemented by 6g fish oil], with patients consuming a diet in which fat constituted < 30% of all calories and saturated fat < 10% of all calories [supplemented by 6g olive oil] (i.e., neither group exactly followed the Swank diet). Recent CDC studies have indicated that the normal American diet includes 33% fat (with 1/3 of the fat being saturated), so the control group with 30% fat was close to the normal American fat intake [a relative 9 % less] except for the olive oil supplement. Of interest, Weinstock-Guttman et al. did not report a statistical comparison of the two groups' relapse rates, noting only that the relapse rate decreased significantly in both groups (as compared

with the patients' histories of relapses during the year prior to the study). This left it unclear whether one approach was better.

6) If, as hypothesized by Dr. Swank, MS is due to damage to the central nervous system caused by embolization of clumps of cells aggregated by dietary saturated fat, why are there no contemporaneous lesions in other organs throughout the body?

7) Why have autopsies and biopsies of MS patients failed to confirm Dr. Swank's suggested pathogenesis?

8) One of Swank's arguments is that MS has increased in prevalence over the past century, suggesting that some environmental change must be responsible. Some recent studies have suggested that increased dietary salt might be predisposing people to autoimmune diseases such as multiple sclerosis. [Kleinewietfeld M, et al. Sodium chloride drives autoimmune disease by the induction of pathogenic TH 17 cells. *Nature*. 2013; 496:518-22.] [Simon KC, et al. Epstein-Barr virus neutralizing antibody levels and risk of multiple sclerosis. Multiple sclerosis. 2012; 18:1185-7.] If salt proves to be the culprit, then saturated fat will presumably be exonerated as the dietary cause célèbre.

Other reasons for doubting the theory could be listed, but, as stated above, this is not meant to be a comprehensive debate, just an effort to let the reader know how much this book differs from the others.

If Dr. Swank's theory was wrong, is it a bad idea to try eating a diet low in saturated fat? No. Why is that?

As the reader learned in Precept 19 of Chapter 1, "there are more things in heaven and earth than are dreamt of in [one's] philosophy..." In this case, the leading cause of death for decades in the United States and other Western countries has been atherosclerotic cardiovascular disease. When physicians don't just write "multiple sclerosis" on the MS patients' death certificates, atherosclerotic cardiovascular disease is the second most frequent cause of death of MS patients. [Redelings MD, McCoy L, Sorvillo F. Multiple sclerosis mortality and patterns of comorbidity in the United States from

1990 to 2001 *Neuroepidemiology.* 2006; 26:102-7.] Eating saturated animal fat is a major risk factor for atherosclerosis. So, eating a diet low in saturated fat makes good sense for other reasons. It has also become known in recent decades that eating animal protein may be a risk factor for cancer, which was the fourth leading reported cause of death among MS patients in Redelings' study. Avoiding animal products in general is thus not unwise.

Are any of Dr. Swank's observations valid? I believe so and will list several examples:

1) Dr. Swank said this in his book: "although the frequency of relapses varied from one person to another, in any one person there was usually a fairly definite pattern and rate of occurrence, as well as circumstances or seasons of the year when exacerbations occurred. The patient also tended to have relapses and remissions that were more or less characteristic for him or her. They were, in fact, predicted with surprising accuracy by many patients. These patterns tended to repeat themselves until late in the disease when the course of the disease became progressive."

This was true of my illness, which recurred at a predictable frequency and tended to affect my left leg and arm far more than my right leg or arm. Rarely I had an attack affecting the right arm and/or leg and twice had attacks that were confined to facial palsy (the two facial palsies differing from one another). A recent study concurred, saying this, "Analysis of prospectively collected data from a cohort of 195 patients suggests that symptomatic demyelinating events in early relapsing remitting multiple sclerosis have a tendency to recur in the same location (e.g., spinal cord, optic nerve, brainstem)." [Mowry EM, Deen S, Malikova I, et al. The onset location of multiple sclerosis predicts the location of subsequent relapses. J Neurol Neurosurg Psychiatry 2009; 80:400.]

Dr. Swank's observation agrees with my experience but creates an additional problem for his hypothesis: embolization through the bloodstream usually occurs randomly. There's no particular reason that emboli of clumps of aggregated cells should land in the same place repeatedly. Pathologic studies in MS patients have not shown disease of the arterial blood vessels that would explain repeated attacks in the same area.

2) For fatigue, Dr. Swank recommends, "pace yourself. Don't rush, don't attempt to be busy all the time, spend time relaxing and even meditating; and if you have a major task to perform, avoid unimportant, tiring tasks, even if desirable. In other words listen to your body. The only effective treatment for fatigue in multiple sclerosis (not due to an infection with fever) is rest by lying down. Rest by sitting up is less helpful.... Rest by lying down restores needed energy far more effectively than rest by sitting. Midday rest is needed by most, and desirable for all MS patient because of the persistence of fatigue in all but a few."

Fatigue in MS patients is often associated with insomnia and poor sleep. Rest has worked for me.

3) Dr. Swank says that the Credé maneuver (applying gentle manual pressure over the bladder) works to help MS patients evacuate their bladders after they start having bladder problems. I agree. But then he says that using the Credé maneuver routinely to evacuate the bladder will prevent urinary tract infections. I'm skeptical of this claim because once it's emptied, it immediately starts refilling. It doesn't stay empty for more than seconds. After 10 minutes, there's more than 10 ml.[Lee SW, Kim JH. The significance of natural bladder filling by the production of urine during cystometry. *Neurourol Urodyn.* 2008;27(8):772-4. doi: 10.1002/nau.20584.] This makes me suspicious that emptying the bladder doesn't really do anything that important. Postcoital emptying of the bladder, also long hypothesized to prevent urinary tract infection associated with coitus, still hadn't been shown to work according to a review. [Hooton TM. Recurrent urinary tract infection in women. *Int J Antimicrob Agents.* 2001; 17:259-68.]

4) Dr. Swank says, "no single medication has been generally successful in alleviating... [MS musculoskeletal] pains. Local heat, however gives most patients relief." It usually helps me.

5) Dr. Swank says, "Constipation may become a problem.... Patients have solved this by adding bran to their diet, by the use of laxatives that, by trial, have proved effective, or by combinations of these methods." I agree.

6) Dr. Swank says, "Urgency and frequency of urination are common symptoms of MS. These symptoms, if not severe, can be managed well by keeping close to the bathroom while at home, but poorly when away from home." I agree.

Dr. Jelinek's Book

If Dr. Swank's book is wrong about saturated fat being the principal cause of MS, can Dr. Jelinek's book be correct? No.

Here is Dr. Jelinek's defense of Dr. Swank's data: "First and foremost, saturated fat must be cut out of the diet. The evidence for dietary change in MS is impressive, as it is for a number of other Western diseases. The evidence is comprehensive, from laboratory bench research, animal research, major epidemiological studies, case-control studies and uncontrolled long-term cohort studies, culminating in randomized controlled trials. The evidence is congruent, consistent and highly persuasive. It strongly suggests that diet is the single most important thing that can be done to facilitate recovery from MS, in that the potential size of the benefit is enormous, at around a 95% reduction in relapse rate with a major effect on progression of disability. It appears however, that it is not enough to modify the diet so that the amount of meat and dairy products is cut down. From the evidence available, that may slow the disease a little or not at all. Swank's work shows that the 'bad dieters' reduced their saturated fat intake by about 75% yet this was not enough to alter the disease course. To really arrest it requires a drastic change to a plant-based, whole food diet supplemented with seafood."

What Dr. Jelinek says in this paragraph is misleading in more than one way. For example, he talks about Dr. Swank's theory having been evaluated by "epidemiological studies, case-control studies and ... cohort studies, culminating in randomized controlled trials" as if these are four different things. Case-control studies, cohort studies, and randomized controlled trials are each types of "epidemiological studies."

Epidemiologic studies are, simply put, those conducted upon people (i.e., not on molecules or tissue slices or laboratory rats). The Greek root words for "epidemiology" are *epi* (upon) *demos* (people) *logos* (study). Classical epidemiological studies focused upon causation and prevention of disease. Clinical epidemiological studies use the principles and tools developed for performing classical epidemiological studies to study other things such as therapy, prognosis, diagnosis, etc.

Dr. Jelinek's sentence is also an exaggeration because Dr. Swank's study was not designed to be a controlled study and there have been no subsequent controlled studies specifically evaluating Dr. Swank's diet. The closest attempt to a controlled study of the Swank diet was a randomized trial published in 2005, which Dr. Jelinek's book notes was "the first RCT on dietary fat in MS..." [Weinstock-Guttman B, Baier M, Park Y, Feichter J, Lee-Kwen P, Gallagher E, Venkatraman J, Meksawan K, Deinehert S, Pendergast D, Awad AB, Ramanathan M, Munschauer F, Rudick R. Low fat dietary intervention with omega-3 fatty acid supplementation in multiple sclerosis patients. Prostaglandins Leukot Essent Fatty Acids. 2005 Nov;73(5):397-404.] Dr. Jelinek cites no other controlled trial evaluating the effect of a diet low in saturated fat on patients with MS, but then says, "I have been unable to find a single clinical study of a low-fat diet in MS that has not shown these strongly positive findings, regardless of methodology. Why then, are such diets often dismissed by doctors?" This is misleading because, as stated above, 5 of 9 published case-control studies reported no association between risk for MS and the amount of saturated fat or animal fat being consumed and because the results of the other four lacked consistency.

Was the 2005 RCT a "controlled" study of the Swank hypothesis? No. As mentioned above, a controlled study of a diet low in saturated fat should require part of the patients (usually half) to eat that diet and the rest of the patients to eat a regular diet for comparison. Instead, the 2005 study included one limb that was intended to be low-fat (i.e., only 15% of all calories ingested could be fat). Unfortunately, the study does not say exactly what percent of all calories could be saturated fat, leaving this important number unclear. Moreover, the other study limb was required to eat a diet that was 30% fat (close to the usual American diet, which the CDC website says is 33% fat with one third of the fat being saturated fat). This second study limb was also required to keep saturated fat down to 10% of all ingested calories. It's unclear which study group ate less saturated fat. Saturated fatty acids in serum measured by chromatography trended down in both study groups, but more in the control group than in the "low-fat" group. This suggests that the control group actually may have been eating less saturated fat than the "low-fat" group. Moreover, making the study still more confusing, the two limbs were given different oil supplements – one fish oil and the other olive oil. Since rates of relapse were the primary data suggesting efficacy of diet in this study and since the baseline relapse rates were determined differently (retrospectively), the significant reductions from baseline in relapse rates in both groups are less easy to interpret than if the prospective portion of the study had been more clearly controlled and if data collected prospectively and contemporaneously had documented a significant difference between the two study groups.

Dr. Swank's diet either worked or it didn't. Dr. Jelinek first argues that it did but then argues that the nonfat milk products that Dr. Swank allowed his patients to consume in unlimited amounts were as harmful to MS patients as saturated animal fat and must therefore be avoided. If the nonfat milk products were as harmful as saturated fat, how could Dr. Swank's patients consuming them have done so well? And if they did do so well, how can Dr. Jelinek reconcile this with their being harmful to MS patients?

As mentioned, the scientific community has, to date, not

accepted Dr. Swank's theory, which is still regarded as "not proven," the term used for it in a *Lancet* editorial in 1991. This is why virtually no neurologists recommend this as a treatment approach to their MS patients.

Dr. Jelinek admits this, but then tries to convince MS patients that it's an "evidence-based" approach to overcoming the disease. In doing so, he cites many publications, but fails to cite many other pertinent publications. This is a problem.

When witnesses take the stand in an American court, they are routinely asked to "tell the truth, the whole truth, and nothing but the truth." I don't believe that Dr. Jelinek is trying to hoodwink MS patients, but his way of writing doesn't reveal all of the relevant facts and is misleading them to believe that Dr. Swank's low saturated fat diet (plus a few of his modifications) is good for what ails them.

Dr. Jelinek spends a few pages talking about how epidemiologists decide that an association is causal (e.g., that a low saturated fat diet could heal multiple sclerosis), but he leaves out some important points. For example, he says that the larger a hypothesized difference, the smaller a study can be to detect that difference as being statistically significant, but then doesn't say that the differences Dr. Swank claimed were so big that confirmation of his results could be achieved with relatively small, relatively brief controlled studies. For example, if one assumes a relapse rate of one per year (the rate observed in Dr. Swank's patients before they commenced eating a diet low in saturated fat) and that the rate will drop by 95% in patients eating a diet low in saturated fat for three years (as claimed by Dr. Swank), then a study of just 14 patients (half eating regular diets and half eating the Swank diet) would have 90% power to detect a statistically significant difference between the two groups. (See Table 2-1)

Dr. Jelinek says, "the results of therapy for the treatment group are compared against what happens to patients in the control group. This is done principally because people taking a therapy for some disease often get some benefit just because they feel that the therapy must be doing them some good (this is known as the placebo response). By using a control group taking just an inactive placebo against which to compare those taking active drug, this effect can be accounted for."

The placebo response is a real phenomenon that must be accounted for, but it's not the "principal" reason for using control groups in epidemiologic studies such as a randomized controlled trial, as Dr. Jelinek maintains. A control group must be used in every type of epidemiologic study because comparing the results between different groups is the only way that the results can be interpreted. In many studies, there is no placebo response to consider, but the control group is as important in those studies as it is in the ones where a placebo response occurs. For example, in the famous study referred to above regarding smoking as a risk factor for death due to lung cancer, the epidemiologic design was a case-control study and, since this was a retrospective, observational study, there was no placebo response, but using a control group made it possible to see that people dying of lung cancer (cases) were 14 times more likely to have been active smokers than controls. [Hill R, Doll AB. BMJ. 1950] The very low calculated probability that this large difference could have been due to chance alone suggested that cigarette smoking was indeed causing lung cancer, a rapidly fatal illness.

Does Dr. Jelinek's testimonial that he had not had a second attack during the 13 years after his first attack suggest that he must be correct that eating the right foods will make MS disappear? No, it proves nothing. As the reader saw in Precept 8 of Chapter 1, testimonials are unreliable in general and this one is more unreliable than most. Why? First, some diagnoses are incorrect. Recent reviews on MS in the *New England Journal of Medicine* and in *Medical Clinics of North America* listed many other illnesses that can be confused with MS and must be considered in the differential diagnosis before diagnosing MS. This means that sometimes physicians get the diagnosis wrong (Alexander Pope said a long time ago, "to err is human...,"). Physicians are human; sometimes they make mistakes. And even if the diagnosis was correct, a review of MS by a group of neurologists at the Mayo Clinic said that 10% of MS patients have a benign form with few to no exacerbations and no progression to disability "for more than 20 years." [Noseworthy JH et al. Multiple sclerosis. *New England Journal of Medicine* 2000; 343:938-952.] If Noseworthy et al. are correct that 10% of patients have benign MS (most of whom are probably eating regular diets), then one can't conclude anything based upon a single patient doing well regardless of what he's been eating. Dr. Lechtenberg's book puts the frequency of benign MS at "about 20%."

Dr. Jelinek says that the benign form of MS couldn't explain the favorable results in Swank's 72 "good dieters" because they were half of the 144 patients who ended up in the publication about the study. But the number of patients Dr. Swank originally assembled for the study was actually 250. Dr. Swank said he selected the 144 patients from the 250 because the 144 were all still working, making the 72 good dieters 28.8% of those present at study onset. [Swank RL, Goodwin J. Review of MS patient survival on a Swank low saturated fat diet. *Nutrition.* 2003; 19:161–162.] This makes it harder to know whether a benign form of MS could have helped confound any of Dr. Swank's study results.

My first MS attack occurred two weeks after I received an injection of hepatitis B vaccine (in the left deltoid muscle; it was a sixth injection – the last of a second series because the first series didn't result in immunity). Does hepatitis B vaccination cause MS? Most studies of this question suggest that it doesn't. Dr. Jelinek's book implies that it does. It says, "there have been many reports of increased risk of MS associated with the [hepatitis B] immunization" without citing the "many reports." He cites three studies reporting a significantly higher rate of MS after hepatitis B vaccine but fails to cite or even mention the larger number of studies reporting the opposite. This may give the reader the impression that this is a fair, balanced representation of all pertinent literature, when in fact it seems to be only the evidence suggesting increased risk after the vaccine.

Dr. Jelinek cites a study by a group of Harvard epidemiologists finding an increased risk of multiple sclerosis after hepatitis B vaccine but does not cite another study by the same epidemiologists finding no increased risk after that vaccine. Nor does he cite what the epidemiologists say about this discrepancy – that this relationship may not yet be well understood. Instead he just says that the study suggests an increased risk and fails to note what the authors said about their own uncertainty.[Hernán MA, Jick SS, Olek MJ, Jick H. Recombinant hepatitis B vaccine and the risk of multiple sclerosis: a prospective study. Neurology. 2004; 63:838-42.]

Dr. Jelinek also failed to cite a review published in *Neurology* in 1997 that had 66 references about diet and the risk of MS [Lauer K. Diet and multiple sclerosis. *Neurology* 1997;49 (Suppl. 2):S55–S61.] even though he says that he started searching for information about this topic in the medical literature right after his own diagnosis in 1999. He cites a study by the same author exploring the possibility that diet could be related to the illness, but not the review. The review concludes that it's too early to know whether diet could help prevent or heal MS – that more data from controlled studies are needed (i.e., the opposite of Dr. Jelinek's conclusion). Here's what Lauer said: "Further studies are needed before any preventive recommendation can be made on a community level. The situation is less consistent for dairy food which might be implicated as a risk factor based on ecological comparisons in different regions. However multivariate testing so far implies that this finding may be due to confounding, especially due to climatic variables although some biological plausibility cannot be denied. A prospective observational study, however, pointed to a beneficial effect of this type of food but randomized trials are needed to substantiate such an effect. The scientific data presently available do not justify any dietary recommendation to patients or on a community level with respect to dairy food, since neither a prognostic effect nor a role as a risk factor have been convincingly demonstrated. Further epidemiological studies with improved analytical methods and more experimental work based on existing hypotheses are urgently needed to assess the etiologic role of nutritional factors in MS."

Because neither of these two topics (the role of diet and of hepatitis B vaccine in MS) seemed to be handled in a balanced way, this leaves me feeling less confident about the accuracy of other parts.

Is there anything in Dr. Jelinek's book that I agree with? Yes. He says that patients should get plenty of sunshine, vitamin D, and exercise and avoid getting depressed. It's hard to argue against sunshine and exercise, but as pointed out in Chapter 1, amounts matter and an MS patient should avoid excessive amounts of either. I agree that vitamin D is important for MS patients. MS patients usually have low vitamin D levels and often get osteoporosis because of repeated methylprednisolone therapy for MS relapses, making them more likely to break bones when they fall. So getting enough vitamin D is rational. Whether vitamin D will affect the prognosis of MS, as Dr. Jelinek implies, is not yet known.[Ascherio A, Munger KL, Simon KC. Vitamin D and multiple sclerosis. *Lancet Neurol.* 2010 Jun;9(6):599-612. doi: 10.1016/S1474-4422(10)70086-7. Review.] A randomized controlled trial of vitamin D therapy of MS patients was reportedly started at Johns Hopkins Hospital to assess this question.

MS patients are more prone to develop depression than the general population, so they should be aware of this risk and take appropriate steps to protect their psyche and seek professional help if they start developing symptoms of depression.

For fatigue, Dr. Jelinek recommends, "energy conservation strategies, cognitive behavior therapy, relaxation therapy and exercise," adding that, "Drugs don't help..." I prefer Dr. Swank's approach, but sympathize with Dr. Jelinek's preference for energy conservation and relaxation as compared with drug therapy for fatigue.

One more thing I should mention before leaving Dr. Jelinek's book: I switched to a diet low in saturated fat 8 years and 4 months before my first MS attack. The reason had nothing to do with MS (I was an epidemiology graduate student and lots of my classmates were doing it). What does this mean? It doesn't mean that the Swank diet couldn't work for MS patients, but it shows that the diet is not a panacea (i.e., it won't prevent or heal MS in every patient).

Dr. Lechtenberg's Book

The *Multiple Sclerosis Fact Book* by Dr. Lechtenberg attempts to provide encyclopedic coverage of the disease, its causes, its diagnosis, its therapy, its prognosis, etc. It's written in language understandable to most patients, but the depth and breadth mean that occasional pearls of advice tend to get lost amidst many pages of general information about the disease. Unfortunately, the latter are not as critically important for patients because they usually don't change anything the patient needs to do.

A principal difference between the book by Dr. Lechtenberg and this one is that his book consists of conventional medical wisdom and lacks the perspective of a patient that has suffered these complications. For example, regarding fatigue, his book recommends trying a medication (amantadine) that is often recommended by neurologists but has been reported to benefit only a minority of patients and to work less well over months. A recent Cochrane meta-analysis said, "The efficacy of amantadine in reducing fatigue in people with MS is poorly documented, as well as its tolerability." [Pucci E, Branas P, D'Amico R, Giuliani G, Solari A, Taus C. Amantadine for fatigue in multiple sclerosis. Cochrane Database Syst Rev. 2007; CD002818.] In the five trials included in the meta-analysis, patients complaining of amantadine side effects ranged from 10% to 57%. Previously reported side effects of amantadine have included nausea, anxiety, hyperactivity, insomnia, difficulty concentrating, agitation, exacerbation of pre-existing seizures, exacerbation of pre-existing psychiatric illnesses, and anticholinergic effects such as dry mouth, blurred vision and constipation. If published data don't show more benefit than risk, I'm not inclined to try the drug and more likely to recommend what Dr. Swank did: "lying down and resting."

Dr. Lechtenberg says, "people with multiple sclerosis do not usually develop serious problems with stomach or intestinal activity, but some problems do result from inactivity and medication side effects. Constipation often develops in people who, either because of pain or weakness, cannot be active.... Fluid restrictions designed to improve bladder control may exacerbate constipation."

I agree with Dr. Lechtenberg that causation of almost everything is multifactorial and that dehydration, medication side effects, and inactivity contribute to the constipation of MS patients. But I disagree with his conclusion that medication side effects, dehydration and inactivity are the primary causes for MS patients because they were not the primary causes of mine. How do I know? When my first MS attack occurred, I became constipated at a time when I was not dehydrated at all and before any MS-related inactivity or medication occurred. It was thus obvious that central nervous system damage from the large gadolinium enhancing plaque in my cervical spinal cord (i.e., in my neck) was responsible. The constipation that started with my first attack never remitted. My constipation also got worse repeatedly with subsequent MS attacks, when, once again, there was no medication side effect, dehydration or inactivity. Dr. Giesser's book disagrees with Dr. Lechtenberg, saying that MS-related demyelination impairs gastrointestinal function. It's possible that my disagreement with Dr. Lechtenberg about this relates to a philosophical or semantic difference regarding the word "serious." I agree that my MS-related constipation is not as serious as intestinal obstruction, but I consider it serious nevertheless because my colon was healthy before the first attack and diseased after it, resulting in my having to eat something different for breakfast every subsequent day for the rest of my life. That's "serious," as I see it. Over the years, my constipation got worse – so much worse that at times I wondered if I might die of terminal constipation. That's serious.

I've seen no studies concluding that gastrointestinal motility isn't affected by MS. Controlled studies showed hyperreflexia, impaired filling capacity, impaired motility, impaired postprandial peristalsis, impaired myoelectrical activity, etc. [Glick ME, Meshkinpour H, Haldeman S, Bhatia NN, Bradley WE. Colonic dysfunction in multiple sclerosis. *Gastroenterology.* 1982;83:1002–7.] [Glick M, Bhatia NN, Bradley WE, Johnson B. Colonometry, cystometry, and evoked potentials in multiple sclerosis. *Archives Neurol.* 1982; 39:698-701.] Another controlled study showed significant slowing of gastric emptying. [el-Maghraby TA, et al. Gastric motility dysfunction in patients with multiple sclerosis assessed by gastric emptying scintigraphy. *Can J Gastroenterol.* 2005; 19:141-5.]

These aren't changes likely to be due to dehydration or inactivity. A normal person at bed rest would not show such abnormalities.

I was most inactive when I suffered three vertebral compression fractures at 15 years of age. I was inactive because a surgeon prescribed bed rest for six weeks after the fractures. I had mild constipation during the first few weeks while taking codeine tablets for pain, but this required no therapy and resolved while still at bed rest after stopping the codeine.

Moreover, at various times following my retirement due to physical disability, I had to use 3 to 5 consecutive partial days of bed rest to heal a herniated lumbar disc. During those weeks of greatly increased inactivity I never experienced a worsening of my MS-related constipation. By contrast, I once took during the same time period one half of an oxycodone tablet because of severe shoulder pain. It relieved the pain, but was followed by a marked increase in constipation the next day.

Intentional dehydration is something most MS patients end up using at some point because of loss of bladder control. I used it with increasing frequency during the 12.5 years that I continued working after onset of MS. During all of that time, I never suffered increased constipation temporally related to the dehydration (e.g., no worsening during the work week or improvement during time off).

I continued using intentional dehydration for social occasions after retirement including severe dehydration for all day travel to and from my 30 year medical school reunion and still had no problems with increased constipation that was temporally associated.

I conclude after years of using intentional dehydration with no ill effects that dehydration contributed little to my M- related constipation. On the other hand, as my MS-related constipation continued to get progressively worse, I reached a point a couple of years later (i.e., after 19 years of having MS) when I was unable to miss a single 13 ounce glass of fluid during the day without suffering an easily noticeable bout of increased constipation that could last for days. So, my comment on Dr. Lechtenberg's conclusion about dehydration contributing to the constipation of MS patients is agreement that it does, but disagreement that it is the primary cause while noting that its contribution varied greatly over the course of my illness.

Dr. Lechtenberg's book says, "Many people become worried when they fail to have a bowel movement regularly, but there is nothing intrinsically dangerous about not having a bowel movement every day. When severe impaction occurs, it can usually be relieved with a soap suds or fleets enema. In extreme cases, manual disimpaction may be necessary, but this type of intervention should be attempted only by experienced personnel." I agree with Dr. Lechtenberg that failure to have a bowel movement every day isn't "dangerous," but constipated feces remaining in the rectum have caused me considerable problems that I will discuss in a subsequent chapter.

Dr. Lechtenberg's book advises that MS patients with vertebral fractures have no weight bearing while the fractures are healing. As mentioned above, I had three vertebral fractures due to an accident at 15 years of age and was prescribed six weeks of bed rest before being placed in a body cast. As a healthy 15-year-old, I tolerated six weeks of bed rest, but a patient debilitated by MS would have trouble tolerating several full days of bed rest, to say nothing of the months required for healing of fractures.

For prevention of urinary tract infection in MS patients, Dr. Lechtenberg recommends 1) cleansing with mild soap and water around the urethral meatus in women (doesn't say what frequency or how long the cleaning should take); 2) acidifying the urine by drinking cranberry juice or prune juice, and eating plenty of meat and poultry [while avoiding tomato juice, orange juice or grapefruit juice]); 3) taking vitamin C supplements—no more than 500 mg per dose and no more often than four tablets per day; 4) and, if the first three measures don't prevent repeated infections, taking long term combination antibiotics like trimethoprim-sulfamethoxazole.

Urinary tract infections (UTIs) are frequent among MS patients (including men) despite using such preventive measures. The recommendation of using cranberry juice is an old, traditional remedy, but a recent Cochrane meta-analysis of randomized controlled trials showed no efficacy in preventing urinary tract infection. [Jepson RG, Williams G, Craig JC. Cranberries for preventing urinary tract infections. Cochrane Database Syst Rev 2012;10: CD001321. doi: 10.1002/14651858.CD 0011321.pub5.] Cleansing with soap and water around the urethral meatus and vitamin C are not approaches associated with much data showing prevention of urinary tract infection. If soap contacts the urethral meatus, this also causes burning pain.

I used a different approach for preventing UTIs that was associated with my getting none during my first 20 years and 8 months of MS. My approach to UTI prevention will be discussed in detail in a subsequent chapter.

Dr. Lechtenberg said that dehydration and hyperventilation can each cause worsening of an MS patient's neurologic deficits. As discussed above, I used intentional dehydration for many years with no ill effects. I hyperventilated one time as an MS patient. I did this because I had a mild rib fracture and, getting up groggy at night, was unsure what the pleuritic sensation in my left chest was; I breathed deeper and felt it more, but was still unsure. Doing that several times didn't seem to worsen any neurologic deficit, but resulted in syncope. After coming to on the floor, the pleuritic sensation in my left chest was clearly pain, the rib fracture obviously worsened by falling on my left side again.

Do I agree with anything in Dr. Lechtenberg's book? Yes. Some examples: I agree with Dr. Lechtenberg that the dietary cure of MS claimed by Drs. Swank and Jelinek is likely inaccurate.

Dr. Lechtenberg says, "Additional fluids may help considerably [with constipation] especially if fruit juices are the major source of the additional fluids. At least 2 quarts of fluid should be a regular part of the daily diet. Increasing fluid intake may be impractical, however, if the individual also has a problem with urinary incontinence. Fluid restrictions designed to improve bladder control may exacerbate constipation, so other changes to the diet must be attempted. Loading the diet with high fiber foods and unprocessed fruits should help to avoid constipation. Bran cereals and whole-grain breads will increase the bulk and fiber in the diet and improve the ease of bowel movements.,,, Sugar, peas, beans, and other foods that produce substantial intestinal gas should be avoided because they can make the individual with constipation even more uncomfortable."

I agree with Dr. Lechtenberg that drinking 2 quarts of fluids would be helpful but also that this can be impractical for patients with bladder control problems. I agree that bran, unprocessed fruits, and whole-grain products help and that foods producing substantial intestinal gas can be a problem in MS patients with constipation; my problem with the gas wasn't bloating and pain as Dr. Lechtenberg seemed to imply, but rather competition with the bladder for space in the pelvis when the colon becomes inflated by gas. I always got "substantial gas" after eating beans but not after eating sugar or peas, but I am sure that some patients have problems from sugar or peas. It's important for each patient to pay attention to what happens after adding something new to the diet.

Dr. Lechtenberg says, "with urinary urgency, the bladder must be emptied within minutes or seconds or incontinence will occur. It is not an illusion that the bladder must be emptied quickly. As the urgency worsens, accidental emptying of the bladder will become more of a problem. The affected individual wets himself or herself because the bladder overflows after it fills to excess or it contracts reflexively before it is filled to capacity."

Yes, this can become a predictable scenario for MS patients, but things can be done to prevent it; I prefer to avoid the anticholinergic medications Dr. Lechtenberg recommends because they can cause constipation, an intolerable complication for me. My approach to preventing this will be discussed in detail in a subsequent chapter.

Dr. Lechtenberg recommends seeing a physical therapist as one approach to controlling spasticity. I strongly agree, but, as mentioned above, his attempt to be encyclopedic means that some "pearls" of wisdom like this don't receive enough emphasis. They tend to get lost among pages and pages of information that changes nothing the patient needs to do.

Dr. Giesser's Book

The book *MS for Dummies* by Dr. Giesser and a couple of co-authors also attempts encyclopedic coverage, but does a somewhat better job of keeping its recommendations separated from the sections of general information and clearly identifiable as such.

For fatigue, Dr. Giesser's book recommends trying the same medication that Dr. Lechtenberg's book recommends (amantadine) or four others (modafinil [Provigil], fluoxetine [Prozac], methylphenidate [Ritalin], and dextroamphetamine and amphetamine [Adderal]). Dr. Lechtenberg's book says the latter is contraindicated. None of these drugs are FDA-approved for MS-related fatigue, and none of the recommendations are based upon positive results of multiple controlled studies. The only drug Drs. Giesser and Lechtenberg both recommended was amantadine, which a Cochrane meta-analysis said didn't work. Dr. Giesser's idea is that the patient should try each of the medications and see which one works the best with the fewest side effects. As stated above, I feel I've already had too many side effects and prefer not to follow this approach.

Dr. Giesser's book recommends three things for preventing urinary tract infections in MS patients: 1) emptying one's bladder completely by urination if possible and, if not possible, by intermittent self-catheterization (it adds that double voiding may help. In order to do that, it says that the patient should move [e.g. stand up if previously sitting down] and try again, reasoning that the movement can "restimulate the urination process.") 2) drinking plenty of fluids (6 to 8 glasses of water per day, specifying that other fluids are okay but avoiding caffeine, aspartame, diet soda and alcohol; it advises that many patients with MS try to manage a misbehaving bladder by reducing fluid intake to avoid an accident but says that that is a mistake); 3) acidifying the urine by increasing daily intake of protein, cranberries or cranberry juice, plums, and/or prunes and by decreasing intake of citrus fruits and juices, milk, milk products, and potatoes; and that, if those measures fail and MS patients get recurrent UTIs anyway, 4) taking a long term, low-dose combination antibiotic such as trimethoprim-sulfamethoxazole.

Does emptying the bladder prevent urinary tract infection as multiple books about MS suggest? The importance of there being 0 mL versus 5 mL in the bladder after voiding has not been clearly documented. I'm somewhat doubtful. I haven't seen data from controlled studies showing the effect. Do those who believe this think that emptying the bladder can cure an early infection? I'm doubtful of that. Do they believe that it can prevent a urinary tract infection about to start by washing microbes out of the urethra? My own guess is that urine left inside the urethra is more of a problem because it can conduct microbes from the urethral meatus to the bladder.

There are also few data available regarding particular fluid volume intakes and the risk of urinary tract infection according to a review by Beetz. [Beetz R. Mild dehydration: a risk factor of urinary tract infection? *Eur J Clin Nutr.* 2003; 52 (Suppl 2):S52-8.]

To manage bowel problems, Dr. Giesser recommends developing a regular bowel regimen: "the keys to comfortable bowel management are preventing the problems in the first place and developing a regular bowel regimen. But remember, regular doesn't necessarily mean daily. Instead, it just means that an interval that's normal for you (probably every one to three days). The following strategies will help you keep things moving along: 1) Drink 6 to 8 glasses of liquid per day. 2) eat a diet that's high in fiber, such as raw fruits and vegetables, nuts, seeds, and whole-grain cereals and breads. 3) pick a consistent time of day for a relaxed bowel movement. The ideal time is about 20 minutes after a meal (breakfast is generally best because you're at home before the start of your busy day), when your natural gastrocolic reflex is working to move content through the bowel. Daily use of a high-fiber product like Metamucil or Citrucel may be sufficient to promote regular bowel movements. Regular use of a stool softener like Colace can help with hard, dry stools. If the first two aren't sufficient, a laxative such as MiraLAX, Peri-Colace, or Perdiem, can help manage constipation. Stronger laxatives should be avoided if possible because they are generally habit-forming. Glycerin suppositories may be sufficient to stimulate a bowel movement. If that isn't effective, a Dulcolax suppository may do the trick. Enemeez Mini -enema is a lubricating suppository that safely stimulates bowel action."

I disagree with Dr. Giesser's recommendation to "pick [any] consistent time of day for a bowel movement." The reason I disagree isn't because of controlled studies but because morning and evening are as different as night and day for an MS patient with severe spasticity and constipation (which are perhaps interrelated problems). The likelihood of success is tremendously higher after breakfast than after supper.

I also disagree with Dr. Giesser's suggestion that a bowel movement every three days is adequate. The reason I disagree is again not that there are controlled studies showing that one frequency is better than another. The reason is that allowing continuation of severe constipation causes me intolerable problems. This will be discussed at greater length in a subsequent chapter.

Dr. Giesser said catheterization of the bladder is "painless (yes, we really mean painless)..." I'm sorry to have to disagree, but having been catheterized one time by a urologist, who assured me that he was using the smallest caliber catheter and being as gentle as possible, I was able to feel a large amount of pain. Blood in the urine that resulted from the catheterization irritated the bladder and caused burning dysuria when I peed it out after getting home. The pain resolved after that one voiding removed the blood. It's possible that women have less pain than men with the procedure, and some MS patients with impaired sensation may feel no pain.

Dr. Giesser said, "people who are experiencing bladder problems tend to cut back on liquid in order to avoid having to pee all the time. However, reducing fluid intake can worsen fatigue and constipation and can increase the risk of urinary tract infections. So do your best to drink eight glasses of liquid per day." As mentioned above, intentional dehydration wasn't associated with increased constipation during my first 19 years of MS; after that, it was. Intentional dehydration was never associated with increased fatigue or urinary tract infection for me, and I was unable to find controlled studies showing that it caused those two things in MS patients. Dr. Lechtenberg said that trying to drink that much could be "impractical" for patients having urinary incontinence.

Dr. Giesser says that, "involuntary "periodic limb movements ... occur only during sleep" and can be controlled with baclofen. I disagree. Periodic limb movements of my spastic extremities do usually occur in bed at night, but often begin in the evening after supper before going to bed and rarely as early as mid-day in my spastic left arm. Even when baclofen was having very powerful effects on my spastic rigidity, it had none on my periodic limb movements. Control of this problem will be discussed more in a later chapter.

Dr. Giesser, who disagrees with Dr. Swank's hypothesis that a diet low in saturated fat can cure or prevent MS, recommended reading another book about MS by a nonphysician entitled *Multiple Sclerosis: 300 Tips for Making Life Easier*, which recommends a low-fat diet for MS patients.

Is there anything Dr. Giesser said that I agree with? Yes.

I agree that the dietary cure of MS claimed by Drs. Swank and Jelinek is likely inaccurate.

Dr. Giesser says that CNS damage causes constipation in MS patients. I agree. Dr. Giesser adds that constipation in MS patients is worsened by reduced mobility due to weakness, fatigue, or stiffness, by relative dehydration, and by medication side effects. I agree.

Dr. Giesser said, "no medication can take the place of adequate rest and exercise." She also recommends energy conservation strategies such as 1) saving energy for the stuff that's most important, 2) not overdoing it, 3) paying attention to the signals one's body sends, 4) making full use of the tools and devices that are available, and 5) maintaining a healthy body weight. I agree.

Dr. Giesser's book recommends seeing a physical therapist as one way of managing spasticity. I agree, but the recommendation was made in the context of discussing how to assemble a team of 15 different individuals to take care of an MS patient, without emphasizing that seeing a physical therapist is vitally important to an MS patient while seeing most of the other mentioned care providers (e.g. a clinical nurse) is not.

The Fifth Book Mentioned Above

A fifth book, *The Handbook of Multiple Sclerosis*, edited by Dr. Stuart Cook, is much larger, more expensive, and written for physicians by a team of neurologists specializing in aspects of multiple sclerosis. This book is the most authoritative reference I reviewed and has the best documentation of the science supporting what it says.

Does that mean that it is invariably correct? No. For example, it says pretty much the same thing that Dr. Lechtenberg says about constipation in MS patients – that it's primarily due to dehydration and immotility rather than a consequence of MS-related damage to the central nervous system. Dr. Lechtenberg may have been influenced by Dr. Cook's authoritative book.

What's to say that Dr. Cook's and Dr. Lechtenberg's books are wrong about this? In the first place, they aren't completely wrong. Dehydration and immotility do contribute to constipation in MS patients. Where they are wrong is suggesting that that's pretty much the be-all and end-all of the problem. How do I know? As stated above, during my first attack, I developed constipation long before any dehydration or immotility, making it clear that these problems were a consequence of the inflammatory lesion and subsequent demyelination in my spinal cord. Studies of colonometrograms in MS patients and healthy controls show significant differences, with hyperreflexia, impaired motility, impaired postprandial gastrocolic reflexes, reduced filling capacity, etc. in MS patients.[Glick ME, Meshkinpour H, Haldeman S, Bhatia NN, Bradley WE. Colonic dysfunction in multiple sclerosis. Gastroenterology. 1982;83:1002–7.] [Haldeman S, Glick M, Bhatia NN, Bradley WE, Johnson B. Colonometry, cystometry, and evoked potentials in multiple sclerosis. Archives Neurol. 1982; 39:698-701.]

The Handbook of Multiple Sclerosis recommends that, "Steady stretching should be done for sustained periods (e.g., minutes) at a force that is sufficient to cause 30 minutes or so of post-stretch discomfort; the stretching should take place several times per day." But the reference supporting this recommendation was based upon a study of stretching the legs of patients with ankle joint plantar flexion contractures after stroke. [Halar EM, Stolov WC, Venkatesh B, et al. Gastrocnemius muscle belly and tendon length in stroke patients and able-bodied persons. *Arch Phys Med Rehabil.* 1978; 59:476-484.] I can stand against a wall or a counter with all of my weight being supported by my spastic left leg for 15 minutes and have no post-stretch discomfort at all. A minute or two of stretching with no post-stretch discomfort usually works to help keep the spasticity in my left leg at bay. By contrast, while stretching, I have caused discomfort in my healthier right leg due to herniation of a lumbar intervertebral disc; this type of post-stretch discomfort is not beneficial, and the MS patient should avoid doing this. This complication and how I prevented it will be discussed at greater detail in a later chapter.

A Sixth Book

I also checked out a sixth book to check for overlap with this book. [*Multiple Sclerosis: 300 Tips for Making Life Easier* by Shelley Peterman Schwartz] Written by an MS patient with no medical training, it mostly talks about nonmedical things like ways of creating a wardrobe for MS patients, ways to make holding a pencil easier by wrapping it with rubber bands, personal care, grooming, dressing, shopping, meal preparation, home safety, kitchen and bath, house-cleaning, exercise, recreation, travel, packing tips, record-keeping, physician appointments, medication organization, speaking and writing.

Her tips and mine thus overlap very little.

I found about a half dozen topics of potential overlap, but we usually had a different point of view even if we started off agreeing (e.g., I agreed with her statement that applesauce or butter can help an MS patient with dysphagia swallow pills that are hard to swallow with water, but that wouldn't lead me to recommend routinely using them for that purpose because a thick, pulpy juice [e.g., Campbell's Tomato Juice] works just as well for me and is logistically easier to use).

Ms. Schwartz's book says, "there is evidence that a low-fat diet might benefit MS patients" and recommends that MS patients consume less than 30 g of fat per day. This recommendation inaccurately portrays what Dr. Swank said, failing to specify that the hypothesis related specifically to saturated fat (which includes hydrogenated vegetable oil). In addition to the 15 to 20 g of saturated fat allowed by the Swank diet, MS patients were allowed to consume up to 50 g of vegetable oil or cod liver oil per day, so the "30 g" limit of fat in Ms. Schwartz's book is incorrect if it's referring to the Swank diet.

Ms. Schwartz's book mentioned using dental floss devices that allow flossing with one hand (without exactly saying this and without discussing why flossing might be more important for an MS patient than for a normal, healthy person).

It said that cordless phones could make it easier for MS patients to answer a landline telephone. I agree, but the Vtech cordless phones we used were inconvenient in another way – they interfered with the Wi-Fi connection of my computer (this was only tried with one brand and model of cordless phone; it's possible that a cordless phone operating on a different frequency wouldn't cause this problem). Cell phones didn't interfere with the Wi-Fi connection to the computers, but they don't allow an MS patient to answer a landline phone. *300 Tips* mentions that headsets are available and can facilitate telephone communication. A wireless Bluetooth headset will allow an MS patient to answer a landline telephone if within 30 feet in the same room. Another type of wireless headset using DECT technology (e.g., Office Runner by Sennheiser) will allow a paralyzed patient in a different room to answer a landline telephone if within 400 feet; that's the type that I use. Sennheiser makes another microphone (DW Pro) that works with the same base and telephone lifter used by the Office Runner. DW Pro is probably more durable. I had to switch to that because the headband used with Office Runner kept falling apart. I had no problems with the Office Runner microphone, base, or telephone lifter.

300 Tips also makes readers aware that dictation programs can be used by those unable to type because of paralyzed hands or carpal tunnel syndrome (e.g., Dragon NaturallySpeaking software). The Office Runner and DW Pro headsets perform very well dictating into Dragon NaturallySpeaking software.

Such dictation software is a godsend for a paralyzed person who can't type anything, and I love it for that reason. As best I can tell, that program is the best dictation program available. But to be completely honest, I would have to admit that my affection for that program (Dragon Premium versions 7-12.5) was tempered by conflicting emotions. Dragon often frustrated me by making the same mistakes repeatedly (e.g., typing "Tuesday" when I said "choose two").

I dictated two pages of text using Dragon Premium versions 12.5

and 13 and had error rates of 4.4%, and 2.5%, respectively. The rate with 13 was significantly lower (p=0.022), implying higher accuracy with the newer version. But dictating the same two pages using Dragon Premium 11 gave an even lower error rate of 1.5%, also significantly lower than for version 12.5. Because I started with version 12.5, I re-dictated the two pages twice more with that version to make sure the higher error rate was not just an order effect (i.e., lower error rates due to my reading better after doing so several times); the error rates actually rose to 5.2% and 6.6%, making an order effect an unlikely explanation for the observed differences. There was not a significant difference between the error rates of version 11 and version 13 (p=0.16). The reason my version of 11 was as accurate as 13 may have been due to more verbal training of the software. Dragon 13 was the only one of three that was able to dictate directly into an email program (Gmail). The other two were incompatible. I dictated the same two pages of text into Dragon Professional (a more costly, reputedly more accurate version), which had an error rate of 2.1%; it also worked with Gmail.

Is there anything Ms. Schwartz says that I agree with? Yes. For example, she says that fatigue can be managed by alternating periods of rest and activity and that "pop-up tissues are easier to grab than the kind that lie flat in the box."

Briefer Comments about 7th and 8th Books

A 7th book about MS was published in 2014 (*The Wahls Protocol* by Dr. Terry Wahls and Eve Adamson). It promotes using a "Paleolithic" diet and percutaneous electrical stimulation (the latter is usually applied to relieve chronic pain). Dr. Wahls reported dramatic improvement of her MS from this therapy (going from being chronically unable to sit upright in a wheelchair to pedaling a bicycle 8 miles a day within eight months). She cautioned that it would take "many years and millions of dollars" for clinical studies to prove that her protocol renders such benefits.

An 8ᵗʰ book (*Navigating Life with Multiple Sclerosis* by Kathleen Costello, Dr. Ben W Thrower and Dr. Barbara S Giesser) was published in 2015. Like a couple of the books for MS patients mentioned above, this 8ᵗʰ one attempts encyclopedic coverage. It discusses a number of MS complications, but has little overlap of coping strategies with this book. Costello et al. say that there are no data from controlled studies of the Wahls Protocol, which thus has "not been proven to positively impact MS."

Can any published data help settle this conflict between the 7ᵗʰ and 8ᵗʰ books? Yes, I believe so. Dr.Wahls published a case report regarding improvement of her own condition with her protocol and 2 case series over the next four years. Like in Dr. Swank's study, there were no concurrent control patients. No patients in the case series showed dramatic improvement like the one in the case report.

One study did report a small significant improvement in subjective fatigue, but subjective improvements can occur due to placebo response, which cannot be evaluated in uncontrolled studies.

Will it really take "many years and millions of dollars" to know if the Wahls Protocol works? Astute readers may remember from Chapter 1 of this book that large differences are easy to detect in small, relatively brief studies. The effects Dr.Wahls reported in her case report were more dramatic than those reported by Swank. They shouldn't be hard to detect.

Paleolithic diets recently have become a fad, and some Paleolithic diet enthusiasts favor Dr.Wahls' idea of curing disease by going back to the diet allegedly eaten by our Paleolithic ancestors. Multiple supportive blurbs in *The Wahls Protocol* were written by authors of other books advocating a Paleolithic diet.

Christina Warriner, PhD, an archaeologist on faculty at the University of Oklahoma with research interest in Paleolithic diets, has commented that the "Paleolithic diets" described by enthusiasts often don't resemble the foods actually eaten by Paleolithic people. She didn't specifically mention *The Wahls Protocol*, however.

Table 2-1. Statistical power to detect the large difference in annual MS relapse rates reported by Swank in patients consuming regular diets versus low saturated fat (Swank) diets as a function of sample size in a three-year study.

% Power *	Sample size ½ on each diet	Annual % relapse rate On regular diet	Annual % relapse rate On Swank diet
90	14	100	5
90	46	90	45
99.9	30	98	5
99.9	112	90	45

*= probability of detecting a true difference if it exists

Chapter 3

Finding a Good Physician That You Are Comfortable with

This makes a difference. ("A difference is a difference if it makes a difference.")

It was a recommendation of the patient who called right after I was diagnosed. But how does this topic fit into a book about coping with complications? A physician you trust can help you cope.

This is important for anyone, but especially so for a patient with MS. The first neurologist who saw me and diagnosed MS told me, "no therapy works for that disease. There's no use doing anything."

Given his statement, which was undoubtedly sincere, I saw no reason to go back for clinic visits. I knew that he was a smart guy and he was my friend. He was leveling with me. For those reasons, I couldn't see much point making an appointment, since he truly believed that nothing would help.

For the first 3 years and 8 months after onset of the illness, I didn't have a regular physician who was focusing on the disease. That was not a good situation.

At that point, I got a third relapse ominous enough that I wanted to try methylprednisolone more rapidly than it was given for the first attack. That was when I found the neurologist who would take care of me for the next two decades.

I don't know why the MS patient who called me didn't trust neurologists, but I believe that an MS patient gets better care from a neurologist. No physician will dispense miracles. No water will turn into wine. No one will say, "pick up your bed and walk." But the patient will get basic assistance for the bare essentials of life with MS.

Although I had been warned about the importance of heat, the first time I experienced a problem with internal heat (fever) the temperature elevation wasn't apparent, being only 37.8°C (100°F). I developed global weakness and staggered. I called my neurologist who suggested that I check my temperature and take acetaminophen if it was elevated. An antipyretic like acetaminophen won't change a normal temperature, but will promptly lower a fever. My temperature quickly dropped, and the global weakness disappeared within a half hour as I sat in front of the television news wondering what would happen next. The mild temperature elevation was apparently due to starting glatiramer acetate (Copaxone) injections several days before and did not recur despite continuing daily injections.

When I fell years later and fractured my spine (vertebral compression fractures) and posterior ribs, I had bad pain. My spasticity ratcheted up markedly, making it hard to move with the walker. When I tried to counter the spasticity with more baclofen (which my neurologist had been encouraging me to try for several years), I got so weak and wobbly that I began to feel unable to move around at all. During that crisis, I began to feel hopeless, like the disease had reached checkmate. My neurologist insisted that I "damn the torpedoes" and take a nonsteroidal anti-inflammatory drug in addition to the acetaminophen to help lessen the pain even though an NSAID had already caused me a peptic ulcer four years before. I did what she suggested, and also stopped taking the additional baclofen and slowly got better, inching past the two crises – the crisis of pain and spasticity and the crisis of confidence.

There will be many reasons to have a physician that you trust. Whenever I needed something, my neurologist was there. MS patients often need something. There are often needs for imaging (e.g., an MRI of the brain and spinal cord, x-rays for fractures, bone densitometry for osteoporosis, a chest x-ray for pneumonia, etc.). Medications are needed for relapses, for osteoporosis, for pain, for insomnia, etc.

Without a physician's order, I wouldn't have been able to get a light, manual wheelchair that was covered by Medicare; this was useful for packing in the car and on an airplane for traveling around. Without a physician's order, I wouldn't have been able to get a rollator walker covered by Medicare. Without a physician's order, I wouldn't have been able to get a motorized wheelchair covered by insurance. Without a physician's order, I wouldn't have been able to get a power lift chair which was helpful for dealing with vertebral compression fractures and for healing pressure related furuncles on my buttocks (more about these topics in a subsequent chapter).

Financial complications of the disease are important to consider. The average patient with MS is able to continue working for 10 years after the disease is diagnosed. Retirement obviously results in loss of one's salary, so this must be replaced in order to keep paying for the essentials – food, clothing, housing, utilities, medications, help with activities of daily living, etc.. The way this is usually done is with disability insurance, Social Security disability payments, and long-term healthcare insurance payments.

Without a physician's involvement, I wouldn't have been able to retire due to physical disability without problems. Without a physician's okay, I wouldn't have been able to get my disability insurance, Social Security disability payments, or long-term healthcare insurance. And without an annual physician visit, I wouldn't have been able to keep getting payments from my disability insurance or Social Security Disability.

A physician can also refer an MS patient for a physical therapy evaluation and therapy, which is very important to help control spasticity. A physician can also refer an MS patient to a urologist for urodynamic testing to see what type of MS problems the patient's bladder has. There is one form of MS bladder that can cause obstructive uropathy and renal failure, which can in turn cause death without medical intervention. When I went for urodynamic testing, the urologist told me this, but said that my hyperreflexic bladder was not the type that did that.

So, if my neurologist helped me cope with complications, what's the point of a book talking about coping with complications? Can't each patient just go to her own neurologist? Yes, but the vast majority of the strategies in this book were not suggested by my neurologist. The complications in this book tend to be those that continue plaguing the patient despite one's neurologist's best efforts to help (e.g., see the 15 examples listed on the second page of the Introduction). It's unlikely that the reader's neurologist will suggest any of these strategies. They didn't appear in other books either.

Chapter 4
Avoiding a Defeatist Attitude

"Worry never robs tomorrow of its sorrow, it merely saps today of its strength." – AJ Cronin

"The best is the enemy of the good." – Voltaire, "*La Bégueule* " (i.e., MS patients are better served by appreciating the good they still have than by pining for what they've lost)

"It's not easy being green." – Kermit the Frog, Jim Henson, creator of the Muppets

"It's not easy being paralyzed." – Barry Farr, corollary to Kermit's postulate

"If you love life, don't waste time, because that's the stuff life is made of." – Benjamin Franklin

"There are compensations in all things." – Ralph Waldo Emerson

"Much is taken, but much abides." – Alfred Lord Tennyson

Attitude is an important place to start because it usually begins as a problem for MS patients. Being handed the diagnosis "multiple sclerosis" is a major downer.

Part of the reason for this is that it's such a comedown for newly diagnosed MS patients, most of whom are relatively young with a normal healthy body that has performed almost perfectly.

Shakespeare described this near perfection in *Hamlet*: "What a piece of work is a man! How noble in reason, how infinite in faculty! In form and moving how express and admirable! In action how like an angel! In apprehension how like a god! The beauty of the world! The paragon of animals!"

Well, the average person may not have a body rivaling that of Nadia Comăneci, the first Olympic gymnast in history to receive perfect scores (she did this at the 1976 Montréal Olympics), but every physiologic mechanism basically works fine (e.g., the excretory systems usually work perfectly and without thinking about it, as if on autopilot).

After a "paragon" becomes paralyzed, however, the body beautiful stops working so well. Some refer to the human body as "God's temple." With the onset of MS, it seems that the Devil is set loose in God's temple, and its approach to perfection ends.

MS is a damned if you do, damned if you don't disease (i.e., "the best laid plans of mice and men [and neurologists] oft gang agley [i.e., don't work]" –Robert Burns). It's about losing control – losing control of one's body and the life one was living up until that time. This change is hard to take. It's such a letdown that it makes developing a good attitude difficult.

I was no Nadia Comăneci, but I did have good hand-eye coordination and could do things that some found difficult (e.g., I had the highest batting average in my town's Little League when I was 10, I shot and killed a running rabbit with a bow and arrow when I was 12, and I killed 12 (flying) doves with 12 shots of a 12 gauge shotgun when I was 17). Some may wonder why I shot animals: I grew up in a rural area where folks used hunting and fishing like they did a vegetable garden—to put food on the table. Anyway, I went from having good coordination before my first attack of MS to basically having none.

If attitude can be a problem from the get-go with MS, the challenge often doesn't get easier as the disease progresses because MS complications can become worse and more frequent. As mentioned,

MS is about losing control, and this results in all sorts of undesirable events that seem to waste an MS patient's time constantly. Enduring for 10 years the pain and other adverse effects of daily injections of 3 different, sequential, disease modifying therapies that never reduced the frequency or severity of my MS relapses didn't help my attitude (two types of interferon and glatiramer acetate [Copaxone]).

These things were as hard for me to adjust to as the initial diagnosis. One reason this was difficult for me was that I dislike wasting anything. This dislike may be "hardwired" into my chromosomes. I was descended from Scottish ancestors who famously abhor waste. I naturally sympathize with Ben Franklin's advice about not wasting time. Ironically, MS occurs at a higher frequency among descendants of ancestors from northern Europe, with Scotland accounting for more than its share geographically. So, MS is like a genetic albatross hanging around the necks of numerous Scottish descendants who despise waste, but have to spend inordinate amounts of time doing things like taking off urine drenched clothes, cleaning up, getting out new clothes, getting redressed, extra washing of clothes etc.

A friend of mine, Thomas Harrison Hunter M.D., was paralyzed by poliomyelitis as a young child and thus grew up accepting his paralysis as a given. He told me that he "never thought about being paralyzed as a problem." Despite paralysis, he lived a full life attending Harvard College and then medical school at Harvard and at Cambridge University. He enjoyed extracurricular activities including being on the rowing teams as coxswain at both Harvard College and at Cambridge University. In medicine, he helped to show that penicillin plus streptomycin therapy work better for streptococcal bacterial endocarditis than what had been tried previously. My father knew and loved Tommy when they were together on staff at Washington University School of Medicine in St. Louis. Tommy then moved to the University of Virginia where he served as Dean of the medical school. It was there that I met him.

An obituary written about Tom by a medical colleague, Dr. R.J. Glaser, said that, "the large number of people who had the good fortune to know him will always remember his wonderful personal characteristics [including] his positive outlook, his warmth, his sense of humor, and his sparkle." I agree wholeheartedly.

Patients with cerebral palsy, a congenital condition, probably grow up the same way, accepting their neurologic deficits as a given.

By contrast, probably no MS patients accept their paralysis as a given. At the time of diagnosis, MS patients tend to think, "My perfect life is over with the onset of this life limiting disease – life limiting in so many ways." We tend to be bent out of shape by this inconvenience. But an MS patient receives lots of punches and over-reacting to an individual punch will make staying on an even keel impossible. It's important to be able to "roll with the punches."

It's hard to find scientific data showing that MS patients adopting a positive attitude will do better than those espousing a negative attitude, but most physicians believe this.

MS patients frequently become dependent upon others, and it's clear that a patient with a positive attitude is easier for caregivers to accept and support (i.e., than one with a sour personality). It's easier for family, friends, and other caregivers to empathize with and care for a patient like Tommy showing "[a] positive outlook, warmth, [a] sense of humor, and sparkle." I believe that a patient manifesting those qualities will probably be happier (with or without the companionship and help of others) than a lonely sourpuss.

Dr. Arthur Guyton, a friend and my first mentor in medical research, was also paralyzed by poliomyelitis, but, unlike Tommy, he was stricken in adulthood. His illness began when he was a neurosurgery resident at Massachusetts General Hospital. When I met him, he was using crutches and a wheelchair to get around, but he didn't seem fazed by his ill fortune. He was President of the American Physiology Society, Chair of the Department of Physiology at the University of Mississippi School of Medicine, and the author of an extremely popular textbook on medical physiology. He told me that he had been asked to serve as Dean at Harvard but that he had refused because he preferred to focus on physiology. He was also the father of a dozen children who all seemed to be graduating from prestigious colleges and medical schools (usually Harvard for both). One of the most resilient and determined people I ever met, he seems as good an example as Tommy of how to overcome adversity with grace.

Thomas Jefferson said, "without health there is no happiness." He was right. Every MS patient would agree that there would be greater happiness with continued health.

But Jefferson was also wrong. Despite all kinds of disease resulting in all kinds of suffering, there can still be happiness. After 24 years of MS, I still enjoy reading a good book as much as ever. Ditto for listening to Beethoven, Bach or the Beatles, for eating a piece of chocolate cake, for looking at a painting by Monet, or for watching a winter sun set in a swirl of silver and magenta clouds. I appreciate a beautiful day as much now as ever.

I was never able to run again after my first attack of MS. As a lifelong runner, this bothered me (a lot). Years later, I once dreamed that I was running again, which felt exhilarating, but my sleeping brain was aware that running was as impossible for me as flying by flapping my arms. This lucidity added a touch of irony to the dream. Running was not the only thing taken from me by this disease. I had to retire prematurely due to physical disability from a profession I enjoyed. Similarly, I had to stop avocations such as photography (operating my old Canon camera became impossible as my left arm became paretic), hunting and fishing.

I could list many other things that I had to stop doing, but I probably don't need to because MS patients reading this book are well aware of what being deprived is like.

One of the points of this book is that MS patients may become helpless, but the situation is often not as hopeless as it first appears. A reason for this is that a strategy for countering a new manifestation of the disease can often be devised. Describing such strategies is a major focus of this book.

Another reason is that MS can have natural variation and seem much worse at some times than at others, as mentioned above. For example, I may fall eight times over nine days but then go eight months without falling.

A third reason is that, there can be "compensations in all things," as argued by Ralph Waldo Emerson. For example, I can no longer go to work, but a silver lining of this black cloud is that this affords me time to do some things I always wanted to do but couldn't (e.g., work on a novel). I can no longer hunt or fish, but I can look at photographs from past hunts (see photographs of me "bringing home the bacon" to my family – a Thanksgiving turkey and several geese with the family Labrador that fetched them out of the water).

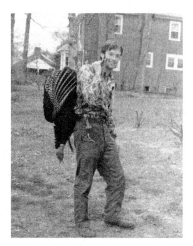

The author bringing home a Thanksgiving turkey before onset of MS.

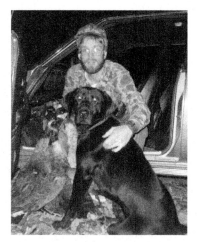

The author bringing home a Christmas goose before onset of MS.

Or I can watch a video about those or other pastimes. I can listen to music, read a book, listen to a book on tape read by someone else, watch a movie, write a letter, or try to write a book. I can't take photographs very well anymore (it's hard for me to handle a camera and it's even harder to move into position to get a good photograph), but I can scan a photograph that I took decades ago and use the digitized photograph to make video presents for loved ones (e.g., with Snapfish online from Hewlett-Packard). I have enjoyed doing this almost as much as I did taking the photographs.

The disabled may begin to feel despondent. Actively seeking a good attitude might help.

MS has reportedly done some very bad things (e.g., caused organic brain syndrome in an 18-year-old patient with his first attack rendering him a human vegetable needing nursing home care; caused paralysis so severe that the patient never walked again after the first attack; etc.), but it doesn't do that to most MS patients and there's no use worrying about every possible manifestation that may or may not occur. That would be like going to war and worrying that every single bullet is aimed at you. There's a philosophical (existentialist) song with French lyrics that won a 1956 Oscar for best original song in the movie *The Man Who Knew Too Much*, "Ce Será Será (whatever will be will be)." That's probably a good way to look at MS – philosophically.

I like to listen to the song "Helpless" by Crosby, Stills, Nash, and Young. Because of its title, I consider "Helpless" to be the theme song of MS. The song is such good music that it almost makes being helpless seem pleasant. After it, I like to listen to "With a Little Help from My Friends" as sung by the Beatles or by Joe Cocker or both, which adds to the same theme. Everybody gets by with a little help from somebody else. This just happens more for the physically disabled. Nobody has to like being physically disabled, but emphasizing the positive aspects seems to help me get by.

After I could no longer do the things mentioned above, I developed an interest in gardening and began tending a patch of 800 daylilies. I was still able to do that for several years and, although I didn't particularly care for weeding when I was young, I came to view weeding these daylilies as therapeutic. As I controlled the weeds that were hampering growth of the daylilies, they sprouted and began growing prolifically, but deer started coming at night and nibbling them to nubs. I heard that deer were like restaurant patrons who don't like finding human hair in a salad, so I started saving clippings of my hair and that of our three sons in Ziploc plastic bags to preserve the human scent. I sprinkled small bits of hair on the daylilies every time a rain washed the hair off. The deer stopped eating the daylilies. They bloomed beautifully all summer for several years until I became too disabled to tend them. After I could no longer tend them, I still enjoyed looking at photographs of them (see photo of my daylilies below and on rear cover).

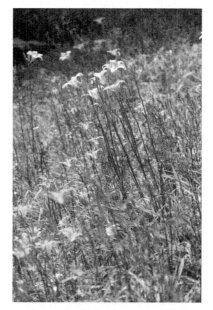

Daylilies prospering with the author's care after he
became too disabled to do much else outdoors.

The only way I could go outside at that point was on my John Deere tractor mower, and I continued mowing through the 17th summer after onset of my MS. Like weeding, mowing was not especially exciting to me as a youth, but I loved doing it as I became more disabled and unable to go outside and feel the ground beneath me and the sun on my face.

Loneliness can become a problem for the housebound, and

constant suffering makes this seem worse. Getting up alone over and over at night for nocturia adds to the misery. There are no easy answers. As mentioned above, I tend to enjoy a number of activities that can be done alone and provide a sense of community with others (e.g., reading a book, listening to music, etc.). It's hard to feel a sense of community getting up to urinate at night, however. I will say that one of our neighbors once hung Christmas tree lights on a small cedar in his front yard and left the lights on all night every night during one Christmas season. Every time I got up for nocturia I saw those lights through my bathroom window and felt a sense of community not only with my neighbor but with everybody who could recognize the value of a Christmas tree –including Charlie Brown's spindly tree ("Maybe it just needs a little love" – Linus). My neighbor never hung lights on that tree again, but I always remembered that they had been there once and felt a sense of community when I remembered how they had cheered me.

It's entirely appropriate to "rage against the dying of the light" as advised by Dylan Thomas and also to "grow old gracefully" as advised by Max Ehrmann in his poem "Desiderata (see below)." While these things may seem to be mutually incompatible, I don't view it that way. As paralysis and spasticity threatened to immobilize me, my approach was to "rage against the dying of the light" by struggling onward as far as I could go with a rollator walker. Because moving around from place to place ends up becoming an MS patient's primary exercise, it's actually this struggle that has kept me going. How does a patient with hemiparesis keep walking? With difficulty. I often feel like getting across the room with my walker seems impossibly far. As I begin to try, I always remember a line by Lao Tzu that, "A journey of 1000 miles begins with a single step."

In this sense, my approach is like that of a basketball coach who says "take what the defense gives you." It also resembles Reinhold Niebuhr's serenity prayer: "God grant me the serenity to accept the things that I can't change, the courage to change the things that I can change, and the wisdom to be able to distinguish the one from the other."

Exasperation with my advancing disability once caused me to snap my wrist angrily [sort of like the motion a Brazilian uses to snap her fingers]. This resulted in stinging pain in the wrist. This leads me to say that it's always better to "get effective" than it is to "get angry." Carpal tunnel syndrome commenced in my wrist right after that stinging pain and has never left. It's possible that it was about to become clinically evident anyway and the angry snapping of the wrist didn't really make much difference, but I'll never be sure. Nevertheless, giving in to the anger probably was not good. Smashing one's fist into a wall is never the right response to feeling angry. The same was true of angrily snapping my wrist.

For the things that are irrevocably gone, I counsel taking a philosophical approach to this – "growing old gracefully." Every reader knows that the family dog seems to age faster than the rest of the family, often reaching old age by the time the family's children are teenagers. It's like that for MS patients. We start using canes, walkers, and wheelchairs long before the rest of our birth cohort. It's difficult at first to accept that. Nobody likes the idea of getting into a wheelchair the first time, just as nobody likes the idea of being paralyzed. Sitting in a wheelchair in front of everyone ("how public like a frog," as Emily Dickinson put it) seems to be a painful admission of personal weakness and failing.

But "honesty is the best policy" and adapting gets a lot easier when the patient is honest with herself about these things. When walking starts failing, a cane, a walker, or a wheelchair can be very helpful and prevent falling, fractures, etc.,

Desiderata

Go placidly amid the noise and haste, and remember what peace there may be in silence. As far as possible without surrender, be on good terms with all persons. Speak your truth quietly and clearly; and listen to others, even

the dull and ignorant; they too have their story. Avoid loud and aggressive persons, they are vexations to the spirit. If you compare yourself with others, you may become vain and bitter; for always there will be greater and lesser persons than yourself.

Enjoy your achievements as well as your plans. Keep interested in your career, however humble; it is a real possession in the changing fortunes of time. Exercise caution in your business affairs; for the world is full of trickery. But let this not blind you to what virtue there is; many persons strive for high ideals; and everywhere life is full of heroism.

Be yourself. Especially, do not feign affection. Neither be critical about love; for in the face of all aridity and disenchantment, it is as perennial as the grass.

Take kindly the counsel of the years, gracefully surrendering the things of youth. Nurture strength of spirit to shield you in sudden misfortune. But do not distress yourself with imaginings. Many fears are born of fatigue and loneliness. Beyond a wholesome discipline, be gentle with yourself.

You are a child of the universe, no less than the trees and the stars; you have a right to be here. And whether or not it is clear to you, no doubt the universe is unfolding as it should.

Therefore be at peace with God, whatever you conceive Him to be, and whatever your labors and aspirations, in the noisy confusion of life keep peace with your soul. With all its sham, drudgery and broken dreams, it is still a beautiful world. Be careful. Strive to be happy.

Max Ehrmann 1927

Chapter 5
The Most Important Attitudinal Question

"There are storms we cannot weather." – *Les Miserables* (the musical)
"I dreamed my life would be so different from this hell I'm living." – *Les Miserables* (the musical)
"To be, or not to be: that is the question: Whether 'tis nobler in the mind to suffer the slings and arrows of outrageous fortune, or to take arms against a sea of troubles, and by opposing end them?"
-- William Shakespeare, *Hamlet*
"Last scene of all,
That ends this strange eventful history,
Is second childishness and mere oblivion,
Sans teeth, sans eyes, sans taste, sans everything."
–William Shakespeare, *As You Like It*
"Come what come may, time and hour run through the roughest day."
–William Shakespeare, *Macbeth*
"Since then – 'tis centuries – and yet
Feels shorter than the day
I first surmised the horses' heads

Were toward eternity."—Emily Dickinson, "Because I could not stop for Death"

The most important attitudinal question routinely faced by MS patients is the most famous one coined by William Shakespeare four centuries ago: "To be or not to be?"

Suicide has been a controversial topic and action for millennia. Some studies say that it occurs two- to three-fold more frequently among MS patients than among the general population, so not mentioning it might be sort of like "ignoring an elephant in the room." It is much more commonly resorted to by patients with depression who feel pathologically that all is hopeless. Because depression is treatable, this is always a mistake for a depressed patient. About half or more of MS patients develop clinical depression. Treatment makes suicide less likely. This is an important reason that depression should be watched for, recognized and treated. Do depressed patients ever commit suicide despite treatment? Yes, but effective therapy can help and should be tried.

International Classification of Diseases (ICD) 10 criteria for a major depressive episode include the following: "the patient usually suffers from a depressed mood, loss of interest and enjoyment, and reduced energy leading to increased fatigability and diminished activity. Marked tiredness is common. Other symptoms include reduced concentration and attention, reduced self-esteem and self-confidence, ideas of guilt and unworthiness, bleak and pessimistic views of the future, ideas or acts of self-harm or suicide, disturbed sleep, and/or diminished appetite." A problem with diagnosing depression in MS patients is that the symptoms of the two diseases often overlap (e.g., insomnia, difficulty concentrating, and fatigue occur with both).

Understanding all of this, can it be said that suicide is ever a rational, right thing for a patient to do?

Many prefer to see this controversial issue as black versus white, but the truth about complicated questions sometimes involves shades of gray. If and when life becomes only suffering, this question can be viewed differently. When I was a medical student at Washington University School of Medicine, an older clinician with a long white coat, gray hair and gravitas, said that it was time to unplug the respirator and allow one of our patients to die. How often does this happen? Is it rare like with Jack Kevorkian?

No, it's actually fairly common. It's usually employed with patients who are about to die anyway, and isn't referred to as "physician-assisted suicide."

Patients can get into very difficult situations from which recovery and meaningful life become impossible. In such a situation, it might be rational. When a physician provides morphine to a patient "circling the drain", this is helping the patient to "get out of this vale of tears" with dignity and without suffering. This is what is done routinely for hospice patients who often have cancer. They may elect to proceed with hospice therapy even though they could live for another 6 to 12 months or more with cancer chemotherapy, but that route involves a lot of painful slogging that they may choose to avoid. I had a friend who recently chose hospice therapy rather than undergo months of uncomfortable cancer therapy.

I will preface my final comments about this thorny subject by mentioning that I was randomly selected to serve as medical school faculty mentor for a freshman medical student starting to learn physical diagnosis. This student and I met over and over throughout the school year discussing how to take a history and how to conduct a physical exam. We went over to the hospital together so he could practice doing both in my presence. We became rather well acquainted. Years later after he finished his postgraduate medical training, he joined the faculty and chose to focus his research on end-of-life management. From this vantage point, he became very involved in the question of physician-assisted suicide that was being used in the Netherlands and Oregon. He always argued vociferously against the practice every time a study or policy statement came out in the news. He became prominent for these views and was frequently in the news himself. By that time, I had been diagnosed with MS and was aware of the bleak circumstances of some of my fellow patients. I knew that suicide was something that crossed the minds of MS patients being paralyzed inside and out, being deserted by spouses, having to retire prematurely, and often becoming housebound and lonely. I never felt that I was in a position to second-guess the judgments of another patient with this disease. So, I wouldn't have been able to oppose the decisions of those in the Netherlands or Oregon in this regard. Oddly enough, "after a' that and a' that," my friend so adamantly opposed to suicide chose to commit suicide himself.

Another friend who was a brilliant physician and head of neuroradiology, the same person who reviewed my MRI with me when I was diagnosed with MS, also chose to commit suicide. It was said that he had developed a brain tumor that was not responding to therapy and he must have been in terrible pain.

There were many details that went into such decisions that were not publicly known. I won't comment upon either case except to repeat that patients can get into very difficult situations from which recovery and meaningful life become impossible. I wouldn't presume to try to judge whether their decisions were "right."

I tend to be a relatively optimistic person. I enjoy reading, writing, listening to music, watching movies − things that can be done alone and yet give me a sense of community with the greatest scholars and artists of all time. I love getting to visit occasionally with family members and friends. I enjoy talking to the nursing aides who assist me with activities of daily living. But having gone through 24 years of this disease and more suffering than most people encounter in a lifetime, it's easy for me to understand how many MS patients could possibly identify with a phrase by John Keats in his "Ode to a Nightingale" about being "half in love with easeful death." At times, struggling with spasticity, weakness and intense pain can become so difficult that giving up seems a reasonable option − "do or die" moments.

When I first was diagnosed with MS, the blow was so devastating that my usual good humor and natural optimism abandoned me. The neurologist who handed me the diagnosis rightly observed that I was bummed out. He suggested that I go for a walk. I said that a walk really wouldn't do the trick. He offered to give me electroconvulsive therapy to jolt me out of the funk his diagnosis had put me in. I said, "no thanks."

There is sufficiently heavy weather for MS patients that pollyannaish bromides like "put on a happy face" often just won't do. I went through stretches of severe pain lasting for months after some vertebral fractures and rib fractures and clavicular fractures, and an undiagnosed right upper quadrant abdominal pain that was apparently due to my trunk flopping forward as I walked holding onto the walker. These were pains not relieved by the only analgesic available to me. At times, I was suffering so much that I wondered whether I would be able to stand going on. It was the sort of pain that forced me to reevaluate that question day after day after day.

When I reached the point of having frank urinary incontinence, at first I had little understanding of what was causing what, and things were seriously out of control. The other books written for MS patients imply that this is just due to hyperreflexia of a spastic bladder, but, as you might guess from Precept 12 in Chapter 1 about cause usually being multifactorial, there are other contributors to the problem. Learning that allowed me to prevent the problem in a way not mentioned in the other books written for MS patients ("there are more things in heaven and earth than dreamt of...").

In one very bad bout, I had to remove wet clothes and put on more clothes resulting in my wearing four different sets of clothes and four different sets of pajamas all during one twenty-four hour period. Some talk about how bad nocturia can be at causing loss of sleep. Urinating on my pajamas and having to remove them, clean up myself, clean the floor, and put on new pajamas takes a patient with hemiparesis like me about an hour. Doing it four times in one night means four hours of lost sleep in addition to the sleep lost due to nocturia. Having to do that four times during the day results in four more hours being lost. And it's more than just wasting time. It's degrading. It's humiliating. In the movie *Groundhog Day*, the main character is perturbed by seeing the same people do the same things repeatedly. With MS, the same things happen repeatedly, but these things seem much worse than what happens in *Groundhog Day*. Being drenched by incontinence one time is awful. Doing this repeatedly is worse than awful.

As mentioned above, when life becomes mere suffering, it's easy to understand a patient wanting to consider options. Being told you have MS is a devastating blow and it seems that more than "a thousand natural shocks" follow that first blow, often in rapid sequence.

At the end, confronting death will be less of a problem after so much suffering. I certainly won't fear "easeful death." But for the first 24 years of my illness, I've always ended up agreeing with what Tennyson says in "Ulysses," "How dull it is to pause, to make an end, to rust unburnished, not to shine in use! As though to breathe were life. Life piled on life were all too little, and of one to me little remains: but every hour is saved from that eternal silence, something more, a bringer of new things...." Or, as George Bailey concludes in *It's A Wonderful Life*, "I want to live again..." I love my family. I always want to see them again. I'd love to see my grandchildren. I always want to see the next sunset, the next sunrise.

For years, when it seemed impossible that I could keep going, I would think of a line in Rodgers and Hammerstein's *The King and I*: "If the Lord in heaven Buddha show the way, I will try to live for one more day..." That's what I usually decide – to try to live for one more day.

Chapter 6
Dealing with Incipient Bowel and Bladder Problems

"A good reliable set of bowels is worth more to a man than any amount of brains." – Josh Billings (Henry Wheeler Shaw), 1818-1885
"In the desert, I learned to keep my bowels open and my mouth shut." – T.E. Lawrence, *Lawrence of Arabia*

Early in MS, my gastrointestinal tract became impaired from top to bottom (e.g., difficulty clearing my throat, spitting or whistling, problems choking on food, drink or saliva, problems chewing food without biting my tongue or cheek, problems defecating, etc.). Those things happened before I started using any medications that could be blamed, making it clear that the MS itself was impairing the function of my gastrointestinal tract. Early in the disease, my urinary tract also became impaired, leaving urine in the urethra that had to be wrung out, blotted, etc. Paresis makes the bowel leave feces in the rectum, just like paresis causes urine to be left in the bladder or urethra.

With MS, many things about the excretory system are impaired and the usual perfection and automaticity of the systems disappear.

A normal healthy person sensing the need to urinate or defecate can postpone this until a socially convenient moment. A paretic, spastic excretory system doesn't allow this. The disease seems to favor whatever is most inconvenient. If I need excretion to be slower, it goes faster. If I want a bowel movement to speed up, it slows down. After years of dealing with this, I decided that an MS patient's colon resembles a snake: it has the shape of a snake (long and tubular) and does whatever it likes whenever it likes with no regard for circumstances.

My first attack began as burning pain and intense itching over the left neck and left shoulder. The neurologist evaluating this said that he believed this was neuropathic pain occurring as a complication of a hepatitis B vaccination given in the left arm two weeks before. The pain continued for two months and was followed by progressive weakness, paresthesias, and numbness of the left arm until the arm was so weak that I could not reach out of the car window to put a card into a slot to drive into the garage at work and had to reach across with my right arm to do it. During those two months, my neurologic exam changed from brisk but normal deep tendon reflexes and downgoing toes when the soles of my feet were stroked with the sharp end of a reflex hammer to pathological (4+) reflexes with clonus and upgoing big toes on both feet (a positive Babinski sign, indicating new upper motor neuron lesion damage). At that point I was admitted to the hospital where an MRI showed unidentified bright objects (demyelination) that didn't enhance in many locations throughout the brain and spinal cord, compatible with a diagnosis of MS and a large gadolinium enhancing (i.e., recent) lesion in the cervical spinal cord.

Although my first attack seemed to focus its fury on my left arm and the left side of my neck, it left me with persistent bowel and bladder problems and difficulty walking securely on my left leg. I could walk for miles (my parking space remained a mile from my office), just not as securely as before.

After my first attack was treated with a several day course of methylprednisolone, I returned to work the following week and tried to go back to "business as usual" as much as possible. I knew there were lingering problems (e.g., residual left arm weakness, numbness and paresthesias, problems with my gait primarily involving the left leg, bowel and bladder problems), but wasn't sure exactly how this would play out since it was my first attack. In the middle of the first morning back at work, I strode to the men's room, walked to a urinal, unzipped my fly and tried to let nature take its usual course. It didn't take more than a few times to know that nature would no longer be taking its former course. Problems I had never had at a urinal before were the following: 1) difficulty initiating urination (especially if someone was standing at the next urinal), 2) markedly reduced pressure of urination, and 3) post void dribbling. By the following week, I had decided that using a urinal was a convenience of the past and that I would always after that have to wait for a stall, sit on a toilet and use a Credé maneuver to initiate urination if needed.

Difficulty urinating or defecating in a public restroom when someone else is present is usually considered a social phobia (paruresis or parcopresis, respectively), [Elitzur B. Psychological treatment for paruresis (bashful bladder). *Harefuah.* 2000; 138:1021-3, 1087.] but physical problems such as obstruction due to prostatic hypertrophy can cause the same symptoms and surgical correction of the obstruction can end the problem. [Rosariao DJ, et al. Urodynamic assessment of the bashful bladder. J Urol. 2000; 163:215-20.] The probability that two diseases would commence at exactly the same time is quite low, suggesting that the new neurologic disease was most likely responsible.

In *Gulliver's Travels*, Lemuel Gulliver extinguishes a Lilliputian palace fire by using his wits and other resources available to him to "make water." This was possible because the palace, like everything else in Lilliput, was tiny. When I was young and vigorous, I'm sure that I could've helped Gulliver. I believe this because when my father would take us deer hunting on a frosty morning, he would stop the car on top of the levee so my brothers and I could "take a leak" before hiking down into the woods to await the dawn. Standing in front of the headlights so we could see where we were peeing, my brothers and I would spout formidable streams of urine, which, falling off the side of a levee top, seemed to fall forever. Sometimes we would "fence" using the streams like Jedi Knights would later use light sabers in *Star Wars*. This prowess at peeing vanished immediately with my first attack, and I'm sure that the Lilliputian palace would've burned to the ground if I was then responsible for saving it like Gulliver.

The incipient bowel and bladder problems were mild compared with what they would become over years of progression, but they were problems nevertheless that had to be dealt with immediately. To keep from wetting my underwear and from leaving urine in the urethra, which could by capillarity conduct microbes from the urethral meatus to the bladder, I began blotting my urethral meatus every time after voiding and thoroughly enough that the last single sheet of bibulous toilet paper was completely dry after the blot. At that time, the volume of urine being dribbled was so small that this only required a minute and just a single sheet or two of toilet paper was adequate. As the disease progressed over years, an enlarging stack of sheets was required and the process consumed more and more time.

My first attack caused constipation and changes to the anal sphincter that required me to use soap and water to clean up after each bowel movement rather than just dry toilet paper. For the constipation, I started eating Raisin Bran each morning to add bulk and fiber to make it easier to have a bowel movement. This worked but resulted in changes in the consistency of the feces that made it still more difficult to clean up quickly after a bowel movement. This made it difficult to get my bottom thoroughly clean after a bowel movement and meant that trying to do this would consume considerably more time than usually devoted to wiping after a bowel movement. Did I find any shortcuts? No. I used soap and water each time until there was no more visible fecal staining on the toilet paper plus one more wipe with soap and water before a couple of wipes with dry toilet paper. If I had fecal staining of any clothes, I undressed, showered and put on clean clothes. That's really my approach in a nutshell – avoiding fecal contamination at all costs, even when it seems tedious and inconvenient.

In addition to walking more slowly to and from the bathroom, these changes (having to routinely blot the urethra and taking longer to clean up after a bowel movement) made using the bathroom at work a problem because it required so much extra time. These changes made me do whatever I could to minimize using the bathroom at work (e.g., intentional dehydration).

Chapter 7
When Constipation Gets Worse

"If you can wait and not be tired by waiting..." – Rudyard Kipling, "If"
"They also serve who merely stand and wait." – John Milton, "On His Blindness"
"They also serve who merely sit and wait." – Barry Farr, corollary to Milton's postulate
"If it be now, 'tis not to come. If it be not to come, it will be now. If it be not now, yet it will come. The readiness is all." – William Shakespeare, *Hamlet*
"Time is different here." – Thomas Mann, *The Magic Mountain*
"My pig won't jump the stile and I shan't get home tonight." English fairytale
"Between the idea and the reality falls the shadow." – T.S. Eliot, "The Hollow Men"
"I'm looking for a miracle" – Jesse Winchester

Normal healthy people often tend to take bowel movements for granted. For most MS patients, bowel movements become too iffy to take for granted.

As mentioned above, constipation began with my first attack of MS, didn't remit much, and often got worse with subsequent attacks (e.g., noticeable exacerbation of constipation with two of the next four attacks).

Also mentioned above, I started dealing with this by eating Raisin Bran each morning for breakfast.

Not long after, when constipation worsened with a subsequent attack, a daily 100-mg capsule of docusate sodium was added with improvement (it's an osmotic laxative that works by bringing more water into the stool).

After that, for each increment of constipation, I added more dietary fiber (e.g., first red grapes, then an apple per day, then blueberries with my daily cereal, then more blueberries with my daily cereal, etc.). Other fruits could be used and work as well, but I got used to using the ones I started with and became well-regulated. Dried fruits could also be used to add dietary fiber (e.g., raisins, prunes, etc.).

After reaching a point of increasing effort with diminishing returns (i.e., the stool kept getting bulkier but stopped helping relieve new increases in constipation), I stopped adding more fiber and started adding more docusate sodium with my neurologist's okay.

As mentioned in Chapter 1 (Precept 16 "Amounts Can Matter"), I came to understand that an increase of insoluble fiber being eaten at one end of the gastrointestinal tract (e.g., raisin bran, blueberries, grapes, apples, salad, broccoli, cauliflower, etc.) resulted in an increase in insoluble fiber coming out at the other end as feces. So, if I was well-regulated eating a certain amount of Raisin Bran cereal, doubling the amount of cereal resulted in more feces and the need for more bowel movements, which is problematic with MS related constipation.

With this approach, I made it through 13 years and 10 months of MS-related constipation before having to add a second daily capsule of docusate sodium to the regimen with breakfast. Three years later, a third daily dose of docusate sodium got added to the regimen, again with breakfast.

Until this point, there was nothing unusual about my approach

to MS related constipation (e.g., trying to emphasize dietary modifications as much as possible before implementing laxatives). The
next paragraph will describe where my path began to diverge from
the approaches the other books describe.

So What Was Different about My Approach?

1) Avoiding Foods That Became Actively Constipating

In brief, I identified and then avoided actively constipating foods
(the other books didn't mention that actively constipating foods
exist; by contrast, they emphasized what was deficient in the diet –
fiber, fluid, etc.).

The constipation discussed above was not related to any recent
changes (e.g., drinking less fluid per day, eating a new food, taking
a new medication, etc.). But after 17 ½ years of MS, I started having
bouts of increased constipation triggered by eating particular foods.
In each case, the food was one that I had eaten many times before
with no ill effects, suggesting that that food may become actively
constipating but only in patients with severe, underlying constipation (e.g., such as that due to increasingly impaired gastrointestinal
motility due to MS).

After this started, these bouts occurred predictably every time
I ate one of the constipating foods, usually beginning the following day and lasting for about a week. The constipation caused by
an actively constipating food also occurred along a dose gradient
(i.e., the more constipating food I ate, the worse the constipation
would be). Before this pattern began, I had heard that certain foods
were constipating (e.g., bananas), but this conflicted with my own
experience, leaving me uncertain what it meant. I had eaten large
numbers of bananas for decades with no problems despite having
MS related constipation.

The first food that caused me a bout of additional constipation
was MorningStar Farms Grillers when I tried to switch to eating
that for lunch as an everyday staple. I had to stop eating it, but then

tried to resume five times. Every time resulted in a bout of additional constipation and excess gas in the colon, which together resulted in increased urinary urgency.

After this pattern became inescapably obvious, I began to notice the same phenomenon with other foods. I ate a single, firm banana to see what would happen. I had a bout of increased constipation that lasted six days. In a different month, I tried eating bananas flambé for dessert with the same result. I wondered whether eating a mushy banana would cause this, but have not tried that.

Eggbeaters, made with egg white, were constipating when cooked in a variety of ways: 1) as scrambled eggs using Pam, 2) when baked as a casserole at 350°F with sliced mushrooms, sliced black olives, artichokes marinated in olive oil, and diced tomato and avocado, 3) when the same casserole was baked at 325°F in a casserole dish sitting in a water bath, and finally 4) when cooked as scrambled eggs using no Pam). I wondered if raw Eggbeaters would do the same, but didn't try that.

Eating vanilla soy ice cream sandwiches with firm chocolate wafers on the side (from the companies So Delicious and Tofutti Cuties) repeatedly resulted in additional constipation, but eating soy vanilla ice cream made by So Delicious with chocolate syrup from Hershey did not. Chocolate chips made by Enjoy Life also repeatedly resulted in additional constipation. Taken together, these observations suggest that chocolate per se is not constipating because chocolate syrup never caused me additional constipation, but the firm, solid chocolate was associated with increased constipation. They also suggest the possibility that undigested portions of certain dense foods flowing downstream through the gastrointestinal tract could serve as a template for formation of more dense, constipated stool. But that certainly would not explain why other foods were actively constipating (e.g., Eggbeaters cooked as soft scrambled eggs).

Other foods that actively caused constipation for me included the following: 1) chocolate cake made by Turtle Island, 2) MorningStar Farms Chik 'n Strips, 3) Portobello mushrooms cooked with oil, 4)

Veggie Patch Portobello Mushroom Burger (apparently no longer available from Veggie Patch), 5) Amy's Bistro Burgers, 6) Jif Peanut Butter, 7) Kroger pizza crust, 8) MorningStar Farms Hickory BBQ Riblet, 9) ratatouille made by sautéeing vegetables, 10) Amy's Roasted Vegetable Pizza, 11) strawberry-rhubarb pie made by Willamette Valley Fruit Company with palm oil as the shortening, 12) chex mix made by baking Chex cereals coated with margarine and spices etc. for a couple hours 13) Tofurkey made by Turtle Island, 14) rum cake made with Crisco or olive oil, 15) sautéed onions, 16) salad cooked down like greens with Good Seasons Italian salad dressing (but not the exact same salad ingredients cooked down the exact same way using ¼ cup of water rather than the salad dressing for cooking, and just adding the same amount of the same salad dressing after the cooking was complete); 17) pesto in which part of the cooking was continued after adding olive oil; and 18) homemade cornbread using olive oil as the shortening.

A Mayo Clinic website regarding constipation advised that, "foods high in fat and sugar and those that tend to be low in fiber may cause or aggravate constipation." I don't believe that my problem with the foods listed above was due to fat per se, sugar, or being low in fiber. I haven't had problems with increased constipation after eating some foods high in fat (e.g., salad with Italian dressing or French bread dipped in olive oil) or sugar (e.g., soy ice cream with chocolate syrup) or low in insoluble fiber (e.g., soy ice cream with chocolate syrup or Cheerios). But I did have problems with bouts of increased constipation after eating multiple foods cooked with fat. For example, vegetables sautéed in fat were routinely constipating for me. This was true whether the fat was olive oil or margarine (hydrogenated corn oil) and was true for a variety of different dishes (e.g., recipes containing sautéed onions and recipes containing other sautéed vegetables [e.g., ratatouille]). As mentioned, I could eat salad with Italian dressing containing olive oil – as much as I liked – without problem. But if I ate the same salad cooked using the same Italian dressing, it was constipating. I could eat a serving of sunflower seeds containing 15 g of fat or more and develop no increased constipation. But if I swallowed a 1 g softgel capsule of flaxseed oil, I developed increased constipation. If I swallowed the 1 g capsule of flaxseed oil every day for a week, the constipation got worse. My best guess is that fat can be constipating when it doesn't get absorbed and flows downstream in the gastrointestinal tract. Of note, when I eat sunflower seeds, I'm certain that small bits of seed don't get digested or absorbed and flow downstream, being incorporated into feces. But the small bits of seed, which undoubtedly contain fat, don't cause bouts of increased constipation for me. Moreover, eating a recipe of canned fruit baked with brown sugar and 1 tablespoon of olive oil never caused additional constipation for me.

Of interest, MorningStar Farms Grillers are made of textured vegetable protein (from soybeans) and MorningStar Farms Crumbles are made of the same thing, but Grillers routinely cause me additional bouts of constipation while Crumbles don't; when I tried to find out what might explain this difference, a MorningStar Farms customer service representative informed me that Grillers were fried before packaging whereas Crumbles were baked. It's possible that there were other important differences in the way that the two products were prepared, but the difference in the way they were cooked (fried versus baked) could be an important determinant of one being constipating and the other not constipating. This seems similar to the observation recounted above regarding cooked salad being constipating when cooked with oil but not being constipating when the same ingredients were cooked only with water.

Bananas contain 0% fat and 1% protein, making it unlikely that fat or protein is responsible for their causing additional constipation in an MS patient like me. What they do contain is small amounts of sugars and considerable amounts of fiber. It seems probable that undigested fiber somehow serves as a template for denser, constipated stool.

Protein shakes can reportedly cause constipation if used with inadequate fluids. I haven't tried them.

I found many publications suggesting that constipating foods are those that lack sufficient insoluble fiber. I agree, but for a patient with MS already taking large amounts of fiber and laxative, eating an occasional low fiber food does not cause additional constipation the way eating a single firm banana does for me. Moreover, constipating foods such as Portobello mushroom and Tofurkey are very dense, so a deficiency of fiber would not appear to be the only explanation. After eating broccoli regularly without problem, a new nurse gave me three times as much as I had been eating. Feeling some trepidation because I had already recognized that amounts can matter, as mentioned in the Introduction, I went ahead and ate it, trying not to make a fuss. The following day I had increased constipation with very dense stools visibly filled with broccoli fiber. Just for interest, a couple of months later, I decided to try eating 1 cup of a high-fiber food – Raisin Bran – as a dry snack to see what would happen. The following day I had constipated stools obviously containing Raisin Bran. So, the high-fiber foods being used to prevent constipation can actually exacerbate constipation if misused (i.e., if used to excess or with inadequate fluid). Eating as little as ¼ extra cup of Raisin Bran in my breakfast was associated with 5 days of increased constipation and 4 days of urinary urgency.

After developing some difficulties with overly bulky, constipated stools and increased urinary urgency while eating a bunch of fresh peaches (several per day, unpeeled), I sympathized with J Alfred Prufrock, the character in T.S. Eliot's poem "The Love Song of J Alfred Prufrock," who says, "Do I dare to eat a peach?"

Can this be true? Can increased dietary fiber cause increased constipation? If extra fiber is ingested without additional fluid, the fiber can reportedly form dense aggregates that can paradoxically lead to dense, constipated stool. As an example, a high-fiber product (psyllium seed husks [Metamucil]), is commonly used as a laxative and stool softener, but when used with inadequate fluid can actually cause intestinal or even esophageal obstruction [according to the National Digestive Diseases Information Clearinghouse of the

National Institutes of Health] . I haven't used Metamucil, but I've had occasional bouts of increased constipation from eating too much of a high-fiber food.

This is an example of there being "truths that are neither for all men nor for all times" because eating excess high fiber foods usually won't cause any problem for a normal healthy person and didn't cause a problem for me until after I had MS related constipation for about two decades.

MorningStar Farms Grillers, which caused me increased constipation, contained 6 g of fat per burger (9%). Raisin Bran, eaten as 1 ounce of a dry cereal, caused me increased constipation and contained only 1 g of fat per serving (2%). A Tofutti cutie vanilla soy ice cream sandwich with chocolate wafers contains 6 g of fat per sandwich. A So Delicious vanilla soy ice cream sandwich with chocolate wafers contains 2 g of fat per sandwich (5%). Hershey's chocolate syrup contains cocoa, but the fat has been removed, so it's fat free. An 81 g (half cup) serving of So Delicious soy ice cream contains 3 g of fat (4%); so, it contains more fat than a So Delicious ice cream sandwich, but it didn't cause me increased constipation. One possible explanation for why one caused me increased constipation and the other didn't could be that the fat in the soy ice cream gets fully absorbed while fat in the chocolate wafers flows downstream into the colon.

When I recognized that particular foods were causing bouts of increased constipation, this didn't require additional laxative therapy for control of the problem, just avoidance of the actively constipating foods. Because I always liked the constipating food, this never was easy. ["Lead us not into temptation." – Matthew 6:13] Benjamin Franklin advised that, "An ounce of prevention is worth a pound of cure." [*Pennsylvania Gazette*, February 4, 1735] This is true regarding all diseases, but with MS related constipation, prevention is probably worth 10 pounds of cure to me.

With the approaches described above, I made it through 19 years and 9 months of MS-related constipation before having to add another laxative (polyethylene glycol 3350 [MiraLAX], also an osmotic laxative). At that time, I tried simply replacing docusate sodium with a daily dose of 17 g of MiraLAX but quickly found that that was inadequate. I tried taking a full dose of MiraLAX with a single capsule of docusate sodium for several weeks, but that too was inadequate. I then tried using a full daily dose of both docusate sodium and polyethylene glycol with better results.

2) Using Enough Laxative

"Use enough gun." – Robert Ruark, *Use Enough Gun*
"To know how much is enough, you have to know how much is more than enough." – Ezra Pound
"Two roads diverged in a wood, and I – I took the one less traveled by, and that has made all the difference." – Robert Frost, "The Road Not Taken"

Neurologists (and the other books for MS patients) usually counsel patience regarding constipation. They advise that a bowel movement every three days is sufficient. Patients who regard that frequency as normal may have no problem with such a recommendation. If bowel stasis doesn't cause intolerable problems, patients used to more frequent bowel movements also may be able to adjust.

In my case, however, a bowel movement parked in the rectum for hours to days (which can hardly be called a "movement") became an extreme problem. I think the rectum should be a launch pad, not a long-term storage area. In normal healthy people, arrival of feces in the rectum indicates the need for defecation. In an MS patient, feces in the rectum can cause constant tenesmus (a distressing but ineffectual urge to evacuate the rectum). This feels miserable, but misery was the least of my problems. A full, distended rectum can cause increased spasticity, which makes falling more likely. At its worst, this resulted in violent myoclonic jerks of the muscles of my more spastic left leg. These violent jerks seemed to occur as hyperreflexia when the leg was stretched by standing on it as I got up and tried to ambulate. Increased spasticity can also increase urinary urgency and urinary incontinence.

For such reasons, I decided that I couldn't accept the approach recommended by the other books for MS patients (i.e., to be patient and wait several days). When increased constipation developed despite my best effort to avoid actively constipating foods (e.g., by encountering yet another constipating food), I decided that something had to be done. One approach to a bout of increased constipation is to alter laxative dosage. It's not as simple as "just use more laxative" because too much laxative can cause significant problems. What's needed is a happy medium, and the correct amount for me changed over and over again.

After eating something actively constipating, I found that a slight increase (e.g., a relative 1%-10% increase in dose) of polyethylene glycol 3350 [MiraLAX] could make things much better. Because actively constipating food remains in the gastrointestinal tract for about a week and taking MiraLAX as a single daily dose could result in episodic constipation (e.g., stools with an appropriate consistency after breakfast but then hard and constipated later in the day), dividing the amount I was taking into three daily doses (with meals) gave me better control of the problem. Instead of suffering with increased constipation, increased urinary urgency, and occasional urinary incontinence in a bad bout, I was able to ameliorate all three problems. Before I took this approach, when I got into such a situation I would have to try to make it to a bedside commode before urinary incontinence, and I might have to use the bedside commode 20 or more times during a week of such increased constipation. After taking the new approach, I stopped having to use the bedside commode at all. I haven't used it in more than three years. If anyone had told me that taking this approach would be associated with such a radical difference, I would have been skeptical.

Are there controlled studies showing that my approach works

better for MS patients? No. Then how do I know that it works better for me? Res ipsa loquitur (i.e., the difference is huge and thus obvious). Will this work for other MS patients? Probably so for those with the problems I have. How common are these problems? Most MS patients suffer from constipation, but remember that I didn't need to add a second laxative, until after 19 years and 9 months of MS related constipation as it got worse and I didn't start increasing MiraLAX dosages to deal with a new bout of constipation until the 21st year of my MS related constipation.

When I said that I increased the MiraLAX dose by "1%-10%," that didn't tell the reader what to do in every possible circumstance (i.e., 1% is very different from 10%). The reason is, as explained above, it depends on the particular situation the patient is facing. Increased constipation can range from mild to severe depending upon the inciting incident (e.g., drinking too little fluids, eating too little fiber, eating a small amount of an actively constipating food, eating a large amount of an actively constipating food, etc.). The amount of increased polyethylene glycol needed depends upon the situation. If the situation is really bad, a relative 7%-10% might be necessary. On the other hand, a mild increase in constipation might be handled just fine by a relative 1%-3% increase. Judgment is required. Careful measurement is required. Amounts matter, as stated above, and this is especially true for actively constipating foods and for the dosage of polyethylene glycol.

Will using extra laxative make my constipation better in the short term, but worse in the long run? The optimal way to decide which approach is preferable would be by making use of controlled trials of MS patients employing the two methods (i.e., using extra laxative to counter a bout of increased constipation or waiting patiently for a bowel movement every three days). Best I can tell, such data regarding MS patients are not yet available. My own experience has been that using this approach for four years has not been associated with greater worsening per year than occurred before taking this approach.

Even though this approach has worked well for me for four years, I'm not sure whether it will be easy for all MS patients to implement. For example, those with visual or cognitive impairment would not be able to see whether feces are becoming too constipated or too loose or able to decide how to adjust the dose of laxative. Furthermore, it's easier to be precise about the dosage of a laxative like docusate sodium that comes in capsules (i.e., so the dose is 1, 2 or 3 capsules per day). With polyethylene glycol 3350 (MiraLAX), the powder form makes a variable dosing possible (e.g., increasing or decreasing the dose by 1-10% if needed). But, having said that, being precise with MiraLAX powder is difficult because it tends to sometimes come out in a gush or as clumps (i.e., more than intended). And even if the patient tries using a graduated cylinder (a tall cylindrical glass vessel with volume markings for measuring substances in a chemistry lab), it's still very difficult to get an exact amount of MiraLAX into the cylinder. A recent study found that medication dose errors were significantly more frequent when using a spoon or measuring cup than when using a syringe. [Ryu GS, Lee YJ. Analysis of liquid medication dose errors made by patients and caregivers using alternative measuring devices. J Manag Care Pharm. 2012; 18:439-45.]

It's possible that a liquid form could be kept in the refrigerator and used for more precise dosing, for making such adjustments. But, to do that, would require some experimentation, which is more than the average MS patient should be required to do. It would be more reasonable for a physician reading this book to try the approach in a small study of 5 to 10 patients to see whether dosage adjustment can be made easier for the patient. Otherwise, it's possible that the great result I had from trying to use the right amount of laxative to control my constipation enough to control urinary urgency may not be doable for most patients.

Store prices for bottles of MiraLAX usually are less per dose for bigger bottles, but bigger bottles are more bunglesome, causing difficulty pouring accurate doses. I have tended to use 30 dose bottles (17.9 ounces), but increasing weakness and spasticity made pouring more difficult so I purchased a funnel and started pouring half of a new bottle into a bottle just emptied and using the half-full bottle for pouring doses. When Sam's Club stopped offering the 17.9 ounce bottle and started selling a larger 35 dose bottle, I tried using a 17.9 ounce bottle of a generic form of MiraLAX (ClearLAX) that cost about half as much but worked just as well for me. The ClearLAX bottle was a bit larger however, so I kept using MiraLAX bottles for storing and pouring my daily doses.

Constipation has been a primary determinant of my crises of urinary urgency for six years. Avoiding ingestion of actively constipating foods during that time has helped me go for weeks to months at a time with no urinary urgency at all. But, over time, my MS related constipation has continued to worsen slowly as it had done since the first year of my illness. Since history tends to repeat itself, I expect my constipation will continue worsening over time. The fact that using laxatives can make the bowel more constipated over time also suggests that I will continue to get worse. Acknowledging that worsening is expected, I can't accept the dogma that a bowel movement every three days is adequate for MS patients like me because I know that that much constipation would cause me terrible problems (e.g., with urinary urgency and incontinence). So, I won't be able to take the old approach of being content with a bowel movement every three days.

I'll keep doing it my way.

3) Figuring out How Much Oral Laxative Is Enough

Juggling MiraLAX dosages to counteract a bout of increased constipation caused by eating an actively constipating food, I have been able to make things better (e.g., lessen the constipation, the episodes of dire urinary urgency, the frank urinary incontinence, the dependence on using a bedside commode, etc.), but it is a constant challenge to try to avoid those things and also avoid the fecal incontinence that increased MiraLAX can cause. I usually know that I am getting closer to too much MiraLAX when I observe the following phenomena:

1) liquid diarrhea.

2) urge to defecate right after waking up in the morning before breakfast

3) urge to defecate after getting to kitchen before I start eating breakfast

4) urge to defecate right after I start eating breakfast

5) urge to defecate right after finishing breakfast so strong that I have to pinch my butt cheeks together to prevent fecal incontinence

6) defecation at the usual time after breakfast but the stools completely falling apart rather than being formed

7) wet farts soiling briefs

On the other hand, I usually know that I'm not taking enough MiraLAX to completely control constipation when these things happen:

1) My morning bowel movement doesn't want to come out.

2) I start having audible farts (this usually is related to constipated stool being in my rectum because with my incontinent rectal sphincter, gas almost always just passes out silently).

3) I have dire urinary urgency after lunch. See the next two chapters for more detailed discussion about why this is so.

4) Gas stops being able to come out of my rectum, as if bottled up by too much constipated stool obstructing the rectum.

5) Borborygmi (i.e., gurgles in bowel audible to anyone nearby) may take on a different tone as they meet an obstruction in the colon preventing emission. In my colon, this can sound high-pitched and whiny or low pitched like a grandfather clock being wound.

Another way to assess how well a laxative dosage is regulating stool consistency is to inspect the feces in the toilet before wiping and flushing. If the stool is hard, stiff and constipated, this is usually obvious. If, by contrast, the stool is falling apart, this is equally obvious. In between these two extremes, the stool may be formed, very firm, but frilly on the outside. To further assess stool consistency, I partially flush the toilet and observe. If the stool is formed, but appears to explode when the toilet is partially flushed, then this demonstrates more laxative effect. Similarly, when the toilet is fully flushed, I watch again for the same signs of whether the stool stays firmly together or falls apart. I estimate how fully the stool falls apart when the toilet is flushed – 0% to 100%. If the estimate is 0%, this means the stool is too constipated and I need to increase the laxative dose. If the estimate is 100%, then I need to decrease the laxative dose.

When feces get very constipated, the amount of stool on toilet paper after a first wipe can be scant. When feces are not quite as constipated, there may be more stool on toilet paper after a first wipe but it tends to be dry and sticky. By contrast, when I've been using too much MiraLAX, there may be plenty of stool on toilet paper after a first wipe and it will be wet.

While seeking an optimal dose of osmotic laxative like polyethylene glycol, an MS patient with severe chronic constipation can pass through days in which feces can alternate between too soft and too hard. Spreading out the daily dosage of osmotic laxative (e.g., part with breakfast, part with lunch and part with supper) helped me gain better control, but there can still be days in which feces alternate between too soft and too hard. Part of the reason is that polyethylene glycol seems to move downstream through the gastrointestinal tract faster than do constipating foods. Another reason is that about half of a 24 hour period is often spent fasting (evening after supper and night for me—the fast that gives "breakfast" its name), which means that there will likely be alternating concentrations of polyethylene glycol in the colon at different times, allowing more constipation to occur during one part of the day than during another part of the day.

Two other variables worth noting are 1) estimated size of a bowel movement and 2) time spent waiting on the toilet. The size is important because a weak, spastic colon usually cannot produce a bowel movement as large as a normal colon does. This means that with adequate food, fluid, fiber, and/or laxative, an MS patient's colon might produce two or three smaller bowel movements to excrete the amount of insoluble fiber ingested per day. And size of a bowel movement can vary at random despite eating the same things for each meal each day, meaning that two relatively large bowel movements in the morning could be all of the defecation for that day, but two relatively small bowel movements in the morning imply that there will be another in the afternoon. It's good to be prepared. Time spent waiting is worth noting because the ideal wait is the minimal. If stool is too constipated, resulting in the patient sitting hours longer than usual, this could be another reason for modest alteration of the laxative dosage.

Is inspecting one's feces getting too anal (excessive)? Shakespeare said, "Nothing is good or bad, except the mind makes it so." My mind believes that getting the right amount of osmotic laxative is critical to doing better (e.g., too little and I can suffer terribly from a really bad bout of constipation and too much and I can suffer just as much from fecal incontinence). Robert Ruark wrote a popular book about African big-game hunting, entitled, *Use Enough Gun* (i.e., don't use a 22 caliber rifle when pursuing a rhinoceros). My approach to controlling severe constipation in the 21st through 24th years after onset of my MS has been to use "enough" osmotic laxative. When I get regulated on a particular dose, I can go for months without feeling additional constipation, without having tenesmus in the late afternoon or evening requiring digital stimulation or a laxative suppository, and without having urinary urgency at night. Being able to free myself from such MS related suffering just by using the right dose of laxative seems wonderful to me.

If the reader understands the way this worked for me, it should be clear why no book and no neurologist can confidently say exactly what regimen will be optimal for every patient without some trial and error. As Dr. Swank put it, "adding bran to the diet, the use of laxatives that, by trial, have proved effective, or by combinations of these methods."

Can this approach be used prospectively to eat a food known to be actively constipating?

"Lead us not into temptation." – *Matthew* 6:13
"Screw your courage to sticking point and we'll not fail." –W. Shakespeare

It can, but this is a little bit dicey (with bad potential outcomes in both directions). My life is generally more peaceful just abstaining, but sometimes temptation becomes irresistible. If I keep trying to find the right dose to counter a particular constipating food's increase in my constipation, I usually succeed.

A principal reason this is challenging is that the amounts of Yin versus Yang (i.e., factors favoring and opposing increased constipation) are hard to quantify. Some constipating foods are more constipating than others. Then there's the amount of the constipating food. Those two variables have to be countered by the right amount of polyethylene glycol (MiraLAX), which is usually provided as a bottle of powder, which is hard to measure exactly even if the exact amount is known (and it isn't). As mentioned above, a recent study found that medication dose errors were significantly more frequent when using a spoon or measuring cup than when using a syringe. [Ryu GS, Lee YJ. Analysis of liquid medication dose errors made by patients and caregivers using alternative measuring devices. J Manag Care Pharm. 2012; 18:439-45.]

4) Using A Laxative Suppository When Extra Oral Laxative Is Insufficient

As mentioned above, my goal was to use enough oral laxative to prevent a desperate situation late in the day with constipation, urinary urgency, etc. But when emerging from a bout of increased constipation by using extra oral laxative, episodic constipation can continue to occur because actively constipating food remains in the gastrointestinal tract for days and such foods move downstream at different rates from the polyethylene glycol, sometimes leaving the undigested constipating foods in areas of the colon where there's no polyethylene glycol. If constipation occurred despite my best efforts to avoid that, a laxative suppository usually remedied the situation (I most often used glycerin [another osmotic laxative], but sometimes bisacodyl [a stronger, stimulant laxative]).

When I had to use a laxative suppository, bisacodyl always worked but frequently took 10 to 30 minutes to produce a bowel movement. By contrast, a glycerin laxative suppository usually worked in the afternoon or evening within five minutes. As midnight approached, the bisacodyl suppository continued to be reliable but the glycerin suppository only worked for me one of six times that late at night. A downside of using laxative suppositories is that the high dosage applied might make the rectum develop dependency on this, which is not good.

5) Using Digital Stimulation When a Laxative Suppository Was Insufficient

If a laxative suppository failed to evacuate the rectum, I then re-sorted to digital stimulation (i.e., inserting a finger into the rectum [or a "digital stimulator" (an instrument shaped like a finger)] that can by creating sensations inside the rectum induce a bowel move-ment). Digital stimulation is most comfortable for me using an index finger inside a latex surgical glove coated with KY jelly as a lubri-cant. The finger has to be moving to cause much stimulation, but the movement should not be aggressive or overly vigorous, which could injure the mucosa (lining) of the rectum. I find that this works best by coupling it with a mild to moderate Valsalva maneuver (i.e., take a breath, hold it, and bear down to create intra-abdominal pressure). In a pinch, liquid soap and water can be used as a lubricant. When this had to be done, I preferred to use a soap like Neutrogena because of its neutral pH, figuring that would be less irritating to the anus and rectum. Also in a pinch, lubricant placed on several sheets of toilet paper can be used to get the anus slippery and slip the index finger inside the rectum. I would never use digital stimulation except in a very clean environment (e.g., my own bathroom).

Digital stimulation always worked for me, but frequently would take 10 to 20 minutes (sometimes as little as two minutes). Being a physician, I knew how to use plenty of lubricant and avoid damaging the rectal mucosa when digital stimulation was needed. A limitation was that a bowel movement stimulated in that manner could not be facilitated by a simultaneous Credé maneuver; this can result in less complete evacuation of the rectum. Another downside of both digital stimulation and laxative suppositories is that physical insertion of a finger into the rectum can traumatize the rectum somewhat despite all the lubricant and care being taken, resulting in a sore anus the following day. This leads me to believe that using enough oral laxative is preferable. As stated above, using an optimal dose of oral laxative has allowed me to go for months without needing a laxative suppository or digital stimulation of the rectum.

6) Shifting to a Different Approach when Constipation Shifts to a Different Mechanism

As mentioned above, MS causes weakness and spasticity of muscles throughout the body. Weakness and spasticity of gastrointestinal tract muscles can cause hypo-motility and hyperreflexia. From what I can tell, from my own case and from reading about the usual pattern for others, constipation usually starts because of MS-related hypo-motility. When the bowel is sluggish at moving feces along, an osmotic laxative may be needed to compensate. During this phase, which lasted from my initial attack until my 23rd year of MS, using enough laxative always guaranteed a bowel movement and using too much laxative usually produced excessively loose stools that could result in fecal incontinence.

A second major way that MS related damage to the central nervous system can cause constipation is by spastic constriction of the external anal sphincter. This happened to me several times when something had caused excessively loose feces (e.g., antibiotic therapy, an excessive dose of polyethylene glycol, etc.) or when there was a major increase in spasticity due to the pain of a fracture.

These two mechanisms both cause constipation, but the two types of constipation feel nothing alike. Constipation due to hypo-motility reminds me of how my ears feel when filled with Murine ear drops (i.e., I can sense that something's in there, but there is a helpless feeling because the external auditory canal, which is filled with drops, is boney and can't do anything to empty itself). Another way to describe what this feels like might be that I ate a hot dog with a generous amount of superglue on it.

Constipation due to spastic constriction of the anal sphincter feels worse because colonic muscles are usually actively trying to expel feces, implying an imminent bowel movement, but this goes on and on as the exit is clamped shut by the spastic sphincter (dyssynergic defecation). It's a desperate feeling. My physician asked if this was painful. I said that it wasn't painful to me, more maddening. When this was happening, my more spastic left leg would repeatedly adduct against the other leg, and I believe that the spastic muscles in my pelvic floor were contracting spastically at the same time. My spastic left arm could join in and contract spastically as well, and when the situation became totally abysmal, it would become a three ring circus because my healthier right leg could start spastic contractions as well.

I seemed to switch from the first mechanism being predominant to the second being transiently predominant after I fell and fractured two bones in my 23rd year of MS. The pain of the fractures caused an immediate surge in spasticity throughout my body, and increased constipation caused me to sit on the toilet seat far too long over a period of weeks. After having had no furuncles on my buttock for over a year, I started having them again on the buttock of my paretic leg where it touched the toilet seat. Because I got four furuncles over a week and simply could not keep up with the large number of warm moist compresses that obligated me to apply, I started taking oral dicloxacillin to see if that would control the problem. It helped but not enough, getting better each night when not sitting on my buttock, but then getting worse again each day after hours of sitting on my buttock, which impaired blood flow and delivery of antibiotic to the site of the infections. The dicloxacillin also caused me to get loose stools even though I was reducing the dosage of my polyethylene glycol 3350 (MiraLAX). The loosened stools seemed to cause the constipation to get worse (i.e., the opposite of what had happened for the previous 22 years of the disease). At that point, I tried laxative suppositories multiple times (first glycerin, and then bisacodyl), but the new form of constipation did not respond to that approach. I tried digital stimulation, which could work but less well than with the other methods I had used in the past because, as mentioned above, digital stimulation with one's only functional hand means that a Credé maneuver can't be used to help expel the bowel movement. The spastically constricted sphincter also seemed to want to clamp shut right after it opened. Doing that several times, I had just a portion of the bowel movement expelled before the sphincter clamped shut again, leaving me in pretty much the same situation I was in before the digital stimulation.

Beginning to feel desperate after a couple of days of terrible constipation, which was causing all of the problems I had observed in the past (e.g., increased urinary urgency, urinary incontinence, increased myoclonic jerks of my left leg when I would stand on it, making ambulation significantly more difficult), I decided to try a 6 mg dose of baclofen (Lioresal) to see if that would relax the spastic constriction of the sphincter. It did. I had a bowel movement about 20 minutes after the dose and another one about an hour and 20 minutes later.

The following day I took a 5 mg baclofen tablet and had the same result. The third day, I took a 5 mg baclofen tablet and had a bowel movement approximately an hour later, but no second bowel movement. There then ensued several days of more natural bowel movements so that I didn't take a baclofen tablet to stimulate defecation. The problem recurred, however, and the fourth time I tried to stimulate defecation with a baclofen tablet (5 mg), it didn't work and I had to resort to digital stimulation. The following day, I had the same problem and tried a 6 mg baclofen tablet with the same result.

For almost 5 years I had been taking a 5 mg dose of baclofen at bedtime only. After I had the prompt cathartic response to baclofen allowing defecation despite spastic constriction of the external anal sphincter, I decided to try holding my nightly dose of baclofen to see whether that would make an occasional baclofen dose more helpful for catharsis when needed. After doing that several days and then taking another 5 mg dose of baclofen, I had a dramatic improvement in leg spasticity. I knew that my legs were both weak and spastic and that they were weaker and more spastic after the two fractures and consequent reduced ambulation, but taking the baclofen tablet after a few days of not taking my nightly dose made it seem that increased spasticity was more responsible for the increasingly difficult ambulation.

Unfortunately, my idea didn't work for making baclofen better at relaxing the spastic external anal sphincter. I tried the same thing six weeks later and the baclofen still did not work, but after six months of not taking baclofen it worked again to loosen up a transient spastic sphincter constriction.

Each time spastic constriction of the external anal sphincter became the predominant mechanism causing my constipation, this would last only a matter of days to weeks before shifting back to hypomotility being the primary mechanism.

7) Trying a Different Tack With the Oral Laxative Dosage To Counter The Spastic Constriction of the External Anal Sphincter

Because the baclofen only worked for a few days and then stopped working to relax the spastic constriction of the external anal sphincter, I felt up a creek without a paddle (i.e., the same way I did before trying baclofen for that purpose).

Because it seemed that I was running out of pharmacological options, I thought maybe focusing on the body's own physiologic mechanisms might somehow help.

Because the loose stools seemed to make the spastic constriction of the external anal sphincter worse, I thought that trying to reduce my oral polyethylene glycol (MiraLAX) dosage enough to make the stool firm enough to engage the rectal vault might reduce the holding reflex that seemed to go into overdrive because of spasticity. I had for years been balancing the oral laxative dose to keep stools from being too loose (causing fecal incontinence) or too firm (causing worse constipation). So, balancing the oral laxative dose between two endpoints was nothing new, I was just modifying the balance point somewhat. This seemed to work. Seemingly out of drugs that could rescue me from this new form of constipation, the new balancing setpoint (causing the stools to be somewhat more firm than they had been but still soft enough that they wouldn't hang up and become immobile) was associated with my coming out of the nightmarish constipation I had been in for weeks. I don't believe that resolution of the fracture pain was responsible for this improvement because the fracture pains had already gotten much better weeks earlier by immobilizing the metatarsal bone in a make-shift cast and reducing ambulation to allow healing of both of the fractures.

8) Using Volitional Control of Timing To Try To Regain Control Of Defecation

After losing volitional control of the anal sphincter, it may be helpful to try to use volitional control of timing of defecation to try to regain whatever control of defecation this might afford.

For example, by pairing my effort to defecate with the time that my bladder would be filling, I could take advantage of the increased sensation that this allowed. The bladder and colon emerge together embryologically and thus share certain innervations that can result in the rectal sphincter relaxing at the same time as the urinary sphincter. I found such pairing to be very helpful as I was trying to achieve a new balance in firmness of the stool with the oral laxative dosage. The Credé maneuver had been helpful to me for 24 years in initiating urination and for a lesser period in initiating and completing defecation. And it was helpful during this most difficult time, adding its effect to those of the pairing and the new balancing of the oral laxative dosage.

9) Avoiding Premature Urination (if Possible) When Trying to Pair Defecation with Urination

At first glance, this might seem to be the same strategy as that mentioned in the paragraph above. It isn't. When trying to pair defecation with urination, there is always a requirement for guesswork. And after sitting on the toilet trying to get the pairing to work, the bladder may become full enough that it wants to empty. I found that allowing the increasingly full bladder to go ahead and empty was a mistake. If I allowed the urine to come out, the increased sensation being generated in the colon by pairing the two would dissipate immediately and opening the rectal sphincter could become impossible until the bladder started approaching full again.

10) Using Applesauce As a Substitute for Eggs and Oil in Baking

As mentioned above, avoiding actively constipating foods worked to prevent bouts of increased constipation, and I was able to go for months at a time without having such increased problems. But there is always a yearning for some favorite food that has become actively constipating (e.g., cornbread, fruit pies at Thanksgiving, etc). An MS patient frequently has to learn to do without constipating delicacies. As also mentioned above, I tried substituting palm oil and olive oil as the shortening for cornbread and pie, but these baked products were always constipating.

But then I saw a book containing all vegan recipes (*The China Study All-Star Collection: Whole Food Plant-based Recipes from Your Favorite Vegan Chefs* by Leanne Campbell, Ben Bella Books, Inc., Dallas, Texas, 2005.) and was intrigued by a recipe for cornbread that was followed by this tip: "Applesauce is a good substitute for eggs and oil in baking – and you won't taste it." I tried the recipe and was very surprised that the cornbread was very good and not actively constipating in the least. Was this the long sought Northwest Passage that had been so hard to find?

I modified a Betty Crocker recipe for peach pie that was always constipating by replacing shortening with applesauce (the only change in the recipe!). The first two times I ate a piece of the peach pie, I fully expected failure with a bout of increased constipation – the full Monty. It didn't happen even though the pie crust was hard and crunchy instead of light and fluffy as in the Betty Crocker pie. To make the pie crust have the usual consistency requires leavening – either baking powder or yeast (both work well if using the right amount).

No baked products using applesauce were constipating for my MS colon unlike those using shortening. This is one of those differences so large that calculating a P value becomes superfluous, but for those unable to see that, I calculated a P value anyway. After eating 16 different products baked with a lipid shortening when I was not in a bout of increased constipation during the five years in which I was susceptible to bouts of increased constipation from eating actively constipating foods, increased constipation started each time within 2 days (usually 1 day). After eating 10 pieces of pie baked with applesauce instead of shortening when I was not in a bout of increased constipation, increased constipation didn't develop. The probability that a difference this large would occur by chance alone was 1.88×10^{-7} (i.e., very low).

11) Adding Extra Fluid When a Supper Entrée Predictably Starts Causing Decreased Nightly Urine Volume Followed by a Bout of Constipation

As mentioned above, measuring fluid volume can minimize problems with both urinary urgency and constipation. But problems can arise despite this because some supper entrées contain less fluid than others. I first became aware of this when particular entrées were consistently associated with fewer episodes of nocturia (e.g., pea soup). This happened many times over several years before a bout of constipation was caused by the same supper entrée; this occurred when the same commercial brand of pea soup was prepared for my supper by a different helper and came to the table more solid than liquid with visibly less soup than usual in the bowl. This was apparently due to the soup being cooked longer and becoming more dehydrated. Eating this more concentrated version of pea soup was associated with a bout of additional constipation lasting days.

After this pattern became apparent, I started trying to notice and drink several extra ounces of fluid with supper when I suspected that my supper entrée was going to cause too much dehydration. I have used approximately 3 extra ounces several times without causing urinary urgency or incontinence problems between supper and bed time; this countermeasure was also associated with increased nocturnal urine volume and no new bout of constipation during the following days.

How can a patient decide the right number of ounces to add? This obviously depends upon the situation. If a bowl of pea soup comes to the table appearing to miss 5 ounces, 1 ounce probably won't do the trick. If a particular entrée is consistently associated with 300 mL (10 ounces) less nocturia per night, then 2 extra ounces probably won't do the trick.

How Bad a Problem Is MS-related Constipation?

It was noted in the introduction that MS patients don't all get the same symptoms. About 70% complain of bowel problems such as constipation and/or fecal incontinence. Of those with constipation, symptoms can range from mild to severe.

When constipation started with my first MS attack, my symptoms were mild. But over the next two decades, the problem became progressively worse.

Constipation can get so bad for an MS patient that many hours of frustration can be spent in the bathroom waiting for something to happen that may or may not happen. I have sometimes gone to the bathroom after breakfast and waited there for hours. The reason I waited was because a bowel movement seemed imminent but wouldn't come (i.e., rectal tenesmus). Tenesmus can occur with more than 20 different illnesses, MS being one. This can be so extreme that the prolonged waiting becomes reminiscent of *"Waiting for Godot,"* a play by Samuel Beckett in which Godot never arrives.

As frustrating as this is, if one chooses to ignore this fickle, capricious call of nature, and defecation occurs before he can make it back to the bathroom, this outcome can be much worse than waiting for an hour or two [because removing soiled clothes, trying to clean oneself despite hemiparesis and then getting out more clothes and getting redressed can be more unpleasant and take more time].

The amount of time I had to spend waiting in the bathroom seemed to increase exponentially as my MS progressed (it didn't, but that's how I felt). After being frustrated by this for years, it got so much worse that the focus on having a bowel movement almost became all encompassing – like Captain Ahab's focus on Moby Dick. For an MS patient, opening one's bowels can begin to seem an impossible dream like Shangri-La, which makes Lawrence's comment about keeping his bowels open in the desert seem luxurious.

When I was young, one of my pastimes with my father was turkey hunting, which entailed a lot of waiting quietly in the woods. Sitting quietly in the woods, there are many beautiful things to see, and something is often changing (e.g., the sky, the weather, different forest animals passing by, etc.). And even so, as a teenager, I once took a paperback book into a turkey blind and read it, being careful to remain still and turn pages quietly. As an MS patient in a bathroom, there's much less to see or do. It would be hard for me to read a book in the bathroom, but I could turn on an audible book and listen to someone else reading or I could listen to music. When I got a turkey, there was a great deal of excitement. As an MS patient, it's hard not to feel triumphant about a bowel movement, which probably sounds ridiculous to anyone who never felt like he might die of terminal constipation.

Reviewing this thin chapter after I completed it, I thought a monograph the approximate size of *War and Peace* might seem more appropriate for such a big problem.

Is Constipation the Only Gastrointestinal Problem Plaguing MS Patients?

Constipation wasn't my only gastrointestinal problem. Spasticity of the rectal muscles made my colon want to empty precipitously as soon as feces arrived there – despite the problem that I was having with constipation. This made fecal incontinence more likely than before (I didn't have it before MS). I had to deal with that at work 6 times before I retired (e.g., rushing home to remove and clean soiled clothes, take a shower, get redressed and drive back to work). Each of those episodes was related to food poisoning, which is also more likely with MS (see Chapter 33 regarding an increased risk for and the prevention of food poisoning).

Chapter 8
Does MS Cause Gastroesophageal Reflux Disease (GERD)?

C an MS related spinal cord damage paralyze the lower esophageal sphincter enough to cause gastroesophageal reflux disease (GERD)? GERD is a condition in which stomach contents leak
backward into the esophagus causing irritation and heartburn. I
haven't seen controlled studies showing that GERD is more frequent
among MS patients than among age-matched controls, but my guess
is that spinal cord damage can do this. My GERD began in my 18th
year of MS.

A review of spinal cord injury says that it causes a variety of gastrointestinal problems, which it referred to as "neurogenic bowel,"
including GERD. [Benevento BT, Sipski ML.Neurogenic bladder, neurogenic bowel, and sexual dysfunction in people with spinal cord
injury. PhysTher2002 Jun;82(6):601-12.] I'm sure that a neurogenic
bowel syndrome exists, but the references offered by the review
were not from controlled studies. Nevertheless, I suspect that the
review was probably correct because I have had impaired reflexes,

spasticity and paresis affecting my gastrointestinal tract from the mouth to the anus since the first year of my MS (e.g., difficulty clearing my throat [second attack], problems chewing without biting my tongue or cheek [second attack], problems choking on saliva, food and drink [second attack], inability to spit or whistle [second attack], problems defecating [first attack], etc.). It seems unlikely that such a disease would spare only the lower esophageal sphincter. Those things happened before I started using any medications that could be blamed, making it clear that the MS itself was impairing the function of my gastrointestinal tract. From early in the disease, my urinary tract was also impaired, leaving urine in the urethra that had to be wrung out and blotted or it would wet my clothes or the floor. Paresis makes the bowel leave feces in rectum, just like paresis causes urine to be left in the bladder or urethra.

A number of risk factors predispose to gastroesophageal reflux disease. [Kahrilas PJ. Gastroesophageal reflux disease. *N Engl J Med.* 2008;359:1700-7.] including delayed gastric emptying, which has been documented in MS patients [el-Maghraby TA, et al. Gastric motility dysfunction in patients with multiple sclerosis assessed by gastric emptying scintigraphy. *Can J Gastroenterol.* 2005; 19:141-5.], decreased esophageal peristalsis and lower esophageal sphincter hypotension. Impaired esophageal motility is a recognized complication of MS. [Richter JE. Oesophageal motility disorders. *Lancet.* 2001; 358:823-8.]

Chapter 9
Increasing Bladder Problems

"There are more things in heaven and earth than are dreamt of in your philosophy...." – William Shakespeare, *Hamlet*
"All animals are equal. But some animals are more equal than others." – George Orwell, *Animal Farm*

In my 14th year of MS, my neurologist referred me (for a second opinion about treatment strategy) to another neurologist who specialized in the care of MS patients. The specialist expressed frank disbelief that I could have gone more than 13 years without frank urinary incontinence (i.e., my bladder "cutting loose" and urinating on my clothes). I had been unable to use a urinal after the first attack because of post void dribbling and the consequent need to be at a commode with toilet paper for blotting the urethral meatus, but had not yet had frank incontinence.

Four years later, I joined the club. Given the specialist's reaction, this may not be surprising, except perhaps the way it happened – after switching to a different food for lunch.

It's important to emphasize in this chapter on bladder problems that eating actively constipating foods didn't just make it harder to have a bowel movement. The resulting urinary bladder control problems were as bad as the bowel control problems. Urinary urgency resulted in wet clothes repeatedly, the need to remove them, the need to clean up, the need to get more clothes, the need to get redressed (which altogether resulted in large numbers of hours of frustration and inability to do other things that I would rather be doing). Each instance of incontinence required about an hour for doing such things with hemiparesis. And, as mentioned in Chapter 5, my worst day of this required me to put on four different sets of clothes and four different sets of pajamas during a 24 hour period. When there was constipated stool in my rectum, I have had to urinate with urgency four times in the two hours after lunch; by contrast, when the constipation was well controlled a week later, I could urinate just once with no urgency during more than five hours after lunch. It's important to understand that these marked differences occurred despite eating the same amounts of the same foods and drinking the same amount of fluids for both breakfast and lunch during those days, suggesting that the presence or absence of constipated stool in the rectum seemed to make a critical difference.

The connection between my constipation and urinary urgency and incontinence was mentioned in Chapter 7 regarding my experience with actively constipating foods – they repeatedly caused me constipation, urinary urgency, and urinary incontinence. Many publications about MS note that constipation, urinary urgency and urinary incontinence are common complications of MS, but none that I found linked these problems together. A recent guideline regarding management of bladder problems in multiple sclerosis said, "A scientific basis for recommending treatment of coexistent constipation as a means of improving bladder function is lacking, but anecdotally many practitioners, and indeed their patients, feel this is important. The effect of anti-muscarinics on exacerbating constipation has not been studied. Further research on the effect of improved bowel management on reduction in bladder symptoms would be valuable." [Fowler C, et al. A UK consensus of the management of the bladder in multiple sclerosis. *Journal of Neurology, Neurosurgery and Psychiatry*. 2009; 80:470-477.]

There are multiple other variables that can affect the urge to urinate: volume of fluids being consumed, amount of salt being consumed, time since last urination, etc. These variables affect urge to urinate in anyone.

Are all drinks equivalent in this regard since they are mostly water? Yes and no. Yes for fluid balance, but some have added chemicals that can affect kidney or bladder function (as in "some animals are more equal than others").

Caffeine can temporarily increase urine output to be more than fluid intake (diuretic action). Alcohol can do the same. Neither can do that chronically, however, because physiology requires a zero balance between fluid intake and fluid output. An old saying maintains that "you can't get blood from a turnip," and the human body, similarly, cannot chronically excrete more water than ingested.

There are some data suggesting that caffeine can also make a spastic bladder more spastic (i.e., feel full and urgent to void earlier despite less urine volume); this would increase urinary urgency and incontinence. But there are also data from other studies suggesting the opposite. And there are data from studies suggesting that chronic caffeine ingestion leads to tolerance and less effect of the caffeine.

So, what should MS patients do, given all of this contradictory data? As mentioned in Chapter 1, a valid causal relationship usually results in studies showing consistent results in different studies of different populations by different investigators. When the results are contradictory, the relationship is usually not causal or may be associated with a smaller relative risk. My approach to caffeine and alcohol is just to avoid them for multiple reasons other than the one being discussed. If a reader is very devoted to a morning cup of coffee, she could try it, being aware of the reported risks and use moderation. If this leads to problems, she could reduce the amount to a half cup or smaller (a demitasse) and still enjoy the taste while imbibing less of the chemical and thereby reducing any associated problems.

Other substances reported to cause problems have been theobromine from chocolate, theophylline from tea, carbonated beverages and artificial sweeteners like aspartame, but again the data have been inconsistent from one study to the next. Carbonated beverages could result in increased gas filling the colon and cause urgency by external pressure on the bladder instead of a direct effect on the urinary tract.

Other books for MS patients referred to such chemicals affecting the urinary tract as "irritants." While this use of the word complies with one Webster's Dictionary definition of irritate (i.e., "to cause an action or function"), it doesn't seem right to me. Urea causes irritation of an MS patient's bottom after urinary incontinence sort of like exposure to a mild form of bull nettle. Vitamin D absorbed from the gastrointestinal tract causes changes in the way the body handles calcium, but most wouldn't refer to vitamin D as an irritant. Likewise, acute alcohol ingestion is believed to cause diuresis by inhibiting release of a hormone called vasopressin from the pituitary gland; this would not usually be called an "irritant."

In a patient with MS, there are other variables that can affect the urge to urinate: bladder hyperreflexia, the amount of fiber being consumed, constipating foods being consumed, foods and drinks that generate increased intestinal gas (e.g., beans and carbonated beverages), swallowing too much air (again resulting in increased intestinal gas), and the amount of edema in paralyzed extremities, which can be absorbed when lying down resulting in extra fluid volume that has to be excreted as urine. Perhaps one reason I found constipated stool in the rectum to be more of a problem was because I had controlled the other variables. Before I started having MS-related urinary urgency, I had noticed that drinking too much liquid caused too many trips to the bathroom, so I cut back. Decades earlier, I had stopped adding salt at the table and generally avoided eating salty foods like pickles. After developing edema in my paretic leg, I tried to avoid salty, processed foods such as Amy's Asian Noodles.

My problem with increased intestinal gas while constipated was that constipated stools occluded the rectum, and the increased intestinal gas didn't just float out through the incontinent rectal sphincter. This meant that gas kept accumulating, inflating the colon, which further cramped the spastic urinary bladder, contributing to increased urinary urgency and episodes of frank incontinence. In fact, during a bout of constipation, gas could sometimes become a problem even if I didn't eat a food causing increased gas (e.g., beans). The excess gas caused by eating beans is due to an oligosaccharide (a type of sugar) that does not get digested or absorbed and flows downstream into the colon where bacteria metabolize it, producing excess gas. This can be controlled by either avoiding such gas-producing foods or by coupling ingestion with an over-the-counter medication – alpha galactosidase (Beano [Glaxo Smith Kline]). Three tablets of Beano is the recommended dose, but the optimal dose for me seems to depend upon the amount of the gas-producing food being eaten. Some gas-producing foods (e.g., milk containing lactose for patients who lack the enzyme lactase) are unaffected by Beano, however. The raisins in Kellogg's Raisin Bran, which are hard and sugarcoated, caused me no perceptible, excess gas. On the contrary, Sun Maid raisins and the raisins in Trader Joe's Raisin Bran, which are soft without a sugarcoating, both reliably resulted in excess gas for me that was unaffected by taking 3 Beano tablets but not if I took 12 tablets. Could those associations be due to chance? Yes, any observed association could be due to chance, as explained in Chapter 1. The P value calculated after a medical study gives the probability that an observed difference was due to chance.

Three tablets of Beano aren't adequate for every food I eat. For example, if my wife makes a pot of vegan spaghetti with 2 bottles of Prego tomato sauce and one package of MorningStar Farms Crumbles, the soybeans always cause excess gas if I use only 3 tablets. For eating a serving of spaghetti sauce that fills 2 "rounded" serving spoons, I found that I needed to use 8 Beano tablets to prevent excess gas.

It's important to understand that before having spastic bowel and bladder problems due to MS, I could eat as many Sun Maid raisins as I wished with no such problem. So, the problem of food-related gas only became a problem for me because of chronic MS complications. I ate Sun Maid raisins more than a dozen times after the gas problem commenced and it happened every time. The problem was bothersome enough that I stopped eating Sun Maid raisins. I later tried eating 1 ounce of Sun Maid raisins with 12 tablets of Beano five times with no problem. The probability that I would have the problem from eating raisins 12 times in a row and then no problem five times in a row due to chance was 0.00016 (i.e., still possible but rather unlikely). Did any of the other books for MS patients say anything about raisins? No. Have there been any medical studies evaluating the use of alpha galactosidase (Beano) with raisins? Not that I could find (my last Medline search was conducted in February 2016).

It's important to understand that most but not all MS patients have bladder hyperreflexia and that those with hyperreflexia usually start off with mild bladder spasticity that can get worse over time. In effect, this makes the bladder seem smaller and smaller, resulting in nocturia and then more frequent nocturia as time goes along. It also means that the patient will need to urinate sooner after ingesting fluids and that increased urgency may accompany the need to void, depending upon the other variables mentioned above (e.g., amounts of fluid and salt consumed, time since last voiding,).

While discussing MS related urinary urgency, I should probably mention that I get an unusual type of discomfort with this. Before having MS, I never experienced this uncomfortable feeling with urinary urgency even when my bladder was very full. For example, on the first day of my medical internship, I urinated after breakfast, went to work and got so busy that the next time I was able to go to the bathroom was at midnight. I was very aware that my bladder was full - very full - but the type of discomfort I got with urinary urgency starting in my 18th year after onset of MS was very different. It's hard to describe the discomfort exactly, but I liken it to a wolf chewing on the bladder. It may be that this unusual discomfort is due to stretching of hyperreflexic (spastic) bladder muscles. I have had discomfort in the muscles in a spastic limb when stretching it. One of the other books for MS patients says that this uncomfortable urgency is indistinguishable from the uncomfortable urgency accompanying a urinary tract infection. I disagree. For me, the uncomfortable urgency with a urinary tract infection is worse. I liken that discomfort to an entire pack of wolves chewing on the bladder.

A urologic study of 225 MS patients with bladder problems reported that 70% demonstrated hyperreflexia on cystometry (9% had flaccid areflexia) and that 82% demonstrated detrusor sphincter dyssynergia (DSD) on coaxial needle electromyography.[Amarenc G, Kerdraon J, Denys P. Bladder and sphincter disorders in multiple sclerosis. Clinical, urodynamic and neurophysiological study of 225 cases. Rev Neurol (Paris). 1995; 151:722-30.] I have both hyperreflexia and DSD.

What is DSD? In normal healthy people, when the bladder contracts to expel urine, the sphincter relaxes (i.e., they work together). DSD is the opposite – when the bladder contracts to expel urine, the sphincter also contracts, preventing urine flow. There are multiple different types of DSD. In Type 1, the bladder and sphincter contract, but then the sphincter relaxes and allows unobstructed voiding; in Type 2, the sphincter contracts sporadically throughout the bladder contraction, and in Type 3, there is a crescendo-decrescendo sphincter contraction causing urethral obstruction throughout the entire bladder contraction.[Chancellor MB, Kaplan SA, Blaivas JG. Detrusor-external sphincter dyssynergia. CIBA Found Symp. 1990; 151:195-206.]

The type I have is Type 2, and the sporadic sphincter contractions can start five seconds after urination begins and occur several times before voiding is completed. This occurred when I went for urodynamic testing in my 14th year of MS and the urologist assured me that stopping and starting wasn't a problem if the bladder could empty the urine. At that point, my bladder could completely empty after multiple starts and stops even though there were four people in the room watching the testing.

When I go to the bathroom feeling the need to urinate and defecate, dyssynergic rectal and urinary sphincters can cause a SNAFU. For example, urination and defecation may start together, but one or the other may stop immediately while the other proceeds to completion. If this happens, the one that paused may seem refractory to any conscious efforts to revive the process (e.g., Credé maneuver), but then want to proceed 10 minutes after I pull up my pants and leave the room.

As mentioned in the introduction, patients with MS tend to be unique, so one can't make summary comments about what will or won't work for all MS patients' bladder problems. Patients can differ. Bladder problems frequently torment but rarely kill an MS patient, but they can cause renal failure and death, so urodynamic evaluation by a urologist is probably a good idea for each MS patient.

I measured the volume of urine excreted when I had to get up with urgency for nocturia several times in my 21st year of MS and found it to be approximately 250 ml at that time (i.e., about half of what a normal healthy person's bladder would usually hold at night). Months later, I had occasion to once again measure the volume present at a couple of times of severe urgency. One time, the volume was 225 mL and the other only 100 mL just a few nights later, suggesting that urine volume in the bladder is only one of the variables determining urgency. Severe urgency with only 100 ML seemed to be related to constipated stool in the rectum. Being a patient with hemiparesis, I couldn't catheterize the bladder, so one could question the validity of these volumes. From other variables, such as how the bladder felt and what the bladder did over the next few hours, I believe the measurements were accurate.

If an MS patient becomes more spastic and paretic over time (as usually happens), it's possible that this could happen to the bladder, as well as the skeletal muscles. If so, it's possible that the patient could choose the right amount of liquid to drink per day and do well for several years, eating and drinking the same amounts of the same things every day, but then get worse despite no change in intake just because the bladder is continuing to get more spastic (and thus effectively smaller).

There are also a variety of conditioned stimuli that can increase urgency for MS patients. One such stimulus is simply moving toward the toilet. This can occur when driving toward home in an automobile; an MS patient may feel perfectly fine for miles and miles passing whole subdivisions of houses, but then, on turning a corner and seeing her own house, she can experience a predictable spike in urinary urgency for the first time. Urgency grows as the house gets closer. Pulling into the garage makes urgency worse. Opening the door to the house makes urgency worse again. Moving through the house toward the bathroom makes urgency still worse. This crescendo of urgency typically reaches maximal one step from the toilet. The first astronaut to step on the moon, Neil Armstrong, described that step as "one small step for [a] man, one giant leap for mankind." Likewise, the last step before reaching the toilet is only one small step for most men, but often seems a giant, insurmountable leap for an MS patient in urinary distress.

This scenario is likely familiar to many MS patients. It's important to understand that the reason this happens exactly this way over and over again is also not due to the bladder suddenly filling up at just that moment. The drastic change in urgency has little to do with the volume of urine in the bladder, which changes very little over those 4 to 5 minutes.

The cause of this is what physicians refer to as "supratentorial" (i.e., a problem in the head) – a conditioned (Pavlovian) reflex.

Pavlovian reflexes work like the salivation that Pavlov first observed in 1901 in dogs with a conditioned stimulus. After Pavlov rang a bell with presentation of supper, the dogs started salivating whenever a bell was rung, even when no supper was presented to them. In addition to ringing a bell, Pavlov used a variety of other conditioned stimuli, all of which worked to stimulate the dogs to salivate: electric shocks, a range of visual stimuli, whistles, metronomes and tuning forks.

Likewise, many conditioned stimuli can cause a spike in urinary urgency for an MS patient sensing urine in the bladder: 1) the sound of moving water (e.g., running from a faucet, in the dishwasher, in the washing machine, rain on the roof, etc.) or the sound of white noise (e.g., a space heater or air conditioner turning on); 2) touching anything wet (e.g., grabbing a squirt of alcohol handrub); 3) turning the corner in the hall nearest to the patient's bathroom; 4) turning on the bathroom light at night when proceeding there because of nocturia; 5) closing the bathroom door at night when proceeding there because of nocturia; 6) nearing the toilet at night when proceeding there because of nocturia; 7) anything untoward (e.g., a spastic foot catching against the bathroom doorjamb impeding progress at night when proceeding there because of nocturia; trying to grab the handles of a rollator walker but a spastic hand misses the handle; trying to sit up in bed and get up for nocturia but losing balance and flopping over onto the bed; 8) rolling the walker around beside the bathroom counter where I often leave it when I urinate; 9) putting the toilet seat down so I can sit on it; and 10) touching anything with my spastic hand or foot (e.g., the handle of my walker) [touching anything cold with my spastic hand or foot causes an even greater spike in urgency]; etc..

Another thing that causes increased urinary urgency for me is pain – or perhaps more specifically, uncontrollable pain. If I am maneuvering toward the bathroom while sensing the need to urinate and experience an unexpected pang of pain, this is usually interpreted by my mind as untoward and followed immediately by a ping of Pavlovian, increased urinary urgency that is often accompanied by increased spasticity of my more spastic left limbs. I said uncontrollable pain because I get a different response to the pain of stretching my contractured second toes on both feet. If I am sensing urine in my bladder as I am removing my shoes before bedtime, difficulty removing one or both shoes can cause increased urinary urgency and decerebration of one or both legs. After I remove the shoes, painful stretching of my contractured toes always is accompanied by a decline in urinary urgency. I assume that this difference is related to the fact that the latter is pain volitionally controlled and considered beneficial rather than untoward.

A patch of flannel (8" x 15") has been important to me for controlling the Pavlovian stimuli that tend to cause urinary urgency in the hour before bedtime. If the bathroom is cold as it often is in winter (and sometimes can be even in summer when the air conditioning goes into overdrive trying to counteract severe heat outdoors), putting my spastic left hand down on a cold bathroom counter can cause increased urinary urgency as I stretch my legs to prevent periodic limb movements. This is a problem because voiding too early before bedtime would mean a problem with urinary urgency when I wake the first time after going to sleep. To keep urgency from occurring while I'm stretching my legs, I thus put my spastic left hand down on a patch of flannel which elicits no Pavlovian urge to urinate. To increase stability of the patch of flannel on the bathroom counter, I had it sewn to a patch of rubbery matting (Easy Liner) that sticks to the counter and helps keep my hand from sliding and me from falling.

A crisis of urinary urgency can cause my spastic left arm and left leg to become increasingly more spastic as I approach the toilet and my spastic leg can seem stiffer and heavier as if switching from flesh to a heavy metal. This change can add to my urinary distress for more than one reason: 1) as stated above, anything impeding progress toward the toilet results in a Pavlovian reflex causing an immediate spike in urinary urgency, 2) the increasing spasticity makes it increasingly difficult to walk, and the increased effort of walking results in a modified Valsalva maneuver (i.e., like when one holds his breath and strains to have a bowel movement) with each step, putting additional pressure on the bladder, further increasing urgency.

I don't have study data confirming this, but I have the impression that an increased blood concentration of zolpidem tartrate may impair my ability to control urinary urgency just as it may impair my ability to get up and walk safely to the bathroom without falling.

Before getting MS, I had no hint of a bashful bladder. But after getting MS, I definitely developed a bashful bladder. The same phenomenon applied to the bowel inside a public bathroom. And years later a new manifestation of the bashful bowel showed up when I was not even inside a public bathroom. After I started having nursing aides help me with ADLs, my daily shower usually took place after lunch. Sometimes after eating something constipating, I would have difficulty with a bowel movement that threatened to come out when I went toward the bedroom to undress for the shower, but would do nothing when I reached the bathroom. Facing this dilemma 6 times, I sent a nursing aide home early because MS related constipation is sort of like "waiting for Godot" who might never come. But each time I did that, as soon as the aide left the house, the bowel movement started moving without my having done anything other than wait just a few more minutes. It seems that even though I was in the bathroom alone trying my best to get the bowel movement to happen before the shower, my brain knew this and knew that someone else in the house was waiting for me to get it done so that we could proceed. As soon as the aide left the house, there was no longer the perception that anyone was around at all, which somehow seemed to free my bowels to move (like a positive Pavlovian reflex for the right thing to happen). At such moments, the MS patient sometimes wonders whether a laxative suppository is necessary. Whenever it seems possible that a bowel movement might want to occur naturally (i.e. without the artifice of inserting a suppository into the rectum), I opt for that approach because a natural bowel movement is always more effective at removing the stool already formed in the colon than is a laxative suppository. In addition, the laxative suppository can cause more problems later (e.g., anywhere from two hours to eight hours later there may need to be an urgent bowel movement containing nothing more than little bits of dissolved bisacodyl suppository and small bits of stool that come out with it. This secondary urgent bowel movement can slip out without the patient even being aware of it while sitting on the toilet (i.e., unlike a normal bowel movement). This can be very disturbing and result in soiling of the underwear, so, after use of a bisacodyl suppository, I always had to be very careful to make sure that such dissolved suppository remnants ended up getting removed. Depending upon the way the rectum felt and the bladder acted, I would sometimes elect to use digital stimulation to remove the suppository remnants. The best way I found to do this was with latex gloves lubricated by KY jelly.

The only stimulus that seems to inhibit my urge to urinate is heating myself. I have done this most often by standing in front of a space heater. I have also done this using a handheld hair dryer, keeping it moving to avoid burning any spot of skin. Heat has worked for me more than 100 times. It always seems to work unless the bladder really is overly full (which is rarely true because I drink the same amount every day due to the history of bladder problems) or the colon is pressing against the spastic bladder. The latter can happen if the colon contains hard constipated feces or is overfull and thus occupying too much space in the pelvis (e.g., from flatus accumulating and unable to exit because of stool blocking the rectal sphincter, excessively bulky stool from eating too much fiber, etc.). I'm not sure whether heat is a conditioned stimulus or if it naturally inhibits the urge to urinate. Being in a warm room seems to inhibit my urge to urinate as well as standing in front of a space heater does, so it may not be merely a conditioned stimulus.

After I started having problems with severe urinary urgency and incontinence and recognized that conditioned reflexes were making the problem worse, I tried talking loudly, or singing to interrupt my own brain's perception of such stimuli. This worked. The first time talking loudly or singing inhibited urinary urgency, it couldn't have been a conditioned stimulus. After it worked a time or two, it may have become a conditioned stimulus that helped calm the urinary urge. But, if I pushed my luck and the strategy failed (e.g., because there was too much in the bladder and/or colon), then singing a particular song could become a conditioned stimulus favoring rather than inhibiting progression of the urge. If that happened, using that particular song was counterproductive.

As I approach the toilet, I try to focus on something other than the uncomfortable urgency in my bladder. For no particular reason, I chose the armpits. As I get up from the wheelchair and take the final steps toward the toilet, the effort causes a modified Valsalva maneuver, which exerts more pressure on the bladder. So, as I take those steps, I try to deal with this problem in the opposite way, by focusing on what the Valsalva is doing; I do this by saying "one Valsalva, two Valsalva, three Valsalva..." as I take those steps.

Direct, sustained pressure on the penis (trying to hold the urethra shut and prevent a desperate urge to urinate) didn't work to calm a crescendo of urgency for me and didn't prevent wet clothes. It's possible that I didn't sustain the direct pressure long enough (being new at trying to interrupt Pavlovian reflexes at the time), but sustained, direct pressure did work to halt a crisis of fecal urgency more than 50 times (i.e., I just pinched the butt cheeks closed and held them for 30 to 45 seconds until the urge to defecate subsided, allowing me to proceed to the toilet with clean underwear).

Since direct pressure on the penis didn't work, I tried alternating pressure on the glans penis, (again trying to interrupt my own brain's perception of such stimuli). Alternating pressure worked the first time I tried it, so it wasn't a conditioned stimulus at that point, but could have become one later. Alternating pressure turned out to be a very useful tool for me to control an episode of dire urinary urgency. I have woken up multiple times with urinary urgency so bad that both of my legs fully decerebrated but managed to avoid incontinence by using alternating pressure on the glans penis long enough to calm the urge (followed by standing up while holding onto a bedrail and then urinating into a handheld urinal).

I later recognized that a crisis of urinary urgency occurring when proceeding toward the toilet in a motorized wheelchair (a Quantum 600 made by Pride Mobility) could be similarly calmed by my rocking forwards and backwards. It's important for me to emphasize that it's not just my upper body that's rocking back and forth – my bottom is actually rocking forward and backward on the wheelchair seat. The same maneuver – rocking back and forth – works very well sitting on the bed. I have woken up with urinary urgency so bad that both of my legs decerebrated and been able to avoid incontinence by rocking back and forth long enough to calm the urge, then standing up while holding onto a bedrail and using a handheld urinal. I can't prove that rocking back and forth doesn't work for me by applying alternating pressure to the glans penis (i.e., like what I was doing directly with my fingers when maneuvering toward the toilet with my walker), but it seems possible that some other sensitive spot on my bottom is more likely responsible for the effectiveness of this rocking motion. After thinking about this, I hypothesized that the sensitive spot on the bottom might be in the perineum. Getting up from my wheelchair during several subsequent episodes of urinary urgency complicating a bout of increased constipation, I tested this theory by trying a brief perineal massage. This seemed to work as well as alternating pressure applied to the glans penis. One caveat is that I have used the latter with success hundreds of times and only tried manual, perineal massage several times. A positive feature is that this should work for female patients, but I haven't had a female MS patient's body to experiment with during an episode of urinary urgency to confirm this. A negative feature associated with this location is that when urinary urgency causes a spurt of urine into the urethra, perineal massage can facilitate excretion of urine from the urethra, which would not be helpful if the woman has already lowered her underpants containing the incontinence pad (i.e., unlike application of alternating pressure to the glans penis).

An experiment that could figure this out would involve male and female MS patients proceeding toward the toilet with urinary urgency and rocking forward and backward on the seat of a wheelchair. If this alternating pressure maneuver works only for male patients, then it may just be an indirect mechanism of applying alternating pressure to the glans penis. If it works as well for female patients, then the alternating pressure must be working at a different spot on the anatomy. A third group could try perineal massage to see if that seems to be the sensitive spot being affected by rocking back and forth.

If I apply alternating pressure for 10 to 15 minutes, the urge to urinate may completely disappear and be hard to restart when I reach the toilet. If I do this, my incontinence pad usually has no drops of urine that can be smelled. If I do it for 10 to 20 seconds, the urge is usually reduced enough to allow me to walk another 5 to 10 steps before I have to repeat the process. Doing this, there may be small spurts resulting in enough drops of urine to smell on the pad, which does not become perceptibly wet if I do this right.

Having mentioned the incontinence pad twice above, I probably should add that the pad is helpful but only a stopgap measure because it has frequent failures for multiple reasons. Some readers might wonder whether an adult diaper might be more effective in stopping the problem of urinary incontinence. It should be, but I was unable to use one because the occlusive nature of the diaper made it unfriendly to the buttock of my paretic left leg (i.e., predisposing it to development of *Staphylococcus aureus* furuncles).

Of note, I have found that most Pavlovian stimuli that cause an unwanted spike in urinary urgency can't be used when I want to stimulate urination (e.g., before going to bed) when I want to encourage my bladder to urinate (e.g., I have tried turning on the faucet at least 15 times, which never works when I want it to stimulate an urge to urinate). By contrast, I have found that a different set of

Pavlovian reflexes can be used. These include flexing my neck which reliably causes Lehrmitte's syndrome with tingling down the spine (I don't know why, but this will usually help encourage my bladder to initiate urination), scratching my head, and yawning (note that this has to be a true yawn, not just opening my mouth simulating a yawn). One exception: sitting down on an uncomfortably chilly toilet seat is a Pavlovian stimulus that increases unwanted urinary urgency but this also sometimes seems to mildly encourage desired urination. Letting my pants droop down around my ankles also makes me chilly and encourages desired urination. If I open my mouth wide and exhale beside my bare legs, my breath comes out warm, but if I blow on my legs through pursed lips, the air is chilly and helps my bladder want to urinate; this has worked for me more than 30 times.

8 Degrees of Misery Associated with a Bout of Constipation Causing Increased Urinary Urgency:

1) mildly increasing urgency on walking toward the bathroom not resulting in spurts of urine

2) moderately increasing urgency walking toward the bathroom resulting in spurts of urine

3) increasing urgency starting before I even start walking toward the bathroom resulting in faster, more copious spurts of urine

4) waking up with so much urinary urgency that there's no way I can make it to the bathroom and have to resort to using the bedside commode

5) waking up with so much urinary urgency that it's difficult making it to the bedside commode without incontinence

6) waking up with so much urinary urgency that it's hard to even sit up in bed without incontinence

7) waking up with so much urinary urgency that my spastic left leg immediately decerebrates making it impossible for me to stand up and thus making it very likely that there will be uncontrolled

urination into the incontinence pad and possibly my pajamas and bed sheets

8) having a bout of constipation so bad that I end up having uncontrolled urination causing me to have to change clothes four times during the day and pajamas four times during the night

Being drenched with water is unpleasant. Being drenched with urine is worse because urea reeks and irritates the skin.

Other Possible Control Measures

When I started having urinary urgency, anticholinergic medications (e.g., oxybutynin) were available for inhibiting bladder muscles and calming the urge, but my problem was self-limited each time it occurred. After the actively constipating foods made their way through my gastrointestinal tract and the bout of constipation passed, I had no more severe urinary urgency. I would have no trouble again for weeks to months until I ingested another actively constipating food. Each time this happened, I would think about the medication that was available, but could not bring myself to use it because anticholinergic medicine inhibits colon muscles as well as bladder muscles and can cause constipation. In a patient like me that had been struggling with constipation for decades that was getting worse each year, not better, an anticholinergic could cause big problems. Oxybutynin can also cause urinary retention. I already had bad constipation and weak urine flow, which made me reluctant to try the drug. Some recommend using oxybutynin only with intermittent catheterization, and a patient with hemiparesis like me cannot catheterize the bladder with one hand.

During the first several years of having intermittent bouts of constipation and urinary urgency, I would suffer through each bout as best I could, without resorting to any extra pharmaceutical agents. Part of the reason for this was that I knew laxative abuse could engender an iatrogenic form of constipation – the colon becoming dependent upon the laxative.

But, at some point, it seemed to me that enough suffering was enough, and that taking a bit of extra laxative might help alleviate some of the suffering. I found that to be correct. After having to rely on a bedside commode as many as six times per day for a week at a time over many months (because the urinary urgency was so intense that I could not make it to the bathroom with my walker without incontinence), using an additional amount of laxative to counter a bout of constipation made it possible for me to stop using the bedside commode. At the time I'm writing this, I haven't used the bedside commode in over 3 years, which seems impossible to believe, given what was occurring previously and particularly because I have taken no medications that inhibit the bladder muscles. This approach has worked well for me, but I saw no studies evaluating its use in MS patients for controlling urinary urgency. None of the other books written for MS patients noted that constipation could cause urinary urgency or recommended controlling constipation to help control urinary urgency. It seems unlikely that I'm the only MS patient with this problem that could benefit from this approach.

There are other medications that can be used to deal with the problem of urinary urgency (e.g., botulinum toxin injections, DDAVP [desmopressin]), but the same thought process applies to them – they have costs and side effects that seemed hard for me to justify for my self-limited problem.

As mentioned above, a bedside commode can be helpful to an MS patient when a crisis of urinary urgency makes it impossible to reach the bathroom. Likewise, a handheld urinal can perform the same function for those with sufficient strength and manual dexterity to do what is required without spilling urine (which, for an MS patient, would be more a disaster than an aesthetic problem because a wet floor could cause a fall and a wet bed would be difficult to sleep in). The advantage of the bedside commode is that there is less probability of a spill. The advantage of a handheld urinal kept at the bedside is that there is less possibility of urinary incontinence resulting in wet pajamas before initiating urination.

Another control measure for urinary urgency and incontinence that could be used is the entrée consumed for supper (i.e., while keeping the type and amount of beverage constant). This may seem obvious to some because of what was said earlier about fluid intake being an important determinant of urine output, but it may seem less obvious to others. I was surprised to find that my eating split pea soup for supper was associated with a much lower urinary output overnight than eating a plate of spaghetti or a vegetable plate (e.g., cabbage, potatoes, carrots, and green beans). The difference was so marked that I often went hours longer between episodes of nocturia and yet woke without urgency; sometimes this resulted in my going an entire night with only one episode of nocturia. Pea soup is thicker than the average soup (hence the expression "as thick as pea soup"), and it's possible that its relative dehydration was at least partially responsible. Another supper entrée associated with decreased urinary output for me was Amy's Vegetable Pot Pie. I saw nothing about such things in the other books written for MS patients.

MS patients suffering repeated episodes of incontinence must heed the call of nature and proceed toward the toilet promptly. Failure to do so is a mistake. For this reason, scheduling social encounters is optimally done at a time just after the patient will be departing the bathroom. Scheduling social encounters just before the time the patient usually needs to go to the bathroom is another mistake. Socializing makes it harder to notice the call of nature and to respond promptly because the patient remembers decades of delaying urination until socially convenient and may think that a couple more minutes shouldn't cause incontinence. Wrong.

Chapter 10
Dealing with Fecal Incontinence

As mentioned above, MS is a disease about losing control and one of the more disturbing features is losing control of one's bowels and bladder. Inability to defecate or urinate is distressing, but incontinence is equally disturbing and more degrading.

Because most of my early episodes of fecal incontinence were due to MS-related food poisoning, preventing food poisoning, as discussed in Chapter 33, is an important part of dealing with fecal incontinence. Most of my later episodes of fecal incontinence were due to an increased dose of laxatives being used in an effort to counter a bout of constipation (others were due to loose stools from antibiotic therapy and still others to solid stools and unfortunate circumstances [e.g., a full bladder coinciding with a gastrocolic reflex following a meal]); urinating before eating a meal is thus wise when that option is available. Knowing how to adjust laxative dosage to avoid fecal incontinence, as discussed in Chapter 7, is also important for preventing fecal incontinence.

But there's more that an MS patient should know and do. Some of this was addressed in Chapter 9 discussing urinary incontinence. But it probably bears reemphasis in a separate chapter because the problems of urinary and fecal incontinence are obviously not exactly the same.

One thing an MS patient should recognize is that an episode of fecal incontinence can often result in less complete expulsion of feces from the rectum for several reasons. During an episode of fecal incontinence, the patient is unlikely to strain and try to help expel all of the feces. This means that another bowel movement may soon be imminent. This can be frustrating when one has to return to the bathroom after spending more than an hour cleaning up and changing clothes.

Pinching the butt cheeks together will effectively halt a strong fecal urge for me 99% of the time, but sometimes this can result in the urge totally disappearing and being hard to restart on reaching the toilet (i.e., similar to the problem mentioned above about totally halting a urinary urge with alternating pressure applied for 10 to 15 minutes to the glans penis). As explained above, halting a fecal urge can be similar to halting a urinary urge in one way, but it is different in other ways. For example, direct pressure (crimping the butt cheeks closed with direct pressure) has worked to prevent fecal incontinence for me scores of times, but direct pressure clamping the urethra shut did not work for me to prevent urinary incontinence while alternating pressure did.

It's also important to know that pinching the butt cheeks together is easier to do when standing up maneuvering with my walker than it is when sitting in a wheelchair. The problem of pinching the cheeks together when sitting in a wheelchair is that it's physically difficult to get hold of them because of the physics involved (i.e. sitting on them makes them harder to gather together). Polyester pants have less friction than cotton and make pinching the butt cheeks together more difficult.

Most of my failures of that maneuver have occurred when I was in a wheelchair motoring toward the bathroom or one step from the toilet– the same as for urinary urgency. I believe that the reason this is true is also the same, that moving toward the toilet while sensing distention of the bowel or bladder causes a Pavlovian reflex that results in an immediate spike and crescendo of urgency.

So it's important to pay attention to early signs (as mentioned in Chapter 9) – more attention than a normal healthy person would ever need because the normal healthy nervous system allows postponement of fecal urges until a socially convenient moment and because the consequences to an MS patient of ignoring the earliest signs can be chagrin and more than an hour of cleaning up. Social encounters just before the time the patient usually heads to the bathroom can make fecal incontinence more likely. Having a full or overly full bladder at a time when a bowel movement is expected also predisposes to fecal incontinence. Delay heading to the toilet in this circumstance is often a mistake.

There's an old saying, attributed by some to Mark Twain, that it's better to remain silent and be thought a fool than to open one's mouth and remove all doubt. Neither possibility is attractive, but one is better than the other. Similarly, when feeling the beginnings of fecal urgency in the presence of other people while maneuvering with my walker toward the bathroom, if the urgency ratchets up and defecation appears imminent within seconds, I believe it's better to set the brake and immediately pinch my butt cheeks closed than it is to try to keep going and hope to get out of the room before having to do something so embarrassing in the company of others. I agree that pinching my butt cheeks closed is embarrassing, but it's much less embarrassing than having a bowel movement in my pants in the company of others. I should mention that this was not an *a priori* decision about which would be better before one or both happened. Rather, this is my advice after experiencing both types of ignominy.

It's also probably important that I distinguish between the constipated MS patient's problem of tenesmus (which can involve feeling like a bowel movement is imminent for hours) and the feeling mentioned in the paragraph above that "defecation appears imminent within seconds." The word "imminent" is used in both circumstances, but perhaps in the latter it should be spelled "IMMINENT" and the words "within seconds" make a critical difference. An MS patient with tenesmus obviously can't sit around for hours pinching butt cheeks closed.

Chapter 9 mentioned a Pavlovian, conditioned reflex increasing urinary urgency when anything untoward happened delaying progression toward the toilet. There seems to be a similar conditioned reflex augmenting fecal urgency. As an example, if I feel that I will need to have a bowel movement after getting dressed and clumsiness with buttoning buttons slows down my progress of dressing and getting to the toilet, this increases my fecal urgency. Fecal urgency and urinary urgency are similar in this way and in other ways (e.g., usually maximal one step from the toilet), but different in other ways. For example, severe urinary urgency often causes decerebrate rigidity of my spastic left leg. Severe fecal urgency never does this for me.

Kermit the Frog said that "being green isn't easy." The same is true of being clean, especially for MS patients who are more likely to have fecal incontinence and are more likely to have contamination of hands and clothes after normal bowel movements because of frequent use of stool softeners and laxatives to counter MS-related constipation. Trying to clean up after a bowel movement also becomes increasingly difficult as the MS patient's more functional hand becomes weaker and more spastic. For this reason, when there is a larger mess to clean, I believe that an MS patient should use more paper (e.g., folded Kleenex rather than a sheet or two of toilet paper) for the initial wipes to avoid contaminating the hand as large amounts of contamination are being removed. The initial wipes should be considered "debulking" (i.e., removing large amounts to begin initial control, understanding that many wipes often are needed to remove the last bits of contagion), taking care to keep the hand clean while doing this so that the process does not have to be paused to wash the hands since trying to clean the bottom with a contaminated hand will likely spread contamination to other clean parts of the bottom. Also avoid overfilling the toilet with paper before flushing. An MS patient without access to a functioning toilet can quickly get into desperate straits.

After gross fecal incontinence, I routinely removed all of my clothes and took an immediate shower until I became too disabled to do that. This approach was associated with no urinary tract infections at all for me over 20.5 years with MS. After I stopped being able to take an immediate shower, I had three urinary tract infections over the next six months, but only one of those infections followed an episode of gross fecal incontinence.

Chapter 11

Is the Credé Maneuver
Helpful to MS Patients?

O nly one of the four books mentioned above that were written by physicians for MS patients discusses the Credé maneuver (applying gentle manual pressure over the bladder to help voiding). Dr. Swank's book says it works but adds that it prevents urinary tract infection. I agree with the former statement but doubt the latter, having seen no data documenting this. Skepticism is healthy.

Why do the other books ignore it? Perhaps because a urodynamic study of the effectiveness of the Credé maneuver reported that it was "an inefficient method of bladder emptying," noting that "relaxation of the external urethral sphincter and synchronous opening of the bladder neck only occurred in 2% of the [207] patients." [Barbalias GA, Klauber GT, Blaivas JG. Critical evaluation of the Credé maneuver: a urodynamic study of 207 patients. J Urol. 1983 Oct;130(4):720-3.]

Another study of 74 paraplegics with flaccid, areflexic bladders using the Credé maneuver for two decades reported that the Credé maneuver worked poorly to evacuate their bladders (93% had post void urine volume > 100 ML and 50% had residual urine volume > 300

ML) and might be dangerous because they had such a high prevalence of urologic complications (pyuria in 82%, nephrolithiasis in 31%,
ureteral dilatation in 60%, hydronephrosis in 35%, and renal damage
in 16% [Chang SM, Hou CL, Dong DQ, Zhang H. Urologic status of 74
spinal cord injury patients from the 1976 Tangshan earthquake, and
managed for over 20 years using the Credé maneuver. Spinal Cord.
2000; 38:552-4.] The frequencies reported may be correct, but knowing
that the Credé maneuver was responsible would require a controlled
study. For example, Mayo Clinic website talked about using only an
alternate approach (catheterization) for areflexic, flaccid bladders,
which might account for lots of pyuria after use for two decades.

A third study reported that 9% of 225 MS patients had an areflexic,
flaccid bladder. [Amarenc G, Kerdraon J, Denys P. Bladder and sphincter disorders in multiple sclerosis. Clinical, urodynamic and neurophysiological study of 225 cases. Rev Neurol (Paris). 1995; 151:722-30.]

My experience using the Credé maneuver during 24 years with
MS leads me to conclude that the results reported by Barbalias et
al are likely correct. But in Chapter 2, I said that I agreed with Dr.
Swank that the Credé maneuver worked to help MS patients with
bladder problems to evacuate the bladder.

So, how can I reconcile these two, seemingly contradictory
statements?

I believe that effectiveness of the Credé maneuver can depend
upon the situation and probably the patient's pathology. If I walked
in off the street at some random moment and Barbalias asked me to
push in over my bladder, probably nothing would happen. In fact, if I
thought it would be nice to urinate because it'd been a couple hours
since the last time and it might be good to do that before going to
the kitchen for my next meal, it might not work then either. The only
times that it reliably worked for me was when I was already sensing
urine in the bladder. When I was already sensing urine, then it would
work every time to initiate voiding. To do that, I would use two
pressure points: the heel of my hand pressing in gently but firmly
over the pubis and my middle finger pressing down gently but firmly

over the base of the penis (don't know exactly why the latter helps, but it may help open the sphincter). It reliably worked for me in the right situation. Whenever there was a pause in urination, which can happen frequently to MS patients, I could press down and reliably get urination started again.

So, for MS patients like me, the Credé maneuver can be very useful. But for patients with a different type of pathology, it might not work. For example, if an MS patient with Type I DSD has a spastic urinary sphincter that clamps shut every time the bladder starts to contract, the Credé maneuver might not help. Likewise, for MS patients with more impaired sensation of the bladder, it wouldn't work as well in the way that I have used it.

As mentioned in Chapter 1, things change over time and there are "truths that are neither for all men nor for all times." This is true of the Credé maneuver being used by an MS patient like me. I had to occasionally resort to using it after my first attack of MS, but didn't always have to use it. When I went for urodynamic testing in the 13th year after onset of MS, I was asked not to use the Credé maneuver because the urologist wanted to see how my bladder functioned on its own. At that time, my bladder was able to completely evacuate urine, but started and stopped micturition several times before achieving that goal. In subsequent years, I had to use the Credé maneuver with increasing frequency and had to use it more frequently to reinitiate urination after a spastic sphincter paused the process.

How can I be sure that the Credé maneuver reliably worked for me when such studies reported ineffectiveness? Bob Dylan famously observed that, "You don't need a weatherman to know which way the wind blows," and a patient with MS doesn't need a urodynamic study to know whether the Credé maneuver is facilitating urination. Urine tinkling into the toilet makes enough noise to be heard in the next room (i.e., *res ipsa loquitur* ["the thing speaks for itself"]).

Similarly, pressing down over the abdomen trying to convince my colon to defecate would virtually never do anything. By contrast, pressing down over the abdomen just over the pubis and slightly to the left of the midline many times helped to initiate defecation or to complete excretion of a bowel movement. The MS colon, like the bladder, can pause and then stop before finishing elimination. A Credé maneuver can help my bladder and colon to more effectively eliminate what is there.

How much pressure is needed to perform the maneuver? I never use a lot of pressure. Sometimes it seems that "less is more" and light pressure may stimulate the bladder or colon to act, functioning more as a biofeedback stimulant than as a pump. It seems to me that selecting the optimal amount of pressure for stimulating the bladder or colon to initiate emptying can be a delicate matter, reminding me of the sensitivity of a safecracker's fingers. For me, too much pressure seems to be counterproductive. For this reason, I prefer to perform the Credé maneuver with skin against skin (i.e., rather than pressing my fingertips against my shirt or undershirt). This also reminds me of the relatively small amount of "activation energy" required to start a chemical reaction, after which the reaction proceeds spontaneously. With a flaccid bladder, more pressure may have to be applied than I usually use for my hyperreflexic bladder. And I do use a bit more pressure when helping the sluggish colon finish expelling stool.

It's obvious that something bulky pressing on the bladder can stimulate the urge to void (e.g., a colon full of bulky constipated stool with or without an accumulation of flatus causes the colon to occupy more than its share of space in the pelvis). So it's not really surprising that light, manual pressure in the vicinity of the bladder and/or colon can stimulate excretion. During a bout of constipation, I decided to try using the Credé maneuver to see how effective it would be. Eight times in a row when it seemed unlikely that my colon would proceed just using things like a Valsalva maneuver, steady gentle pressure using the heel of my hand pressing in over the left lower quadrant stimulated a bowel movement [as quickly as would be expected with a laxative suppository]. But then, two of the next three times I tried it, the same, sustained, light pressure didn't work at all when my constipation switched to a different mechanism being predominant after I fell and broke two bones as discussed in Chapter 12 (i.e., a spastic anal sphincter clamped shut, "dyssynergic defecation"); in that situation, I had constipation despite having unformed stools due to the antibiotic therapy.

For stimulating defecation, alternating pressure with no pressure (trying to simulate a wave of peristalsis) has generally worked better for me than applying steady pressure. Another thing that seems to work better for me to stimulate defecation is to envision the colon descending through the left lower part of the abdomen and grasp the left flank and try to give the colon a gentle squeeze.

So, is the Credé maneuver useful for MS patients like me? It's not a panacea. It won't work every time. But it's often helpful for an MS patient with bowel and bladder problems like mine.

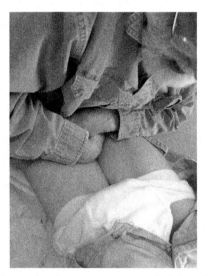

Figure 11-1 The author's spastic, paretic left hand usually gets in the way, as shown, and is usually thus tucked inside a T-shirt while the functional right hand reaches below it to apply light, judicious pressure over the urinary bladder and/or base of the penis for the Credé maneuver to facilitate urination.

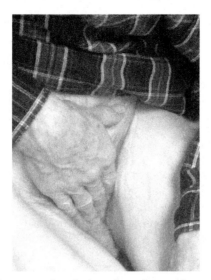

Figure 11-2 The functional right hand performs the Credé maneuver as shown with fingertips applying any needed pressure over the base of the penis and the heel of the hand applying pressure over the bladder to facilitate urination, and the thumb applies any needed pressure over the descending colon and/or rectum to facilitate defecation.

Chapter 12
The Bother Room

"Oh, bother!" – AA Milne, *Winnie the Pooh*
"If you love life, don't waste time, because that's the stuff life is made of." – Benjamin Franklin
"If anything bad can happen, it will." – Murphy's Law

As implied by Chapters 6-10, MS patients spend an inordinate amount of time in the bathroom experiencing all sorts of bother and frustration. A weak, spastic bladder and a weak, spastic bowel ensure this. The patient can sometimes have to get up every hour all night long for nocturia (e.g., if (s)he pushed fluids at bedtime because of the onset of symptoms of a new kidney stone) and even on a good night, nocturia may require visiting the bathroom several times.

During the day, drinking liquids necessitates frequent visits for urination and after breakfast and lunch additional possible visits for bowel movements, which don't always occur in a timely, convenient fashion. The patient may thus go to the bathroom when it seems reasonable, but the MS patient's colon is not reasonable and the patient may thus remain there for hours waiting for something to happen. When a bowel movement seems imminent, a normal healthy person usually heeds this "call of nature." For an MS patient who has had incontinence multiple times, this is even more important. But there are times when a bowel movement seems imminent but stubbornly won't move out of a constipated colon. Hence, the prolonged waiting.

Sometimes this gets so long that it seems reminiscent of a barnacle attached to a wharf. I have spent the entire morning waiting in the bathroom for a bowel movement that never arrived. Because there is so much bother in the MS patient's bathroom, I call it "the bother room." In the board game Monopoly, one penalty is "Go to jail, don't pass Go, don't collect $200." That's how I feel when arriving in the kitchen for breakfast only to receive an urgent summons to the bother room.

Having said that, I must add that despite all the hours of frustration in that room, there are many times when there is nowhere else that an MS patient would rather be. As Dr. Swank's book says, "Urgency and frequency of urination are common symptoms of MS. These symptoms, if not severe, can be managed well by keeping close to the bathroom while at home, but poorly when away from home."

Because MS routinely wastes large amounts of the patient's time on such waiting, it seems ironic that the disease occurs at a higher frequency among descendants of ancestors from northern Europe and especially Scotland because Scots traditionally abhor wasting anything.

Impairment of the autonomic nervous system and of blood flow to a paretic limb make maintenance of a normal body temperature in that limb impossible. My paretic limbs thus often seem as poikilotheremic (cold-blooded) as a fish. This is uncomfortable in more than one way. In cold weather, the paretic limb feels uncomfortably cold and year-round feels unpleasantly cold when it touches other parts of the body. Sitting on the toilet, my paretic left arm is always a problem and I manage the problem by wearing T-shirts a size larger so that I can tuck the paretic hand into the T-shirt and get it out of my way while my other arm does everything else needed for toileting (e.g., applying pressure for the Credé maneuver, blotting the urethra, wiping after a bowel movement, etc).

Chapter 13
Dealing with MS
Pain In General

There's a lot of pain. As mentioned in Chapter 6, my first symptom was pain in the left side of my neck. Ten years and multiple pains later, I started having a new one – in the butt.

That's right. MS can be "a pain in the neck" <u>and</u> "a pain in the butt."

And it can cause a lot of pain in a lot of other places (e.g., tooth and tongue pain due to trigeminal neuralgia, breast pain due to mastitis commencing weeks after a fall on the left chest, toe pain due to spasticity so bad I couldn't stand up, and the excruciating pains of a broken elbow [worst at full extension and full flexion] and broken coccyx that made sitting anywhere at any time uncomfortable, etc.). The diversity and severity of MS pains remind me of those torturing Caliban in Shakespeare's *The Tempest*.

It isn't unique in causing pain. Many diseases do it (e.g., cancer, heart attacks, angina, arthritis, etc.). But it's relatively unusual in a) making it so difficult to tolerate analgesics, b) causing so many different types of pain, and c) causing so many epiphenomena (e.g., increased spasticity, increased likelihood of falling with increased risk of fractures and still more pain, increased urinary urgency, increased urinary incontinence, increased constipation, etc.).

Inability to tolerate narcotics can mean continual, severe suffering for months. And when an MS patient tries to stand by grappling awkwardly with the handles of a walker, this motion can intensify the pain and make the epiphenomena acutely worse (e.g., a sudden spike in urinary urgency). At times, this constellation of symptoms can be so overwhelming that it seems impossible to go on. The frequency of such predicaments is why I think of MS patients as *les miserables* (the miserable ones).

If pain is described with an ordinal scale ranging from 1 (minimal) to 10 (so bad it causes you to pass out), I have experienced the full spectrum with this disease. Unfortunately, MS patients often battle constipation so bad that it would qualify for the word obstipation. This is one reason why constipating medications can be out of the question, making first line, narcotic analgesics unavailable to treat severe pain. Another reason is that one dose of a narcotic can make a patient feel as tipsy as a stiff cocktail, and patients already prone to fall become more likely to fall.

Stuck with second and third rate approaches to pain relief, MS patients often end up taking combinations of drugs like acetaminophen (which alone reduced one of my severe fracture pains from 8 to 7) and a nonsteroidal anti-inflammatory drug like naproxen (which gave me a peptic ulcer that started hurting on the 13th day after I began using it to relieve the pain of a clavicular fracture [broken collarbone]). Until it became clear what was causing the abdominal pain, I had to suffer for a couple weeks with no analgesic for the fracture pain. During those two weeks, I held my weekly dose of alendronate given for osteoporosis because it can exacerbate a gastric ulcer. When I had been asymptomatic for two weeks, I presumed incorrectly that the coast was clear and resumed alendronate therapy. The first dose of alendronate made clear that the twinge of abdominal pain had been an ulcer. The ulcer then caused pain for seven months despite immediately stopping the alendronate and taking daily stomach acid suppression therapy with a proton pump inhibitor (omeprazole).

Pain due to complications of MS such as fractures or a gastric ulcer due to medications used to treat the fractures is referred to as "secondary" pain. By contrast, pain caused by MS damage to the central nervous system is referred to as "primary" or central pain. Because the latter type of pain is due to damage to the nervous system, it's also referred to as neuropathic pain. Central, neuropathic pain can be manifested focally (e.g., in an arm, half of the mouth, etc.) or globally (i.e., all over the body) and doesn't tend to respond to regular analgesics like those mentioned above (e.g., narcotics, acetaminophen, aspirin, NSAIDs). For that reason, other types of drugs are often tried to control neuropathic pain. I had a transient, neuropathic (burning) pain with my first attack and transient, neuropathic (lancinating) pains with several subsequent attacks but never required analgesics for these pains because each attack promptly responded to methylprednisolone therapy. I have had transient, trigeminal neuralgia (a pain in the face[left maxillary branch]) hundreds of times, usually when I'm bending forward (e.g., to brush my teeth, to apply a warm moist compress to a furuncle on the buttock, to hold my walker, etc.).

A couple days after fracturing two bones, I developed trigeminal neuralgia of the left mandibular branch with pain in my teeth that at first made me worry about a dental problem. It hurt to chew food. When I realized all of the lower teeth on the left side were hurting, I knew that this was very unlikely to have any relationship to the teeth themselves. When I stuck out my tongue and it hurt, it was clear that the pain was trigeminal neuralgia affecting the mandibular branch for the first time. All previous times my trigeminal neuralgia had always affected the left maxillary branch and would last for seconds to minutes. This time it affected a different branch and recurred repeatedly for 10 hours without slacking up. At that point, the pain stopped for a while but then resumed at a lesser intensity and recurred repeatedly for about another day. Every time I yawned during that interval, the yawn would be interrupted by a stab of sharp pain, which would stop the yawn, leaving me in nearly constant pain with a feeling of dissatisfaction.

In my 25th year of MS, I developed trigeminal neuralgia in the maxillary branch of the right trigeminal nerve for the first time. Once again, this neuralgia always started when I was bent forward, but it caused more severe pain than the earlier manifestations of the problem (i.e., about 8 of 10 on a 10 point ordinal scale). Gabapentin (Neurontin) didn't control the pain and caused 7 side effects (additional weakness that persisted for days, blurred vision, amnesia, drowsiness, daytime somnolence, ataxia, and dizziness) but also reduced periodic limb movements and urinary urgency. Oxcarbazepine (Trileptal) prevented the pain and caused no noticeable side effects.

Because I haven't had continuing neuropathic pain, I don't really have a personal strategy for controlling it, but, as a physician and epidemiologist, I will offer a few comments at the end of this chapter based on medical studies regarding the problem.

So, what are my recommendations for dealing with pain in general? 1) Analgesics are very important for MS patients. 2) For this reason, it's important to try to keep them usable. 3) A patient using a nonsteroidal anti-inflammatory drug (NSAID) should always use a full dose of a proton pump inhibitor (e.g. a dose every 12 hours of omeprazole) and take the NSAID only with food in the stomach, to try to prevent peptic ulceration, which can make NSAIDs unavailable to MS patients. 4) An MS patient relying on acetaminophen for pain relief should avoid using any other hepatotoxic drug (e.g., rifampin, isoniazid, etc.) or beverage (e.g. alcohol) because acetaminophen can be toxic to the liver and swallowing multiple hepatotoxins simultaneously makes liver toxicity more likely, which would make acetaminophen unavailable to the MS patient. Needles of pain over the right upper quadrant of the abdomen were my only symptom when my liver became inflamed (hepatitis) from taking interferon injections for MS. Enzymes from the liver measured in the blood went up 25-fold, but I didn't develop nausea, queasiness, anorexia, vomiting, dark urine, etc.. It's important to recognize the onset of hepatitis quickly so that any hepatotoxic drug (such as acetaminophen [Tylenol], statins, NSAIDs, etc.) can be stopped immediately. If an offending drug is continued as the hepatitis gets going, the process may reach a point of no return – like an avalanche. 5) When in a lot of pain and relying on acetaminophen, it's important not to overdose because that could make hepatotoxicity more likely (sometimes it can occur even on the recommended dosage). 6) For controlling pain, it's important to stay on the acetaminophen dosing schedule, but this can become tricky at times (e.g., at bedtime, it may not be time for the next dose, but waking for nocturia after that dose time, the patient may suffer worse pain which can result in additional epiphenomena as mentioned above. To deal with this, one can split the difference and take half of the dose at bedtime (an hour before the scheduled dose) and half of the dose when waking for nocturia an hour after the scheduled dose (i.e., bracketing the dose time; mathematically, this results in the patient staying on the recommended dosage, and avoiding intensified pain and epiphenomena from missing a dose because of bedtime). An equally important reason to avoid getting hepatitis from acetaminophen is that the patient who can't tolerate other analgesics is prone to feel desperate because of the frequency and severity of pain endured by an MS patient. So even if the analgesic is relatively wimpy (e.g., reducing the severe pain of my anterior rib fractures from 8 to 7 on an ordinal scale), I still feel that it's extremely important to have something that will do anything to lessen such pain. 6) Physical therapy can be as important as pharmacotherapy for some types of pain (e.g., local heat, extension exercises for mid thoracic back spasms, lying flat in the bed with knees up for the pain of a herniated lumbar disc, bed rest for an hour or two in the morning and again in the afternoon for 3 to 5 days for a herniated lumbar disc; lying flat on the back without a pillow under the head or being strapped into a wheelchair vest that straightens the spine for as little as a half hour in the morning and a half hour in the afternoon has provided me more pain relief than acetaminophen for a thoracic vertebral compression fracture or a thoracic back spasm).

The importance of watching for the pain of hepatitis while taking a variety of drugs such as statins, which can be given to MS patients as immunomodulators, is mentioned above. Drugs can also cause multiple different painful side effects. For example, statins can cause pain in the liver due to hepatitis but can also cause pain in skeletal muscle, which can range from a benign nuisance to a life-threatening emergency (rhabdomyolysis, which can cause acute kidney failure). Pains in the arms and legs can develop in MS patients for a variety of reasons (traumatic injury from falls, overuse syndrome, and muscle pains due to statin therapy). Each of these is managed differently so it's good to pay attention to whether pain is in the joint (as in overuse syndrome), the bone (as in fracture from a fall) or in the muscle (as in statin related muscle problems [myopathy]). With statin problems, it is usually best to hold the statin dose and watch for improvement. A blood test showing very high muscle enzymes would indicate rhabdomyolysis, and, with that, statin therapy should not be resumed.

Lying flat on my back without a pillow really helps relieve the pain of thoracic vertebral compression fractures and also helps alleviate adjacent muscle spasms, but can bother my neck if I do this night after night for weeks. When I had a large sacral abrasion and had to lie flat on my back because of a compression fracture and adjacent muscle spasm, the abrasion also took unusually long to heal. It's possible that lying flat on my back all night every night for weeks was impairing wound healing of the sacral abrasion. If I hadn't had the back pain, I could have slept on my side, removing the continual pressure on the abrasion.

I developed a frozen shoulder three times – the first time due to MS related weakness and increasing immotility and the next two times after clavicular fractures. Stretching a frozen shoulder causes pain but "thaws" the frozen shoulder and minimizes pain if repeated regularly. As spasticity of my paretic left arm increased, spastic muscles began to hurt with stretching, but, again, stretching helped to keep the spasticity from advancing and to minimize pain if repeated regularly. I never took pain pills for either of these types of pain because the pain was not constant.

Different types of pain may respond differently to a particular drug such as acetaminophen. For example, as mentioned above, acetaminophen provided minimal relief for the pain of vertebral compression fractures. But when I had considerable pain an hour after a toenail biopsy, acetaminophen provided almost total relief. The point of this is that MS patients can barely get around as it is and need analgesics when moderate to severe pain makes this even more difficult, such as after the toenail biopsy. The black, subungual hemorrhage that caused me to have the toenail biopsy (because my dermatologist said the possibility of melanoma had to be ruled out with a biopsy) was not a complication of MS, but the pain caused by the biopsy was more difficult to deal with because of MS.

Using antiepileptic and antidepressant drugs to control neuropathic pain can result in a significant reduction in pain, but the reduction remains relatively small. For example, in a placebo-controlled, randomized trial comparing venlafaxine with imipramine, the placebo was associated with no reduction in pain scores and the two antidepressants were associated with relative 20% and 23% reductions, respectively. [Sindrup SH, et al. Venlafaxine versus imipramine in painful polyneuropathy: a randomized, controlled trials. Neurology. 2003; 60:1284-9.]

When I developed intolerable pain in a torn rotator cuff, I started methylprednisolone 40 mg by mouth each day and took that for six days followed by a taper over a week. That was coupled with resting the shoulder by avoiding activities that had been bothering it (e.g., reaching up into a cabinet, reaching up to put food into the microwave, etc.). This worked like a charm. I found out about the need to rest the torn rotator cuff by reading abstracts of medical studies, and I found out about calming down the inflammation with methylprednisolone from my wife – a rheumatologist. Many MS patients will probably be startled that the low dose (40 mg) was so powerful since MS patients frequently get pounded with much larger doses (the writer Flannery O'Connor referred to this as "riding the rocket," with which she was familiar because of therapy for systemic lupus erythematosus). [Most readers of this book are probably well aware that moderate to high dose steroids like methylprednisolone can cause an ulcer and simultaneous stomach acid suppression treatment with a proton pump inhibitor like omeprazole is thus indicated to prevent this problem – just like with an NSAID.]

When I developed intolerable pain in the right upper quadrant of my abdomen, my liver enzymes were normal, making a disease in the liver unlikely. The only analgesic available to me – acetaminophen – provided very little help, but when I lay down flat on my back in bed, I had no pain. The pain was due to a mechanical problem from flopping over as I walked holding onto my walker with my ribs presumably digging into my liver as I did so. This got much better after I started "practicing" standing upright as much as possible – so much better that the chronic right upper quadrant pain eventually, completely disappeared. But I occasionally still experienced a sudden stab of that same pain (i.e., same quality, same location) for months just by suddenly flopping over forward, probably compressing my liver with my rib cage jabbing it.

What about Neuropathic Pain?

Neuropathic pain usually doesn't respond to conventional analgesics and thus often gets off label treatment with an antiepileptic drug or antidepressant. Should a patient with neuropathic pain use one of those as an analgesic to control the pain? As discussed in Precept 11 in Chapter 1, the patient will need to balance the risk of adverse effects with the probability of benefit from a proposed medication. My feeling about chronic, unrelieved pain is that it's one of the worst problems MS patients face. If a patient has bad, chronic, neuropathic pain, an effective drug should be sought.

But it's kind of tricky figuring out which one is likely to help this type pain because MS patients tend to get more side effects than benefits with these drugs. A Cochrane review of this topic said, "There is no firm evidence to answer the important pragmatic questions about which patients should have which drug, and in which order the drugs should be used." [Wiffen PJ, Derry S, Moore RA, Aldington D, Cole P, Rice AS, Lunn MP, Hamunen K, Haanpaa M, Kalso EA. Antiepileptic drugs for neuropathic pain and fibromyalgia-an overview of Cochrane reviews. Cochrane Database Syst Rev. 2013 Nov 11;11:CD010567.]

Trial and error may be required. For example, with the drug gabapentin, which the Cochrane review cited above said was one of the better options for treating neuropathic pain, 4 to 10 patients had to be treated in controlled studies to find one with a 50% reduction in pain intensity. By contrast, the same authors said this about the prospect for side effects with gabapentin in a different publication: "Persons taking gabapentin can expect to have at least one adverse event (66%), withdraw because of an adverse event (12%), suffer dizziness (21%), somnolence (16%), peripheral edema (8%), and gait disturbance (9%). " [Moore RA, et al. Gabapentin for chronic neuropathic pain and fibromyalgia in adults. Cochrane Database Syst Rev. 2011 Mar 16; (3):CD007938. doi: spell 10. 1002/14651858.CD007938.pub2.] So, even if a drug works, it may not be usable if it causes an unacceptable side effect. This means that trial and error and careful observation will be needed to find an optimal approach and that the patient's neurologist will be indispensable for helping select and prescribe these medications.

For severe trigeminal neuralgia pain, there seem to be more data supporting the use of carbamazepine (Tegretol) or one of its metabolites oxcarbazepine (Trileptal) than for other drugs. [Gronseth G, Cruccu G, Alksne J, et al. Practice parameter: the diagnostic evaluation and treatment of trigeminal neuralgia (an evidence-based review): report of the Quality Standards Subcommittee of the American Academy of Neurology and the European Federation of Neurological Societies. Neurology 2008; 71:1183.] So that might be a good first option. My own better response to oxcarbazepine (Trileptal) than to gabapentin mentioned above would support that notion.

Chapter 14
Severe Rib Fracture Pain

In the 21st and 22nd years after my diagnosis with MS, I had a lot of falls, a lot of fractures and a lot more pain. The worst pain caused me to black out, which made me fall and fracture more ribs. That worst pain resulted from a combination of vertebral fractures and posterior rib fractures located close together. The next fracture affected anterior ribs and hurt almost as bad as the fractures that caused me to pass out. The pain of the anterior rib fractures felt like I was being stabbed with a knife, which was then being twisted.

Over the next three weeks, I suffered severe pain from both sets of fractures taking only acetaminophen, which reduced the pain but only minimally. I had seen a study reporting rib fracture pain relief with lidocaine patches, but also another study reporting the opposite and I was told that insurance companies were routinely denying coverage for lidocaine patches for that reason (and because the FDA refused to approve usage for this indication).

At that point, I didn't think I could stand such severe pain much longer, so I called my neurologist to see if she could think of a way to convince the insurance company to let me try using lidocaine patches. She ordered it, but my insurance company immediately denied coverage of her prescription, saying that a randomized controlled trial had shown the drug to be ineffective. After that, I suffered for another five days and then called my neurologist back to see whether she could appeal the denial. She said she would, but suggested that in the meantime I buy and try a patch. I did. They cost over $20 apiece, but within 20 minutes the severe pain that had persisted for 27 days completely disappeared.

The patch is supposed to be left on for a half day and then removed. The pain didn't start coming back until 2 ½ hours after the patch was removed the next day, and took more than a day to build back up to maximal.

After waiting six days until it was convenient for my wife to apply the patch again (using tape this time because the once used patch was less sticky after being stored on wax paper in a Ziploc bag), we observed the same results. It seemed that the study reporting efficacy of the patch was correct and the other study was false-negative

The two studies that evaluated lidocaine patch therapy of rib fractures didn't consider body mass index, but a very obese patient might not get effective relief because a different study of lidocaine patch therapy found that lidocaine penetrated only about 8 mm through the skin (i.e., if there is a large layer of fat beneath the skin, lidocaine might not reach a broken rib). My body mass index (BMI) was 19.2 (low normal), and the patch may be more effective in patients with my body habitus.

Studies haven't been published regarding effectiveness of the patch for clavicular fracture pain (broken collarbones), but I believe it will work. By contrast, it seems unlikely that the patch will provide meaningful pain relief for fractures of larger bones such as vertebrae or hips because of inadequate penetration of the drug to the site of the larger fractured bone.

Chapter 15
Fatigue

The other books written for MS patients by physicians note that fatigue is among the most frequent and bothersome symptoms of MS and routinely recommend pharmacotherapy. As mentioned above, I had 23 different unpleasant side effects of 10 medications prescribed because of MS and its complications, giving me a different point of view.

For managing fatigue, Dr. Giesser s book recommends trying five different drugs, including amantadine, and Dr. Lechtenberg's book recommends only amantadine for fatigue, but admits that it only appears to benefit "some" patients without mentioning that studies have reported response by only 20 to 40% of patients, and Dr. Lechtenberg also admits that the effect in this small proportion of responding patients "lessens after a few months." By contrast, Dr. Jelinek says this about using such drugs for treating fatigue in MS patients: "fatigue is very common, affecting over 80% of people with MS; it is often the most troublesome symptom and can significantly affect quality of life. Energy conservation strategies, cognitive behavior therapy, relaxation therapy and exercise have been used to effectively manage fatigue. Drugs don't help; some commonly used MS medications worsen fatigue."

Fatigue has been repeatedly associated in multiple studies with insomnia, which can occur for multiple reasons in MS patients (e.g., methylprednisolone therapy, pain, nocturia, CNS lesions, etc.). In one such study, 15 MS patients with fatigue were compared with 15 MS patients without fatigue and 15 normal healthy controls; the study concluded that, "There is a significant correlation between fatigue in MS patients and disrupted sleep or abnormal sleep cycles." [Attarian HP, Brown KM, Duntley SP, Carter JD, Cross AH. The relationship of sleep disturbances and fatigue in multiple sclerosis. Arch Neurol. 2004; 61:525-8.] Some talk about how bad nocturia can be in causing loss of sleep. Urinating on one's pajamas and having to remove them, clean up myself, clean the floor, and put on new pajamas takes about an hour for a patient with hemiparesis. Doing it four times in one night means four hours of lost sleep in addition to the sleep lost due to nocturia. When fatigue is due to insomnia and inadequate sleep, a nap seems better to me than a new medication.

But, as mentioned above, patients with MS don't all share the same problems. For example, not all patients have pain and those without pain may find other problems more troubling such as fatigue. So it's important that each patient balance the risks and benefits of proposed therapy based upon her own problems.

Fatigue was one of multiple symptoms that led me to consider retiring when I did – 12 ½ years after onset of MS (the average MS patient reportedly works for 10 years before retiring). Retiring allowed me to get a little extra sleep at night and also occasionally a nap after lunch when needed. Unlike what Dr. Giesser said about naps being counterproductive because they disrupt the normal sleep wake cycle, I didn't find that an occasional nap prevented me from falling asleep at night. And, perhaps as a result, I've felt less fatigue since retiring.

An exercise session obviously can produce fatigue in anybody, but regular exercise makes an MS patient more fit and reduces the patient's overall sense of fatigue according to several recent studies. What type of exercise is optimal? Both resistance training (e.g., lifting small weights) and endurance training (aerobic exercise) have reported benefits. Most important is doing exercise safely to avoid falling. For example, exercising beside a grab bar or with one's strong leg braced against something stable can prevent falling. Similarly, avoiding getting overheated because of the ambient temperature or an excessive amount of exercise can avoid heat induced weakness (Uhthoff's phenomenon), which could make falling more likely.

Chapter 16
Insomnia

"Sleep that knits up the ravell'd sleave of care,
The death of each day's life, sore labour's bath,
Balm of hurt minds, great nature's second course,
Chief nourisher in life's feast. " – William Shakespeare, *Macbeth*
"Whatever gets you thru the night – It's alright..." – John Lennon

Sleep is important. This is nothing new. It was known long ago, as evidenced by Shakespeare's comment from the 17th century regarding the importance of sleep. Humans don't seem to be able to live without it.

It isn't just important to humans. It seems vital to the entire animal kingdom (e.g.,"Birds do it, bees do it..." Even fish do it.). When laboratory rats in an experiment weren't allowed sleep, all died within two weeks.

So, it's easy to understand why insomnia is an important problem for anyone. It's an even larger problem for MS patients because they often have a diurnal rhythm of spasticity and weakness getting worse through the day and better at night with sleep. If unable to sleep, the much-needed daily improvement does not occur.

Before onset of MS, I never suffered insomnia except once on

Christmas Eve when I was five years old (probably due to sugar plum fairies dancing in my head).

For the first 21 years of MS, I rarely needed a sleeping pill except when taking high dose methylprednisolone. At those times, I would take a 10 mg zolpidem tartrate tablet, which would allow me to sleep five hours. After that, I was wide awake again and had to take more zolpidem tartrate to sleep more.

Sometimes during those years I had severe pain unrelieved by the analgesics available to me and couldn't sleep because of pain (because MS patients generally can't use first line, narcotic analgesics without developing severe worsening of constipation and/or having a higher risk of falling). Other times, periodic limb movements related to MS spasticity made sleep impossible. For such situations, I usually resorted to zolpidem tartrate. Sleeping with this drug, I got the usual benefits of sleep (e.g., feeling refreshed, getting stronger, becoming less spastic, etc.), and it provided an additional benefit – inhibiting the involuntary motions caused by spasticity when stretched out in bed trying to sleep (periodic limb movements, clonus, spasms in the calf and arch of the foot, decorticate posturing, etc.). It was also possible using this drug to take a dose that would allow me to sleep for an appropriate amount of time, given whatever was going on in my colon and bladder that evening (e.g., on a good night, I could routinely take a dose that would keep me asleep for three hours and on a bad night I could take a dose that would allow me to wake up after 1.5 hours if necessary).

As discussed in the Introduction, there are usually risks as well as benefits for each therapy and zolpidem tartrate has risks. It causes increased weakness, increased falls, and increased fractures. In a cohort study, patients taking zolpidem had a 2.55-fold increase in the rate of fall related fractures (of hips and bones other than vertebrae). This increased risk significantly exceeded the risk seen with a couple of other hypnotics (alprazolam and lorazepam), and was similar to the risk observed with diazepam (Valium). [Finkle WD, et al. Risk of fractures requiring hospitalization after an initial prescription for zolpidem, alprazolam, lorazepam, or diazepam in older adults. Journal American Geriatric Society. 2011; 59:1883-90. doi: 10. 1111/j.1532-5415. 2011.03591.x. Epub 2011 Sep 21.]

Some studies suggest that zolpidem tartrate works well as a hypnotic [Nowell PD, Mazumdar S, Buvsse DJ, Dew MA, Reynolds CF, Kupfer DJ. Benzodiazepines and zolpidem for chronic insomnia: a meta-analysis of treatment efficacy. JAMA. 1997;278:2170-7.] and may be safer than the benzodiazepine hypnotics (sleeping pills), which can make a patient feel tipsy like a glass of whiskey does and can addict the patient like alcohol.[Buscemi N, VanderMeer B, Friesen C, et al. The efficacy and safety of drug treatments for chronic insomnia in adults: a meta-analysis of RCTs. J Gen Intern Med. 2007; 22:1335-50.] Two studies that followed thousands of patients reported that use of hypnotics appeared to be safe and that increased mortality was due to confounding. [Jaussent I, Ancelin ML, Berr C, Pérès K, Scali J, Besset A, Ritchie K, Dauvilliers Y. Hypnotics and mortality in elderly general population: a 12 year prospective study. BMC Med. 2013 Sep 26;11:212. doi: 10.1186/1741-7015-11-212.] [Rumble R, Morgan K. Hypnotics, sleep, and mortality in elderly people. J Am Geriatr Soc. 1992; 40:787-91.]

Others reported that all hypnotics are dangerous for patients with chronic insomnia, finding a significantly higher mortality, significantly higher risk of falls and fractures, significantly higher risk of developing depression, significantly higher risk of cancer, and significantly higher risk of infection. [Kripke DF, Langer RD, Kline LE. Hypnotics' association with mortality or cancer: a matched cohort study. BMJ Open. 2012 Feb 27;2(1):e000850. doi: 10.1136/bmjopen-2012-000850.] [Kao CH, Sun LM, Liang JA, Chang SN, Sung FC, Muo CH. Relationship of zolpidem and cancer risk: a Taiwanese population-based cohort study. Mayo Clin Proc. 2012 May;87(5):430-6. doi: 10.1016/j.mayocp.2012.02.012.] [Kripke DF. Greater incidence of depression with hypnotic use than with placebo. BMC Psychiatry. 2007;7:42.] [Joya FL, Kripke DF, Loving RT, Dawson A, Kline LE. Meta-analyses of hypnotics and infections:eszopiclone, ramelteon, zaleplon, and zolpidem. J Clin Sleep Med. 2009;5(4):377-83. Review.] [Huang CY, Chou FH, Huang YS, Yang CJ, Su YC, Juang SY, Chen PF, Chou P, Lee CA, Lee CC. The association between zolpidem and infection in patients with sleep disturbance. J Psychiatr Res.2014;54:116-20.doi:10.1016/j.jpsychires.2014.03.017.]

Some studies concluded that drugs that bind gamma-amino-butyric acid (GABA) receptors can stimulate growth or metastasis of cancer. Many different hypnotic drugs used for insomnia bind to those receptors. Other drugs that also act by binding with these receptors such as baclofen have also been reported in some studies to increase risk of cancer growth and spread. [Zhang D, et al. GABAergic signaling facilitates breast cancer metastasis by promoting ERK1/2-dependent phosphorylation. Cancer Lett. 2014;348(1-2):100-8.doi: 10.1016/j.canlet.2014.03.006. Epub 2014 Mar 18] [Azuma H, et al. Gamma-aminobutyric acid as a promoting factor of cancer metastasis; induction of matrix metalloproteinase production is potentially its underlying mechanism. Cancer Res. 2003; 63:8090-6.]

So, is using zolpidem tartrate to deal with chronic MS related insomnia and periodic limb movements a good idea or a bad idea? This depends upon a number of things, and each patient should balance the risks and benefits of each proposed form of therapy. What's good for one patient might not always be good for another. For example, not all MS patients complain of constipation. For those who are spared that affliction, a narcotic analgesic might be possible to relieve severe pain from fractures; in that situation, the patient's balance might be the critical issue because a dose of narcotic analgesic can make a patient feel intoxicated like alcohol does. My own preference has been to continue using zolpidem tartrate despite knowing of its risks because I'm not yet aware of a better hypnotic and because of its ability to suppress the periodic limb movements ("better the devil you know than the devil you don't know").

What should an MS patient do if she feels the onset of rectal fullness while preparing to take a bedtime dose of zolpidem tartrate to induce sleep? This is an important question, and the answer, like those to many questions, depends on the situation. If the rectal fullness feels like a definite and imminent bowel movement, then bedtime should be delayed until after defecation and cleanup. If, on the other hand, the sensation is vague, implying that it might develop into something after an hour or two, then my approach is to go ahead and take the zolpidem tartrate dose and go to bed.

Why is that approach not foolhardy? What if this sensation is followed by development of an urgent need to defecate after an hour or two? I wondered the same thing the first 10 or 12 times that occurred for me. But slowly over time, I got the impression (despite the absence of pertinent data from clinical epidemiologic studies) that taking zolpidem tartrate in that situation seemed to have a calming effect not only on the spasticity of my limbs but also on my colon. This seemed to be so reproducible that I stopped worrying about this question.

Many times my swallowing sleeping pills with tomato juice was followed immediately by a sensation of rectal fullness, implying a gastrocolic reflex, but the sensation was always subdued or gone when I woke up for nocturia hours later.

Zolpidem causes the patient to fall asleep. If the patient is up walking around too long (e.g., 20 or more minutes) after taking a dose, sleep may start at that time and cause the patient to black out and fall. For that reason, it's important to get in bed quickly after the dose and stay there until sleep occurs. If the patient is lying in bed awake and not feeling particularly sleepy at that time wondering whether the zolpidem tartrate tablet was swallowed into the stomach or got stuck on the esophageal mucosa, it's not safe to get up and walk back to the bathroom for a couple more swallows to be sure it gets washed down. It's better to wait for a full hour. If the patient falls asleep during that interval, the question is answered. If not, it's probably safe to proceed back to the bathroom at that point. It's a problem though because waiting that long before getting the tablet swallowed into the stomach means that the bladder will likely be full requiring nocturia when the zolpidem tartrate blood concentration is still higher than desirable for getting up. This is hazardous and is the reason that I believe choosing the optimal liquid for swallowing tablets at night is important (see next chapter).

One way to avoid having a sleeping pill get stuck in the esophagus is to hold it in the mouth long enough for it to dissolve. It certainly won't get stuck in the esophagus, but it will be absorbed into the bloodstream faster and it thus becomes imperative to get into bed immediately (i.e., swallow the pill while sitting on the bed and then get into bed right after doing that).

After sleeping for an hour or two, I typically feel stronger and less spastic (due to sleep) and the blood concentration of zolpidem usually will also have declined enough to make it safer to get up if necessary for nocturia. It's important to take an appropriate dose so that the concentration won't be too high at that time. An appropriate dose depends upon the situation. In a bout of constipation, I predictably wake up sooner for nocturia (because the constipated stool in the rectum takes up more than its usual share of the pelvis, cramping the spastic urinary bladder). If I know that I'm going to have to wake for nocturia an hour and a half after going to bed, I take a smaller dose of zolpidem tartrate than if I'm not in a bout of constipation and can expect to sleep for three hours without waking up for nocturia.

When taking a dose of zolpidem tartrate, I try to get into bed within 10 to 15 minutes because if my zolpidem tartrate level gets too high, I also can get too weak to get into bed; my wife has had to rescue me multiple times by lifting my legs into bed when the zolpidem made me too weak. When I wake up for nocturia a couple hours later, the drug concentration is always low enough that I'm stronger and able to maneuver to the bathroom with the walker. But it's important to pay careful attention to dosage because this could be a big problem.

If on occasion I took too much zolpidem tartrate and woke up having difficulty sitting up or standing on my left leg, I would prop myself against the bed, use a handheld urinal, and go back to bed rather than maneuvering with the walker to the bathroom (e.g., for stretches).

For completeness, I should probably mention that zolpidem inhibits penile erections, so usually I have none while taking doses to sleep through the night. The next erection usually occurs when waking in the morning after I let the zolpidem concentration decline and that erection subsides after I urinate. In addition to inhibiting erections, zolpidem tartrate usually seems to shrink penile size. I mention this because a handheld urinal needs to encompass my full genitalia to ensure that the tip of the penis is inside (i.e., to avoid urine leaking down the leg). Patients wearing a condom catheter measured to fit the daytime penile circumference also could possibly have more problems with leakage at night if zolpidem tartrate causes penile contraction.

Chapter 17
What Is the Best Liquid for an MS Patient for Swallowing Pills at Night?

I s this an important question? I believe it is.

Why? Chapter 16 made clear that sleep is vital for an MS patient like me in part because I get stronger and less spastic with sleep and I get none of these improvements if I can't sleep.

So, if a sleeping pill adheres to the oral or esophageal mucosa and doesn't wash down into the stomach, I may not fall asleep due to MS related insomnia (e.g., involuntary, periodic limb movements make it hard for me to sleep).

When I first go to bed, this is most critical because my paretic left leg swells during the day and the edema fluid starts being re-sorbed when I lie down. This means that more fluid will be in the blood vessels, resulting in formation of an increased amount of urine, which in turn means the bladder getting full faster. So, if I have to get up after waiting to see whether the sleeping pill will work to go take more swallows of the fluid, I get behind and I am in danger of waking up later with a bladder too full to make it to the toilet without an accident. There is also the matter of when it is safe to get back up to go for more liquid because that first dose of zolpidem tartrate (2-2.5 mg for me) can make me suddenly black out while walking and fall. For that reason, I have to wait a full hour to make sure that doesn't happen. So, failure to get the sleeping pill washed down into the stomach is a major problem for me that can ruin the night and make the next three months agony if I fall and fracture vertebrae.

Many patients with MS suffer from osteoporosis because of corticosteroid treatments given for MS relapses. Gastric acid suppression, which many MS patients end up using, can make osteoporosis worse. Osteoporosis patients taking an alendronate tablet to increase bone density are instructed to take the tablet with an 8 ounce glass of water. This volume of water is recommended because it's very important that the alendronate tablet gets swallowed into the stomach. If it doesn't get swallowed, the tablet could cause an esophageal ulcer.

MS patients with nocturia wouldn't do well using that approach for taking pills through the night for multiple reasons (he, using that volume would cause more nocturia). This is true even though it's very important that certain pills (e.g., sleeping pills like zolpidem tartrate) get swallowed into the stomach. If they don't, it could be a very bad night for the MS patient. For example, the patient might not fall asleep, and staying awake would make the normal diurnal increase of weakness and spasticity remain bad, making getting back up at night more dangerous because of the possibility of falling. If the patient has to get back up an hour later to drink more liquid to get the pill to go down, this would mean that the last urination was further back in time, making the next nocturia dangerously close and likely to occur when the zolpidem blood concentration is still too high to get back up to maneuver safely back to the bathroom for more nocturia.

The optimal drink for taking pills at night for me was tomato juice because it was thicker than water and thus made swallowing pills easier. It's important that I mention that some commercial brands of tomato juice are as thin as water and thus no more helpful for a patient with dysphagia. The Campbell's brand was suitably thick. Because tomato juice was not sweet, it did not tend to spoil when left out on the bathroom counter overnight (I always put a plate over the top of the glass to keep any insect that found its way to the bathroom from descending into the glass for a drink).

Chapter 18
What Is the Optimal Number of Swallows to Assure That a Sleeping Pill Is Washed down into the Stomach?

This is another important question for multiple reasons and the answer depends on several things such as the volume of the glass being used, the frequency of nocturia, and the urinary urgency being experienced at the time. It's important for me to make it through the night, which means that I can't afford to drink all of the juice the first time I get up for nocturia. For the MS patient, the next nocturia may be 2 to 3 hours after the last. If the sleeping pill doesn't make it to the stomach (i.e., just sticks to the esophagus), the patient may not fall asleep due to various types of MS related insomnia and can get behind the eight ball if it becomes necessary to go back and take more swallows of juice later (because this means that the duration of sleep after the sleeping pill will make the bladder fuller and more likely to be a problem with dire urinary urgency). So, a thick drink (like tomato juice) works better for washing a pill down with fewer swallows. If I'm going to need to take Tylenol, baclofen and zolpidem, I take the first two with one swallow of tomato juice. I then put the zolpidem tartrate in my mouth and take 3 to 4 swallows.

Chapter 19
The Hazards of Heat
(Uhthoff's Phenomenon)

Ambient Heat

Several years after being warned that heat was a problem for MS patients, I was able to confirm the truth of the warning. Because the mind can have a powerful influence over what someone "sees" or "feels," the reader may wonder whether the warning was a self-fulfilling prophecy, causing the author to decide that heat must be a problem. But it wasn't like that.

As mentioned above, there was no confirmation for several years, perhaps because the amount of heat is important but also the amount of neurological damage wreaked by the disease also appears to be important for an MS patient to be able to recognize the heat effect. For several years I watched for but recognized no important exacerbation at any time during the summer despite mowing the yard regularly from March through October.

But then, while at work in my office on a humid, 90° day during summer, I stepped outside of the air-conditioned building at noon wearing a clinician's white coat and began walking down a sidewalk toward another part of the University of Virginia Hospital. Within 30 seconds, I was perceptibly weaker – globally weaker (i.e., this was not a pseudo-exacerbation involving weakening only of the left arm and/or leg prominently involved in the first attack, but rather a general weakening of all four extremities). The speed of onset of the global weakening by intense ambient heat made me think of fiction – Superman's reaction to exposure to kryptonite. But this was clearly real. I observed this multiple times after that and began taking care to spend less time outside when it was very hot and humid. I continued mowing the yard with a John Deere tractor from 1992 the year of diagnosis of MS until the autumn of 2008. During 2007 and 2008, I tried to mow early in the morning because the heat was exacting a higher toll on my body as the years passed. When I stopped mowing at the end of the 2008 mowing season, it wasn't because of the heat but because of severe pain in my right shoulder due to a torn rotator cuff and the need to rest the shoulder from any activities that might be contributing to the pain.

Sitting too long or too close while enjoying the warmth in front of a space heater (or roasting chestnuts on an open fire) can cause Uhthoff's phenomenon and make an MS patient too weak to stand up.

Like every other occurrence of Uhthoff's phenomenon that I have experienced, the weakness from sitting too long in front of a space heater has been global, not focal, so it's been typical of my episodes of Uhthoff's phenomenon and very atypical of the MS attacks that I've experienced (always focal). Other MS patients have had other manifestations (e.g., visual problems).

Climatic extremes

The other books for MS patients emphasize problems related to hot weather, but don't mention anything about cold weather being a problem. But as I became more debilitated and feeble, it got harder for me to tolerate climatic extremes in either direction. It's often said that arthritis patients can feel a coming change in the weather in their joints. An MS patient can do this as well – not in the joints but in the entire body. I came to sense the onset of a new heat wave before the temperature went up and I felt weaker despite staying indoors in the air conditioning when heat and humidity soared outside. During a severe heat wave (100°F each day for 10 consecutive days), I actually felt physically ill during the hottest part of each day despite remaining indoors in the air conditioning the entire time.

When young and healthy, I didn't mind a winter storm causing a power outage. My family wore long underwear and coats indoors, and it seemed sort of romantic warming a single room with a crackling fire in a wood stove where we would all sleep and heat cans of beans on top of the wood stove. But as MS disability progressed, it also got harder for me to adjust to extreme cold and inability to use the toilet; my spasticity would always get worse even inside a heated house. Floors and counters would become cold and cause vigorous startle reactions when touched. When a patient can barely stand up and move with a rollator walker, such extreme reactions to cold can cause a fall. Every successive winter and summer seemed more difficult for me to endure. The return of biting cold weather every November began to remind me of a line in the musical *Les Miserables*: "Winter's coming on fast, ready to kill."

Power outages can leave the temperature inside broiling hot or freezing cold for more than a week before utility crews get to our neighborhood for repair. For that reason, a generator that turns on automatically when power to the house is interrupted seemed a valuable investment for an MS patient like me with trouble tolerating extreme weather and inability to use the toilet because the electrical power went out and with it the pump, etc.

Inability to tolerate climatic extremes is not unique to MS – many patients with chronic illnesses feel this way. But with MS, the problems are not just a matter of discomfort. With extreme heat, the patient may become profoundly weak and be more likely to fall with all the pain, fractures, etc., that that may entail. With extreme cold, I predictably became more spastic and was again more likely to fall.

Internal Heat (fever)

On the sixth day after I began daily, subcutaneous injections of glatiramer acetate in my 11th year of MS, I was still working in my office in the early evening but noticed that I seemed to be moving slowly doing everything. After struggling to finish what I was working on at the computer, I decided to head home. When I picked up my briefcase and started for the door, I realized that I was unusually weak and wobbly. As I progressed out of the building, I seemed to get weaker, so weak that I felt the need to hold onto a handrail going down a ramp towards my car, which I held onto until I got to the car door. This continued driving home and getting into the house where I immediately called my neurologist. She told me to take my oral temperature. It was 37.8°C [100°F] (almost, but not quite a fever). She suggested that I take acetaminophen (Tylenol). I did that and sat down. Within 30 minutes, the feeling of being weak and wobbly was completely gone and did not return during that night or the next day. There were no other symptoms. Sometimes there can be systemic symptoms with onset of glatiramer acetate injections. Presumably this was one, but, regardless of the etiology of this mild temperature elevation, it showed that internal heat can be even more enervating than ambient heat. One other time, I developed a similar mild temperature elevation with a gastroenteritis acquired as food poisoning at a Cracker Barrel restaurant in North Carolina as my wife and I drove home from a week at a beach house on Hilton Head Island. As this second malady began, the first symptom was the same feeling of being weak and wobbly. Because of feeling weak, I decided to lie down. Just after lying down, I answered the telephone ringing beside the bed. It was my sister, but I told her that I felt too weak to hold the phone (I know this probably sounds ridiculous, but that was how I felt). Because of the similarity to the apparent reaction after starting glatiramer acetate injections, I measured my temperature and once again found it to be near, but not quite a fever. A dose of acetaminophen had the same effect as before, confirming once again the powerful effect of internal heat on an MS patient like me. Very quickly after that, the gastrointestinal manifestations of the illness began, suggesting that the mild temperature elevation was its prodrome.

The similarity of the weakness observed and of the oral temperatures measured in these two episodes four years apart makes it seem probable that a mild increase in body temperature can have a major effect on the strength of an MS patient with my degree of neurologic impairment.

After these two episodes had occurred, I asked my neurologist what she believed would happen if I got a true fever – perhaps due to influenza. She said that if I got the flu, which could result in high fever for five days, that I might be so weak that I would be battling for life on a ventilator in an ICU.

Chapter 20
What's the Best Way to Keep from Getting a High Fever?

A void infections in general because many types of infection can cause fever, (see Chapter 29) and be careful to avoid drug-related fevers. For example, high dose baclofen can be complicated by fever if the dose is suddenly reduced according to the following publication, which reported resolution of the fever after increasing the baclofen dose. [Mandac BR, Hurvitz EA, Nelson DS. Hyperthermia associated with baclofen withdrawal and increased spasticity. Arch Phys Med Rehabil. 1993;74:96-7.] Low doses of baclofen, like what I have taken, have not been associated with fever that I can find. Antibiotics (especially penicillin drugs) are frequent causes of drug fever.

Chapter 21
The Benefits of Heat

"I have only one burning desire. Let me stand next to your fire."
   – Jimi Hendrix, "Fire"

O ne other thing I should mention is that there can be beneficial effects of heat for MS patients. MS patients are often advised of the danger heat poses to MS patients, but may not hear that it has benefits.

For example, when I have pain poorly relieved by the only analgesic available to me, if I get into the shower, which has a hose so that a disabled person can optimally spray where needed, I often point the warm water at the place that is hurting the most at the moment (e.g., vertebral fractures, herniated lumbar discs, herniated cervical discs, rib fractures, torn rotator cuff, wrist sore from carpal tunnel syndrome, etc.). It has been surprising to me how much relief a minute or two of warm water on such a sore spot can provide and moreover how the relief can persist for an hour or more after the shower.

In addition to warm water in the shower, there is the soothing warmth of a heating pad. Putting a warm heating pad over the same places of maximal pain mentioned above can be very soothing. Some might worry about the danger of using heat in either of these situations, and it's true that it can be a problem, but for me the balance of risk and benefit often motivates me to use it for alleviating pain.

Finally, there is a small space heater in my bathroom that I turn on regularly in the winter because getting cold makes me feel more spastic which can increase pain and add to Pavlovian reflexes that increase urinary urgency. So, a small space heater also can be soothing even when its heat can't be directed at a sore spot. Disabled, relatively immobile folks also often have poor blood circulation and cold hands. Holding cold fingers next to most any source of warmth can help. The same is true for a paretic leg that often feels so uncomfortably cold in winter that it almost seems cold blooded. Putting my cold paretic hand or leg in front of the fireplace or a space heater feels almost too good to believe. In the words of Gershwin, "S' wonderful." But as wonderful as this feels, there are risks as well as benefits. As stated in Chapter 1, amounts matter. Too much heat can cause Uhthoff's phenomenon. Moderation is important.

Are all space heaters equally good for such purposes for MS patients? No. MS patients like me tend to lunge unpredictably against the counter and against a space heater sitting on the counter, which poses a risk for burns if the space heater has metallic surfaces. The type that I use is an Optimus H-1322 space heater. This has multiple advantages: 1) it's inexpensive (in 2013, Lowes was selling this Optimus heater for less than $15), 2) it's light and easily maneuvered by a weak, awkward MS patient, 3) its surfaces are all plastic, so lunging against it doesn't pose a risk for burns, 4) it has a sturdy on-off switch, which makes breaking the switch less likely, 5) it can be set so that it won't turn off, which would be counterproductive when the space heater is being used to counter a bout of urinary urgency, and 6) the switch being located at the bottom makes it easier for me to reach with a torn rotator cuff.

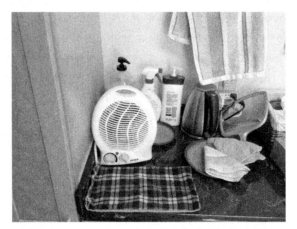

Figure 21-1 The Optimus space heater is light and easily moved by a disabled MS patient and completely covered with plastic so lunging against it doesn't cause skin burns like space heaters covered with metal. The patch of flannel is used for a place to put the spastic left hand when stretching the left arm and left leg by leaning against the bathroom counter.

Warm moist compresses are the conventional, accepted therapy for *Staphylococcus aureus* furuncles and they have worked well for me for years.

I have seen no data showing that warm moist compresses at the site of excessive pressure on the buttock (e.g., pinching the butt cheeks closed to prevent fecal incontinence) will prevent onset of a new furuncle at that site, but I believe that it will, based upon my having had that complication multiple times until I started trying immediate application of heat after applying the excessive pressure.

I also believe that a small hairdryer providing heat for 2 to 3 minutes in a circular pattern to avoid burning the skin can work well to treat and prevent furuncles in the same way that warm moist compresses work, only faster and more easily. With a hairdryer, a broader area can be quickly warmed to ensure that the furuncle isn't missed. This would be difficult to do with warm moist compresses and it has gotten harder for me to apply warm moist compresses to a precise spot as I have gotten weaker.

The hairdryers I have used were a small Gillette and a Vidal Sassoon 1875. Like the space heater mentioned above, these dryers were useful for an MS patient because they are inexpensive and light, they have sturdy switches, and the exterior surface is entirely plastic. I purchased the second one for $13 in 2015. The Vidal Sassoon has a lint filter that should be regularly cleaned because accumulating lint can obstruct airflow and even catch fire, which can quickly destroy a hairdryer; an old toothbrush (no longer useful for cleaning teeth) has worked well for cleaning my lint filter.

A hairdryer can also be useful for dealing with small leakages of urine into underwear or clothes. A major caveat is that they tend to be noisy and could wake your spouse if you do this at night. The advantage is that a small leakage can be dried with a hairdryer in five minutes and allow avoidance of a complete change of clothes, which usually takes an hour for a patient with hemiparesis.

Sitting on a wet shower chair after the shower is turned off is usually not comfortable because it quickly becomes clammy. What's the best way of dealing with the cool, clammy feeling of sitting in a shower chair? Hot towels can help. I put several bath towels in the dryer on high heat so that they will be warm for drying off after the shower. One of those towels is placed over the top of my head extending down to my sacrum. The next towel is placed over my front from ankles up to umbilicus (taking care to avoid allowing the towel bottom to drag through water on the shower floor, which makes for uncomfortable moments in drying off). A third towel [which doesn't need heating] is spread out on the floor so that the shower chair will wheel up to it after the head, back, abdomen, groin, underarms, sides and arms have been dried with the first two towels. The towel on the floor is important for catching lots of drips from the wet chair as hair combing and drying of legs is done. The fourth hot towel we use for the nurse aide to place around my waist so that I can dry my bottom. She holds on to my hips through the towel so that I won't teeter over onto the floor. I've now done this for 3.5 years and never fallen using this approach.

Chapter 22
Dealing with Weakness

"The spirit is willing, but the flesh is weak." – Matthew, 26:41
"If you can force your heart and nerve and sinew
To serve your turn long after they are gone
And so hold on when there is nothing in you
Except the will which says to them: "Hold on!""
   – Rudyard Kipling, "If"
"We are not now that strength which in old days moved earth and heaven, but that which we are we are, one equal temper of heroic hearts, made weak by time and fate, but strong in will to strive, to seek, to find and not to yield."
   – Alfred Lord Tennyson, "Ulysses"
"Beware the power of the Dark Side." –*Star Wars*

M S related destruction of the central nervous system typically causes upper motor neuron lesions which are associated with a variety of problems, weakness and spasticity being two hallmarks. These are common afflictions for MS patients and seem to be as inextricably linked as the words "horse and carriage"– often starting together early in the disease and getting worse together for decades.

   Robert Frost wrote, "Some say the world will end with fire,

others say ice." MS patients like me often wonder whether life will end when I'm unable to get out of bed because of too much weakness or too much spasticity.

For a patient with hemiparesis, walking across the room becomes an extreme effort. When a world-class athlete like Monica Seles serves a tennis ball, she exerts extreme effort, often grunting loudly. I sometimes grunt trying to cross the room – more after a hot shower, which makes me weaker and more spastic, and less during the night after sleep makes me stronger and less spastic.

Weakness causes falls, which cause fractures so painful I have to avoid using the involved anatomic part (e.g., with a left clavicular fracture, I had to avoid using my left arm for months). That fracture resulted in increased spasticity due to pain and due to inability to perform the usual active or passive stretching of the involved limb. This in turn meant that a frozen shoulder originally incurred because of MS related weakness of my left arm (and subsequently rehabilitated with physical therapy exercises and stretching) relapsed and got much worse.

I suffered two clavicular fractures and with both I got much weaker much faster (i.e. like a step function in mathematics). I also lost the ability to do a number of things that I had managed to keep doing for years despite the slow progressive increase in disability (e.g., after the first left clavicular fracture, I had to stop raising my left leg with my stronger right arm and placing it into the grip of my weaker left arm to allow me to wash the bottom of my foot with soap and water). Once I stopped doing something, like washing the bottom of my left foot, I often was unable to resume doing that again.

Different episodes of MS related weakness can be different in type and severity. Some the patient can alter, others not. If someone doesn't say that to you (and no one did to me), the patient can feel blown away and helpless to do anything against fate, which seems in charge. If your physician tells you that "nothing works for that disease," (as the physician diagnosing my MS did) that doesn't help the patient to understand that some things can and should be done to counter weakness.

During my first attack of MS, my left arm became mostly paralyzed over a couple of months (January and February). Before a diagnosis is reached, there's nothing a patient can do to counter this process. Being paralyzed, one feels "the power of the Dark Side" (i.e., something sinister). Its power over your previously healthy body is impressive and unsettling.

At the time, I was coaching my oldest son's basketball team. In one practice I was standing beneath the basket demonstrating moves of the low post when my assistant coach fired me the ball. My brain told my left arm to reach out to catch the ball, as it always had before. The signal wasn't received. The ball kept going and bounded off a wall so hard that a player had to run after it. I was as surprised as everyone else at this disobedience of my arm. Things got worse from there (e.g., inability to hold a fork, which made cutting meat with a knife impossible; inability to reach my left arm out of the car window to stick a card into a slot for access to the parking garage at work, etc.).

During an acute MS attack in which a limb becomes paralyzed, all a patient can do is wait for a remission or take a course of medication that halts the attack and speeds up the remission (e.g., methylprednisolone). The weakness of an acute attack can't be countered by exercise.

But increasing chronic weakness in the latter part of the disease due to neurodegeneration and especially due to accompanying deconditioning can and should be influenced by exercise. During the first 13 years of my illness, I felt like the illness was in control and I had to just accept whatever happened. ("Events are in the saddle and ride mankind." – Ralph Waldo Emerson)

Shortly after that I saw a physical therapist who quickly convinced me that regular stretching and exercises were important for preserving whatever muscular functions I still had.

The physical therapist I saw was not very knowledgeable about

MS, but gave me photocopied pages from a physical therapy book showing exercises and stretches that MS patients should consider doing. That was very valuable, not because every one of the exercises and stretches was helpful, but because it gave me the idea that a patient could do something helpful.

Some of the PT exercises were clearly useful. One of those was using my paretic left hand to squeeze putty. The putty deteriorated quickly, but I substituted a more durable, soft rubber ball, which seemed to work better than the putty. I try to squeeze the ball with my weak left hand multiple times per day.

The physical therapist advising me about exercises and stretches didn't mention that I should practice opening my weaker, more spastic hand, perhaps because in the 14th year after diagnosis of MS, that hand was still doing relatively well. But within several years, it became clear that that arm was losing function faster. So I began trying to practice opening the hand. When I first started, I was only able to open the hand 13 times. I then discovered that I could open it 20 times if I did so right after I woke up in the morning. I began doing it every morning when I woke up and then added the same exercise every time I woke up for nocturia at night. After doing that for a couple of weeks, I was able to increase the number of replications dramatically – from 20 to 200.

Some of the other exercises I started using had to be discontinued after I fell and fractured a bone. And after a couple months of convalescence, I was more disabled and unable to go back to doing those exercises.

A few things I was encouraged to do by the therapist were harmful (e.g., one exercise was supposed to be performed while kneeling on a floor mat, which quickly resulted in a painful bout of pre-popliteal bursitis in my paretic leg requiring antibiotic therapy). One or two exercises probably helped injure the rotator cuff in my only functional shoulder and also had to be abandoned.

After six weeks of evaluation and therapy, the physical therapist was unable to make any impact on my worsening limp and discharged me (probably because six weeks was the limit allowed by my insurance). But the experience had been helpful, and the knowledge that stretching and exercises could help counter weakness and spasticity encouraged me to develop other stretches and exercises beyond the ones that I saw demonstrated. At this point, 10 years later, most of the stretches and exercises I do every day are different from the ones the therapist taught me, but I wouldn't have known that I needed to devise them if I hadn't seen the therapist.

Types of MS related weakness:

fatigable: patients with myasthenia gravis are famous for having fatigable weakness that can be quickly demonstrated by having the patient repeatedly use the same muscle. The same phenomenon occurs in MS, but the onset of the fatigability is slower in me than in a myasthenia gravis patient (e.g., I practice opening my weak left hand after waking in the morning because that's the only time I'm able to do it because of diurnal variation in strength and I can sometimes open that hand 300 to 400 times; a myasthenia gravis patient usually has demonstrable weakness much faster).

debility: this type of weakness can occur with anyone including those with a completely normal nervous system; all that's required is the absence of exercise (e.g., patients put at bed rest for any reason can develop debility depending upon the time they are left lying in bed). There is an old maxim that applies to muscular strength: "use it or lose it". This type of weakness is an important problem for MS patients because their ability to exercise becomes limited because of damage to the nervous system causing weakness. The weakness caused by damage to the nervous system probably can't be undone, but the additional weakness caused by debility from lack of exercise can be improved using physical therapy exercises.

diurnal variation in strength: this varies with the duration of MS. At the outset, after my first few attacks, there was no perceptible variation during a day or from day-to-day. Decades later, there was dramatic variation within each day and sometimes from day to day. The most important variable returning strength in this diurnal variation is sleep. If I go to bed at bed time but can't sleep, not much strengthening occurs just from lying in bed even if the room is cooler (e.g., because of a lower set-point of the air conditioner at night). I always feel weakest at the end of the day and feel worse the day after missing a couple of extra hours of sleep; the symptoms of such a sleep deficit increased over time for me as the MS progressed (e.g., in the 23rd year after diagnosis of MS, I missed an extra couple of hours of sleep one night [i.e., beyond those regularly lost due to nocturia] and the following evening at about 8 PM I experienced a feeling of increased weakness accompanied by malaise and increased spasticity with a 3- to 4-fold increase in clonus. These symptoms were considerably more than I had gotten after missing a similar amount of sleep a year or two before that. After I went to sleep the next night, these additional symptoms all vanished.).

weakness caused by an acute attack from damage to the central nervous system: Some medications such as high-dose steroids (e.g., methylprednisolone) can cause a much faster onset of remission because of decreased inflammation at the site of a new MS plaque. For most MS patients, the early attacks are followed by partial repair of the central nervous system even if no therapy is given.

This repair can occur over weeks to years. For example, I had trouble walking after my first attack, and that trouble persisted for much of the first year but then remitted and I was able to walk pretty well up and down mountains for miles until the next attack affecting the spinal cord. After that attack, I didn't get as much remission and my problem walking began to grow.

weakness caused by chronic neurodegeneration (more damage to the central nervous system): there's nothing known that will stop this neurodegeneration. But during that phase, weakness due to debility occurs and can be countered by regular exercise of the affected muscle. Each time I remove my pants, I rock back and forth, sitting on the bed holding my left shin with my left hand until the pain in my left biceps and shoulder diminish, and, at that point, the paretic left arm starts acting as an arm again and can lift the left leg many times. The physical therapist didn't tell me this could be done. I discovered I could do it through desperation and serendipity. This regular exercise has helped me to keep using this paretic arm for years longer than I would have been able to use it without such exercise.

drug induced: the prescription drugs zolpidem tartrate (Ambien) and lioresal (Baclofen) have both caused me to have transient, increased weakness. The prescription drugs gabapentin (Neurontin) and tizanidine (Zanaflex) were associated with more severe weakness for me that each lasted for days. Alendronate doses always were associated with transient weakening of my urinary muscles and decreased urinary pressure.

heat induced (i.e., Uhthoff's phenomenon): this reportedly occurs because an increased temperature results in slower conduction through demyelinated nerves. With increased ambient temperature, the onset can be very rapid after stepping out of an air-conditioned building into a hot summer day with temperatures exceeding 90°F. With me, the effect was a global rather than focal weakness and slowing. With increased internal heat (i.e., fever), the effect was more dramatic with again global rather than focal weakness. The first time it happened to me I still had been able to walk without anybody seeing a limp, but the mild fever made me stagger and hold onto the wall trying to get out of my office.

protein deficiency: Protein deficiency can cause weakness. Could that happen in America where the most common nutritional problem is eating too much – not too little? A review of malnutrition in elderly people cited three studies reporting protein deficiency in 2%-16%. [Whitehead C, Finucane P. Malnutrition in elderly people. Aust NZ J Med. 1997; 27:68-74.] A popular fad among some in the MS community for several decades has been avoiding saturated animal fat. One way to do that is to switch to a vegan diet (i.e., a plant-based diet including no animal products). But another common practice by MS patients mentioned above is restricting fluids when having bladder control problems. When combined, these two practices can make calcium oxalate kidney stones more likely (because plant products rich in protein are usually also rich in oxalate [e.g., beans, nuts, etc]. An MS patient with a kidney stone trying to limit dietary oxalate might thus ingest too little protein.

Measures to Counter Advancing Debility

Exercise is the most important measure for countering weakness due to advancing debility. The exercises I have used have changed repeatedly. For example, when my left arm was still able, it could participate more actively in exercises. As that arm became more paretic, I had to use whatever function remained as much as possible (e.g., using it to help put on socks, tie shoes, tie ties, put on clothes, etc.). As the options dwindled, I continued to use the remaining functions as much as possible.

My hand continued to be able to squeeze a soft rubber ball, so I kept doing that as much as possible.

The same hand was losing the ability to open voluntarily, so I started trying to do this repeatedly as an exercise.

The weakening arm didn't want to lift my weak left leg, but if I persisted in trying to force it to do that, as described above, it would somehow reawaken like Rip van Winkle and start working well enough for me to not just hold the leg up, but lift it 200 times (even though the first 10 to 20 times I tried, it might not be able to lift the leg at all). I could usually tell when it was about to "switch back on" because the spastic muscle pain would ease.

These sorts of exercising of the left arm proved to be very helpful for allowing me to keep using the arm for other purposes such as walking with my walker. After exercising the arm by lifting the leg, it was always easier walking with the walker. And walking with the walker became my main exercise.

Chapter 23
Spasticity

"Diseases desperate grown by desperate appliance are relieved, or not at all."
  – William Shakespeare, *Hamlet*

What Is It?

Spasticity is increased muscle tone, manifested by rigid stiffness. It also causes a variety of involuntary movements.

Where Is It?

For me, it seems to occur in all my muscles. My first, recognized MS attack prominently affected my left arm, leaving it severely spastic. But that first attack also left me with spasticity of both legs. Deep tendon reflexes in both legs converted from normal to pathological, 4+ reflexes with clonus. There was also conversion from negative to positive Babinski signs in both feet. My left leg also started adducting against the stronger, right leg (i.e., scissoring together).

Since that first attack (and following many others), I have had evidence of spasticity affecting muscles throughout my body (e.g., both legs, both arms, colon muscles, the external anal sphincter, bladder muscles, bladder sphincter, muscles of respiration, muscles of deglutition [swallowing], muscles of mastication [chewing], muscles of phonation, and muscles of articulation [speaking]). As spastic dysarthria gets worse, it can be difficult to talk at all when feeling stress.

When Is It?

The chronic spastic stiffness generally increases over time after an upper motor neuron lesion (i.e., like weakness due to the same lesion). So, for the last 24 years, my spasticity has generally gotten slowly worse every year. At first, the annual worsening spasticity may have been the cumulative result of each year's attacks, but after the disease switched from relapsing remitting to secondary progressive, it probably just increased constantly.

But there are also fluctuations in stiffness that occur constantly as well. Each day, I become less stiff with sleep and more stiff as the day goes along. Pain of any type usually makes my stiffness worse.

My spastic left leg can also become suddenly stiffer due to decerebrate rigidity. This can happen because the bladder is overfull, or when the bladder is not overfull but there is external pressure on the bladder from constipated stool filling the rectum, or when a Pavlovian reflex causes increased urinary urgency (e.g., when switching on the bathroom light at night). It can also happen when anything untoward happens when proceeding toward the toilet for urination (i.e., anything impeding progress toward the toilet is another Pavlovian reflex for me, and it's important to understand that the specific type of untoward event is immaterial, so this happens immediately regardless of what the untoward event happens to be, even if that specific event had never happened before). It can also occur when removing a shoe if something untoward happens repeatedly even if there is no sensation of fullness in the bladder (and this is not due to the motion of removing the shoe, which is the same for me every day). Decerebrate rigidity in my spastic left leg also occurs immediately due to the "fight or flight" response whenever I start to fall.

When I'm in a bout of additional constipation, I can develop dire urinary urgency four times during the two hours after lunch, and, each time, my more spastic left arm and left leg become noticeably more spastic as I approach the toilet. This can get so bad that the left leg will decerebrate and stick straight out like the leg of a Nazi soldier goose-stepping as I sit down on the toilet. If it gets even worse, the less spastic right leg can decerebrate as well at the same time. So I may sit down on the toilet and have both legs sticking straight out in front like the double prow of a ship – an unusual sailing ship. The other books for MS patients say that bladder distention can cause increased spasticity, which is correct, but the increased urinary urgency and spasticity four times during the two hours after lunch is not primarily due to bladder distention after only 30 minutes of bladder filling each time. The reason for the dire urinary urgency after a half-hour is the combination of the bladder starting to fill and the external pressure on the bladder from the rectum already filled with constipated feces (as mentioned above). And when I try to sit down on the toilet, the spastic left leg often adducts against the right leg preventing the penis from pointing down into the toilet. In an urgent situation, this contretemps can cause urine to get all over me and the floor. During a bout of constipation, lying in bed also becomes a problem because fluid gets reabsorbed from a paralyzed leg, increasing urine volume and making dire urinary urgency more likely. If that happens, my spastic left leg can decerebrate as I try to sit up, preventing me from standing up and thus making it very likely that there will be uncontrolled urination into the incontinence pad and possibly my pajamas and bed sheets

Of interest, my spastic left leg can often decerebrate in a crisis of urinary urgency (as discussed above), but doesn't when I am in a crisis of fecal urgency only.

A sudden, pronounced increase in stiffness can also be caused by an interaction between the patient's conscious mind and the disease (one that's not due to a Pavlovian reflex). For example, after having MS-related weakness and spasticity for 13 years and attending the same church that full-time, I was starting to have a noticeable limp and, as I returned from the altar after communion, I realized that I was walking in front of about 200 people facing me and that my limp was undoubtedly obvious. My spasticity suddenly got much worse. Why did it choose that precise moment? Probably because it was what I REALLY didn't want to happen (i.e., a self-fulfilling prophecy that Murphy's Law would prevail against this MS patient – "if anything bad can happen, it will"). After that first embarrassing worsening in church with 200 witnesses, the same marked accentuation of my spasticity occurred at exactly that same place every time I returned from communion to my pew. In all those subsequent times, the worsening could have been due to a Pavlovian reflex.

As mentioned above, spasticity generally worsens and adds new problems over time. A new problem in my 23rd year of MS was something that I will refer to as "sympathetic spasticity," for want of a better term. In my first attack, an increase in spasticity in my leg was noted after stretching that leg with a reflex hammer. In my 23rd year, spastic contractions started happening in other spastic muscles in response to my stretching my spastic left arm (e.g., I could feel my spastic bladder muscles contract and create a false sense of urgency, and my spastic left leg would simultaneously decerebrate). The same sort of thing began occurring repeatedly when I would stand up and pull up my pants (i.e., if my knees were fully extended, the spastic muscles in both legs would be maximally stretched and my left hand would become more spastic and less helpful for raising pants and underpants). By contrast, partially flexing my right knee made my left hand less spastic and more helpful for raising pants and underpants (initially, I only had to resort to this device in certain evenings when my cumulative spasticity got bad enough). Likewise, if I stood beside the toilet with both knees fully extended, my spastic bladder muscles would contract and this could stimulate a desire to urinate.

It has long been recognized that distension of an MS patient's bowel or bladder is associated with increased spasticity of muscles in the limbs. Urine stretching spastic bladder muscles or feces stretching spastic colonic muscles may result in tensing of other spastic muscles ("sympathetic spasticity") and explain the observation. If sympathetic spasticity accounts for increasing spasticity of limb muscles with a distending bladder or colon, then this would be the first example of sympathetic spasticity that I encountered due to MS (i.e., years earlier than the examples cited above). If I am unavoidably delayed in moving toward the bathroom to urinate, the sympathetic spasticity increases. Stretching of my spastic bladder muscles due to accumulating urine also can cause one or both of my spastic legs to decerebrate. The decerebration resolves as I finish voiding, but the general increase in spasticity of my legs persists for about a half hour and causes me to be more wobbly when I rise from the toilet, increasing my risk for falling.

How Bad Is It?

Spastic stiffness reminds me of the rusting Tin Man in *The Wizard of Oz* (before he gets help from an oil can). Muscles become stiff, and joints can be very difficult to bend. Being so rigidly confined can make me feel like a prisoner in my own body, unable to get up and go for a walk, much less a jog. The stiffened muscles can sometimes also hurt to move.

And it's not just stiffness and pain that are problems. Spastic rigidity also makes me so awkward and clumsy that food, drink, pills, pill bottles, etc. often spill on clothes, the dinner table, and the floor. Putting a glass down and trying to pull a spastic hand away from it, the hand often refuses to let go, causing the glass to tump over. This non-volitional act reminds me of snakes reflexively biting a hand touching them after death. To give the full flavor of what this is like, I'll share an incident: I spilled a bowl of cereal containing milk and blueberries onto the floor and then fell into the mess. When I was rescued, my clothes were wet and stained and I had not yet started to eat breakfast. Cleanup required more than an hour, delaying breakfast. And it's not just when something is spilled that time is wasted. Everything seems to take forever (e.g., putting on a sock, buttoning a button, etc.). Frustration becomes a way of life.

Decerebrate rigidity can make it hard (and sometimes impossible) to get up from the bed or from a chair or to walk and get to the toilet. Arriving at the toilet, decerebrate rigidity at the knee and hip joints can make it impossible to sit down on the toilet, which can result in soiling the floor, one's clothes, etc. And if the patient is able to sit down on the toilet, spastic adduction of one leg against another can prevent the penis from pointing down into the toilet, again resulting in soiling of the floor, one's clothes, etc. These are degrading outcomes even when the patient is housebound and alone. Cleaning up such a mess can take hours that an MS patient struggling to perform ADLs can ill afford.

Decerebrate rigidity of a spastic leg gets worse over decades with MS (like most of my MS complications have) and, like a 20 pound anchor, can prevent getting back up from the floor without assistance.

I first noticed decorticate rigidity was affecting my more functional right arm (clenched fist with flexed wrist) on waking up one morning after 21 years of MS. After that, the same rigidity was present in that arm frequently when I woke in the morning. The spastic flexion of that wrist caused mild carpal tunnel syndrome discomfort. I believe that the same decorticate rigidity occurred in my left arm, but was not as obvious because the arm was relatively immobile because of weakness and spasticity; instead, I would waken in the morning in the morning with a spastically clenched left fist.

Spastic stiffness can cause an MS patient to fall in multiple ways. For example, it can cause the patient to be so awkward that falling becomes more likely. It can make my spastic left arm too stiff to reach or hold the handle of my walker, which can cause a fall. And it can make my spastic left leg too stiff to walk safely, making it more likely that the foot will fail to take a full safe step.

Control Measures for Spastic Stiffness
Drugs for Spasticity

Unfortunately, there is no oil can to loosen the terrible MS rigidity. The closest I ever came to finding "an oil can" was my first 5 mg dose of baclofen. The response to that first dose was amazing. After years of becoming slowly more stiff and spastic, I felt suddenly freed from my fetters and loose. Anybody with spasticity should try at least one dose. You can feel the power of the medicine in more than one way. I didn't break into a sweat but felt like I was going to. I also felt weaker and more wobbly and became so groggy that I fell asleep every time I tried to read after taking a dose with supper. Because these side effects persisted, my nighttime dose was switched from supper time to bedtime.

But what it did to the chronic stiffness was hard to believe. I wasn't able to walk like a normal healthy person, but that first 5 mg dose of baclofen made my walking so much more fluid that I almost felt like it was normal. Its effect persisted for 24 hours. I don't know if it would have persisted longer than that because that's when I took the second daily dose as prescribed by my neurologist. Within the first few days, that very powerful effect started eroding as my body developed tolerance to the medicine, which had less and less effect. Webster's dictionary defines tolerance as "the power of enduring or resisting the action of a drug, poison, etc." After the first week or two of daily dosing, there was so much tolerance that it was sometimes hard for me to tell that there was any therapeutic effect at all (although the drug's side effects remained obvious). This is true for patients who "chase their tail" by continually upping the ante by raising the baclofen dose to try to overcome the body's rapid and progressive development of tolerance. It has been reported that such patients may need to sometimes stop the drug for a couple of months and start over to experience the drug's therapeutic effect again. It's important to understand that a high baclofen dosage often has to be tapered before being stopped because a sudden reduction or sudden cessation of therapy can cause bad side effects (e.g., malignant hyperpyrexia [high fever], which can be unpleasant for anybody, but especially devastating for an MS patient who can become very weak with even a mild increase in body temperature). [Mandac BR, Hurvitz EA, Nelson DS.Hyperthermia associated with baclofen withdrawal and increased spasticity. Arch Phys Med Rehabil. 1993;74:96-7.] The drug also has more side effects at high dosage.

Fourteen months after starting a daily dose of baclofen, I had a terrible problem with increased spastic rigidity after some vertebral fractures and tripled my daily baclofen dose to 5 mg three times per day to see if that would help. It didn't. The side effects of the higher dose per day were much worse (e.g., weakness, imbalance), but the increased spastic rigidity really wasn't helped much by my tripling the baclofen dose.

It's probably important that I note that my long-lasting muscle rigidity and my episodes of sudden decerebrate rigidity are both due to spasticity caused by the upper motor neuron lesions from multiple sclerosis damage to my central nervous system. It's also important to note that baclofen's powerful effect on my spasticity relieved the chronic rigidity, but did not prevent the sudden decerebrate rigidity accompanying a bout of urinary urgency.

As mentioned above in Chapter 7 regarding constipation, baclofen worked great the first three times I used it to relieve spastic contraction of the external anal sphincter when I had unformed stools due to dicloxacillin therapy, but then it did nothing at all the next six times I tried it for that purpose.

The Introduction said that this book would make no attempt to provide encyclopedic coverage and that applies to the topic of MS related spasticity, which, like MS related constipation, could easily be the subject of an entire book. Other books already attempt encyclopedic coverage of MS (and leave out things that are in this book). So the effort seems both unnecessary and unattainable.

As mentioned in Chapter 10 regarding insomnia, some data suggest that drugs that bind gamma-aminobutyric acid (GABA) receptors can stimulate growth or metastasis of cancer. Many different hypnotic drugs used for insomnia bind to those receptors as does baclofen, a commonly prescribed drug for MS-related spasticity.

Does that mean that baclofen should not be used?

Chapter 1 advised that an MS patient needs to balance the potential risks and benefits of each proposed form of therapy (with help from her neurologist).

When doing this, the best choice is obviously the safest and most effective drug for treating a particular problem. The optimal drug would be one works perfectly in all patients and causes no side effects. Unfortunately, most drugs used for MS don't approach that ideal, usually providing marginal benefit and posing risk for a variety of side effects.

So how effective and safe are the drugs for treating spasticity? I can't provide personal comment on the other drugs for spasticity because baclofen is the only one my neurologist prescribed for me. That may be because baclofen is the most frequently prescribed drug for spasticity. [Rizzo MA, Hadjimichael OC, Preiningerova J, Vollmer TL. Prevalence and treatment of spasticity reported by multiple sclerosis patients. Mult Scler. 2004 Oct;10(5):589-95.] In my 25th uear of MS, tizanidine was tried but hallted after 2 days because of increased weakness.

Some of the other drugs used for spasticity also bind to GABA receptors (and thus may share some of the putative risks of GABAergic drugs) and can also be intoxicating and habit-forming (i.e., like alcohol), so these are not easy, slam-dunk decisions. I was so compromised by weakness, spasticity and imbalance that taking any intoxicating medication seemed out of the question for me.

Taking oral baclofen during the day was also associated with too many persistent side effects (e.g., increased weakness, increased imbalance, somnolence), so I chose to take it only at bedtime as my neurologist suggested.

One's view of the utility of drugs for MS-related spasticity may depend on one's philosophy (i.e., is the glass half-empty or half-full?).

This may explain why some allege that these drugs work very well and others maintain the opposite.

For example, a review of tizanidine reported positively that randomized trials showed that it reduced the spastic increase in muscle tone by "21 to 37% versus 4 to 9% for patients receiving placebo." [Wagstaff AJ, Bryson HM. Tizanidine. A review of its pharmacology, clinical efficacy and tolerability in the management of spasticity associated with cerebral and spinal disorders. Drugs. 1997; 53:435-52.] This modest improvement was documented in 60% to 82% of tizanidine recipients.

That may give an accurate depiction of how well tizanidine worked in the short term, but doesn't reveal how well it does over the long haul. For the 18% to 40% with no short-term improvement, it's unlikely that there will be later improvement. For those with short-term improvement, there could be problems over the long haul. There are at least two reasons for this: 1) spasticity increases over time, and 2) the body develops tolerance to both baclofen and tizanidine, making them less effective.

A recent survey of neurologists treating MS patients implied that these drugs' effectiveness was only so-so, saying, 'Numerous antispastic agents such as baclofen and tizanidine, as well as others, are available for the management of MS spasticity but, overall, they offer limited clinical benefit.' [Collongues N, Vermersch P. Multiple sclerosis spasticity: "state-of-the-art" questionnaire survey of specialized healthcare professionals. Expert Rev Neurother. 2013; 13 (3 Suppl 1):21-5.doi: 10.1586/ern.13.10.]

And a recent review of the same topic by a neurologist reported a similarly negative conclusion: "Despite the difficulties experienced by MS patients with spasticity, the condition is largely undertreated because current treatment options do not provide adequate control of MS spasticity." [Berger T. Multiple sclerosis spasticity daily management: retrospective data from Europe. Expert Rev Neurother. 2013; 13 (3 Suppl 1):3-7.doi: 10.1586/ern.13.3.]

How about safety of the drugs used to treat spasticity? The MS

Society website lists the following potential adverse effects of baclofen and tizanidine (without stating the relative frequency or
saying that these side effects occurred significantly more often with
the drug than with a placebo):

baclofen side effects: "drowsiness, increased weakness, dizziness, confusion, worse constipation, increased bladder problems,
insomnia, unsteadiness, clumsiness, fainting, hallucinations, mood
changes, skin rash, itching, and several others with an overdose
(blurred vision, double vision, convulsions, shortness of breath,
vomiting). If taking more than 30 mg of baclofen daily, do not stop
taking this medication suddenly. Stopping high doses of this medication abruptly can cause convulsions, hallucinations, increases in
muscle spasms or cramping, mental changes, or unusual nervous-
ness or restlessness."

tizanidine side effects: "dryness of mouth, somnolence increased weakness, fatigue, dizziness (especially when getting up
from sitting or lying down), increased muscle spasms, increased
muscle cramps, increased muscle tightness, back pain, burning sensation, prickling sensation, tingling sensation, diarrhea, fainting,
fever, anorexia (loss of appetite), anxiety, pain or burning during
urination, skin sores, stomach pain, vomiting, yellow eyes or skin,
and blurred vision."

Other websites listed hallucinations or delusions as an occasional
side effect of tizanidine (reportedly observed in five of 170 tizanidine recipients in two controlled, North American clinical studies)
and some important drug interactions (e.g., hypotension, brady-
cardia and/or excessive drowsiness when taking tizanidine with
ciprofloxacin). A recent review of tizanidine adverse effects said,
"Serious adverse events were substantially less frequent in children
than adults (19.2% vs 45.9%) in the clinical adverse event database.
" [Henney HR 3rd, Chez M. Pediatric safety of tizanidine: clinical
adverse event database and retrospective chart assessment. Paediatr
Drugs. 2009;11:397-406. doi: 10.2165/11316090-000000000-00000.] But

I saw no data suggesting a predisposition to cancer from taking tizanidine (unlike baclofen).

Using Gravity to Control Decerebrate Rigidity of My Spastic Leg

If, while sitting on the bed, my spastic leg starts developing de-cerebrate rigidity as part of a crisis of urinary urgency, it may be impossible to pull the foot of the stiff leg close enough to put on my slippers or shoes to walk toward the bathroom. Moreover, it also may be impossible to pull the stiff leg close enough to stand up in order to start walking barefoot toward the bathroom. As the crisis of urgency worsens, it may seem inevitable that there will be incontinence while sitting on the bed which would be terrible in multiple ways.

How can this problem be controlled? Using my one strong arm, I have been unable to wrestle the decerebrated leg into submission, but I can grab it and lift it up over the other leg (i.e., crossing my legs). After I lift my stiff, decerebrated leg over the other leg, it initially sticks out like the prow of a sailing ship, but it can't stay like that. Gravity won't allow it. As gravity pulls the leg down, the crescendo of urgency that was swelling is also reduced so much that I can usually then put on a slipper or shoe and stand up and walk toward the bathroom with the crisis temporarily dissipated. I often get better results by grabbing the popliteal fossa to do this (the hollow in back of the knee). After the rigidity yields to gravity I then grab the top of the sock on my left foot to move the leg back (rather than by grabbing the popliteal fossa or the end of my pants). Conventional sock lengths (6 inches above the shoe line) are probably best for this purpose because they afford plenty of sock to grasp close to the bottom hem of one's pants. Knee socks that cover the entire calf don't work because the top of the sock is hard to access, especially when needed in a hurry. Low-cut socks (that are not visible inside the shoe) also don't work because the top of the socks are similarly hard to access and don't have enough material to grab hold of conveniently even if a shoe is removed.

If the crisis starts to rebuild as the toilet is approached, grasping the glans penis and applying periodic pressure 5 to 20 times (until the crisis is once again defused), has almost always (> 100 times) allowed me to reach the toilet with dry clothes and without my bladder cutting loose into the incontinence pad.

What Can Be Done When Decerebrate Rigidity Prevents Wheelchair Access?

What can you do if your spastic leg decerebrates because of dire urinary urgency when trying to get into the motorized wheelchair to proceed toward the toilet? In this circumstance, the decerebrated leg is so stiff that it cannot be flexed at the knee to get my foot onto the wheelchair foot rest. To circumvent this obstacle and proceed toward the toilet, I simply grab the spastic decerebrated leg and lift it onto my other leg (i.e., crossing my legs) as described above. When doing this, the decerebrated leg will again stick straight out like the prow on a sailing ship, so special care has to be taken if maneuvering the wheelchair before the leg comes down. As also described above, the spastic stiffness is ameliorated over 10 to 15 seconds by gravity, allowing me to place my foot on the foot rest and proceed toward the bathroom more safely.

What Can Be Done When Decerebrate Rigidity Prevents Sitting down on the Toilet?

What can be done if decerebrate rigidity at the knee and hip joints makes it hard to sit down on the toilet during a crescendo of urinary urgency? What I try to do is to hold onto something stable like a grab bar and slide my left spastic leg further to the left and, leaving my left foot where it is on the floor (i.e., with a larger than normal space between my two legs), I spin to the right and try to bend my left knee as I do. This usually works for me to unlock the decerebrate rigidity of the knee. Once the decerebrate rigidity of the knee is unlocked, still holding onto the grab bar, I can sit. That usually allows me to sit down on the toilet, but if the crisis of urgency is too severe and the leg won't bend, then I try to lower myself onto the toilet as best I can despite the leg being completely stiff. This is difficult and never works very well, but it's better than remaining standing and allowing urine to fall on the floor, my legs, my clothes, the toilet seat, etc. In this desperate circumstance, I don't usually end up sitting on the toilet correctly (e.g., my butt may be all the way back against the toilet lid, requiring repositioning ASAP).

Sleep

As mentioned above, sleep seems to be an important ally in combating spastic stiffness, but, spasticity generally gets worse over time and, perhaps for that reason, the benefit of sleep declines somewhat.

Over most of my 24 years with MS, I was maximally stiff at bedtime and had less spasticity in the morning. I started using the head of the bed for stretching my spastic left arm when I got into bed at night and did it every time I got up for nocturia for years. This was always hardest when I first got into bed (even if I had taken a daily dose of baclofen 30 minutes before trying this) and easiest after a nighttime of sleep. But, over years of doing this, it got harder to do as the arm became more spastic. As the arm became more spastic, I often had to stretch my hand and wrist before trying to stretch the arm. Over still more time, I also began having to stretch the shoulder and elbow joints before I could stretch the entire arm. And over more time, the spastic stiffness got so bad that it subsided more slowly through the night until I could only do this after a full night's sleep. Then it got worse again and I had to do extensive stretching of the hand, wrist, elbow and shoulder before trying to stretch the arm on waking in the morning.

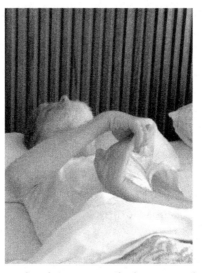

Figure 23-1 The author has to stretch the spastic left hand, wrist and forearm as shown before the entire arm can be stretched.

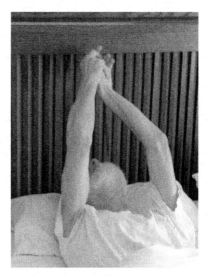

Figure 23-2 The functional right arm lifting the spastic left hand up to the head of the bed where it can be temporarily lodged in order to passively stretch the spastic arm.

Stretching
Stretches: active and passive

A Wikipedia article about spasticity available online in June 2014 said that exercise was beneficial for spastic muscles but that the available evidence did not show stretching to be effective, citing two systematic reviews. [Ada L, Dorsch S, Canning C G. Strengthening interventions increase strength and improve activity after stroke: a systematic review. Australian Journal of Physiotherapy. 2006;52(4):241-248.] [Bovend'Eerdt TJ, Newman M, Barker K, Dawes H, Minelli C, Wade DT. The effects of stretching in spasticity: a systematic review. Arch Phys Med Rehabil. 2008 Jul;89(7):1395-406."],

My response to these two claims is both agreement and disagreement, based on my own experience as well as the data in the two reviews. Because the article focuses on spasticity, many readers probably assume that it meant that exercise was beneficial for spasticity, but that's not what the review said; Ada et al said that, "Across all stroke participants, strengthening interventions had a small positive effect on both strength and activity. There was very little effect on spasticity." Likewise, many readers probably inferred that the data showed that stretching was not beneficial. Again, that's not what the other review said; Bovend'Eerdt et al said that "The methodologic quality of the RCTs was low" and that "all studies show[ed] great diversity at the levels of methodology, population, intervention, and outcome measures making a meta-analysis not feasible." They concluded that there was "some positive evidence supporting the immediate effects of one stretching session," but that it was unclear how long these effects persisted and whether there were "long term consequences."

My own experience has been that exercise has a small beneficial effect on the strength of my paretic limbs, so I can agree with the meta-analysis by Ada. Regarding my spasticity, my experience has been that it gets much worse when I'm unable to exercise and stretch. Because exercise of limbs usually actively stretches muscles of the limb, it's hard to know how much of the benefit of exercise comes from this stretching. For me, these things, emphasized by physical therapy, have been as or more valuable in countering my spasticity than baclofen. They don't seem to make my spasticity less the following day, but they seem to keep it from getting worse the following day, which tends to happen when I have to avoid exercise and stretching (e.g., because of a fracture).

This is not to say that baclofen is not a powerful drug with remarkable activity against spasticity, but its most wonderful effect occurs after the first dose. With continual administration, so much tolerance develops that it is sometimes hard for me to tell that there is any effect at all. By contrast, if I stop the drug for several days and take a dose, I can tell that it is having an effect on my stiffness. The drug also can have powerful adverse effects.

Spastic rigidity increases over time and an MS patient has to keep a mental list of body parts that need to be regularly stretched to counter this process. Walking around during the day stretches the legs naturally, but extra stretching of the legs became necessary for me after 13 years of the disease. Over the years, I had to increase the frequency of the leg stretches. Similarly, I had to add regular stretching of my spastic arm and two spastic toes.

What are spastic non-volitional movements?

These are movements that occur because of MS related spasticity that are not intentional. The first non-volitional movement that I had due to MS was clonus (rapid jerking of a muscle [occurring several times per second and usually lasting for five to 25 jerks for me]). It occurred during my neurologic exam when my neurologist was eliciting deep tendon reflexes two months after my first attack started. Within moments of seeing that change, the neurologist informed me that he had changed his diagnosis of my new neurologic illness to MS.

I have had other non-volitional movements that can occur after stretching but also can follow other stimuli (e.g., a single drop of tap water fell onto my spastic leg while I was being rolled into the shower on a shower chair and the leg kicked out violently due to myoclonus like Charlie Brown trying to kick a football). For me, myoclonus is usually a sudden single contraction of a muscle or group of muscles in my spastic left leg. Spasms of the pedal arch and calf occasionally occur when I roll onto my back and stretch my legs in the morning. My other non-volitional spastic movements usually haven't followed stretching (periodic limb movements, adduction of my spastic left leg against the other leg, spasms of the back muscles, full spastic flexion of my arm at the elbow, spastic contraction of chest wall muscles, decerebrate posturing of my spastic left leg, and decorticate posturing of my arms).

I also have restless leg syndrome (RLS), which doesn't exactly qualify as a non-volitional spastic movement, but seems related to one (periodic limb movements). RLS is a vague discomfort in the lower leg coupled with an inclination to move it that gets worse at night in bed or lying down in a recliner and gets better when standing up and walking. It occurs significantly more frequently among MS patients than among the general population, and MS patients with RLS usually have periodic limb movements. RLS can occur at increased frequency for a variety of reasons (pregnancy, kidney failure, iron deficiency, etc.), but also occurs in patients with spinal cord lesions who have periodic limb movements that mimic the triple flexion (i.e., Babinski) movement that is a hallmark of upper motor neuron lesions characteristic of MS.

My restless leg syndrome and periodic limb movements commenced at the same time, which was 13 years and three months after my diagnosis of MS. At first they affected only my more spastic left leg. Three years later, periodic limb movements started happening in my more spastic left arm as well. Nineteen years and four months after diagnosis of MS, RLS and periodic limb movements started happening in my right leg. After 24 years of MS, I've not yet had periodic limb movements in my right arm.

My periodic limb movements usually recur four times per minute, and can continue for hours.

The Medscape website said this about the periodic limb movement disorder: "The movement simulates triple flexion with knee flexion, ankle dorsiflexion, and great toe extension; it lasts approximately 2 seconds and thus is not consistent with the rapid jerk that defines true myoclonus." I have never seen the periodic limb movement of my more spastic leg, but I have seen the periodic limb movement of my more spastic left arm and believe that the movement does involve multiple different muscle groups and that the assertion that this contraction is sustained for seconds is correct.

The first time I experienced myoclonus was in the 14th year after my diagnosis of MS. I was still able to walk around the house without a cane or walker, and I was standing in the kitchen looking out the window when myoclonus occurred in my more spastic left leg like an unexpected rogue bolt of lightning out of a blue sky, causing me to fall to the floor.

An NIH website said this about myoclonus: "myoclonus describes a symptom and not a diagnosis of a disease. It refers to sudden, involuntary jerking of a muscle or group of muscles. Myoclonic twitches or jerks usually are caused by sudden muscle contractions, called positive myoclonus, or by muscle relaxation, called negative myoclonus. Myoclonic jerks may occur alone or in sequence, in a pattern or without pattern. They may occur infrequently or many times each minute. Myoclonus sometimes occurs in response to an external event or when a person attempts to make a movement. Most myoclonus is caused by a disturbance of the central nervous system (such as multiple sclerosis)." Normal, healthy people can get mild myoclonic contractions (e.g., a hiccup, and the jerks or "sleep starts" that some people experience while drifting off to sleep).

In the 21st year after my diagnosis of MS, I started having spastic flexion at the elbow of my more spastic left arm after a fall resulting in very painful vertebral fractures. I call this spastic flexion my "chicken wing spasms" because the spastically flexed arm reminds me of the way chicken wings look in a plucked chicken in the grocery store.

Spasticity can cause non-volitional movements of muscles attached to middle ear bones, which can result in an unwanted, repetitious sound (tinnitus) in the ear; the sounds have been described in many ways (like a heartbeat, clicking, etc).

When do spastic non-volitional movements occur?

Clonus: as mentioned above, this occurs after stretching, which can be a deep tendon reflex in a neurologic exam or just stretching a spastic leg after rolling over prone in bed, or lifting a spastic leg onto a foot rest, which stretches the ankle tendon. A myoclonic jerk of my spastic left leg is often followed by clonus.

Periodic limb movements: at first, in my 14th year after diagnosis of MS, I had these only in bed at night while asleep, but over years they became more frequent and started occurring after supper in the evening and then sometimes as early as mid-day. They never occurred in the morning after a night's sleep. Movements during the day usually involved my spastic arm, but if I lay down in my recliner after supper, I could have periodic limb movements in my more spastic leg as well within 20 minutes.

On a bad night, periodic limb movements have sometimes begun before I could get to sleep using a sleeping pill and continued for 2 to 3 hours until I woke up for nocturia. How did I know that the periodic limb movements continued while I was asleep? When I had severely painful anterior rib fractures, I woke multiple times with the left spastic arm repeatedly striking the fractured bones, which hurt much more than when I went to bed.

Adduction of my more spastic left leg against the right leg: this tends to occur when I sit down and gets worse when spasticity in general is increasing such as when bowel or bladder is distended, when sitting down on a cold clammy shower chair, when sitting down on the toilet due to urinary urgency, or when sitting on the toilet because of an unusual bout of constipation due to spastic constriction of the external anal sphincter (e.g., when having unformed stools due to antibiotic therapy).

spasms of the pedal arch muscles: I've only had these in bed at night,

spasms of the calf muscles: I've only had these in bed at night

spasms of back muscles: I've only had these during a 2 to 3 month period following a vertebral compression fracture. These tend to be worse as the day goes along after I've been up and the weight of my body on my vertebral column has been stressing the fracture. When I lie down in bed at night flat on my back, I usually can't feel the pain at all.

spastic contraction of chest wall muscles: I've only had these at the site of very painful anterior rib fractures and they occurred intermittently as long as the pain of those rib fractures continued (two months).

decerebration of my spastic left leg: this occurs most often for me during an episode of urinary urgency. It also occurs every time I start to fall.

myoclonus: a sudden single rapid jerk of a muscle in my more spastic leg (e.g., the quadriceps [thigh] muscle): I tend to have these when in a bout of increased spasticity, usually due to pain, but have also had this happen when I was about to shower and a nurse touched me with a cold antiseptic at the site of an abrasion or when grabbing the shower nozzle and a single drop of chilly water fell on my spastic leg. A sudden itch has done the same. The sudden violent jerk can cause a fall and trigger clonus (i.e., a series of less forceful contractions).

spastic full flexion of the arm at the elbow (which I refer to as "chicken wing spasms") first started when I was in a bout of increased spasticity after a fall with very painful fractures. The same thing then happened after multiple other falls with painful fractures. And, as the disease got worse over time and the spasticity progressed, I started having chicken wing spasms later in the day when the usual diurnal increase in spasticity was giving me more trouble (i.e., without requiring a very painful fracture). If I have to reduce my ambulation, the chicken wing spasms become worse and more frequent.

tinnitus: I have had several episodes of transient, unilateral, pulsatile tinnitus, usually following what amounted to "extreme exertion" for me.

How bad are spastic non-volitional movements?

Periodic limb movements were the first non-volitional movements that really bothered me. They reminded me of an internalized form of Chinese water torture, making sleep impossible without a pill. When I had severely painful anterior rib fractures, periodic limb movements of my more spastic arm would repeatedly thrash the fracture site at night, making it more painful when I woke up. Spastic contraction of chest wall muscles at the site of that same severely painful rib fracture continued off and on for six weeks, causing me to suffer more pain from the fracture. The pain of these contractions also prevented sleep.

When I step on a cold floor in the winter, this can cause spastic withdrawal of the foot that can cause a fall, and the toes of that foot try to curl under. The second toe does this the most and can do it so much that I am actually walking on the back (dorsum) of the toe, which is painful. Strangely enough, the floor can also be cold in the summer due to air conditioning running to keep up on a hot day, causing the same problem.

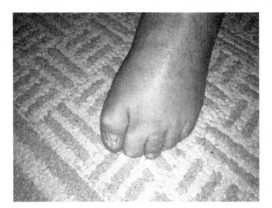

Figure 23-3 The spastic left foot reacts to a chilly sensation with spastic "white knuckle" flexion of the first two toes after clothes are removed for a shower. The spasticity is so pronounced that the end of the second toe curls under so that the foot is walking on the usual top (dorsum) of the toe, which is very painful.

When I was sleeping in a recliner because I was wearing a shoe as a makeshift cast to immobilize a metatarsal fracture, the periodic limb movements were able to remove the shoe from that foot three times, causing me difficulty getting the shoe back on without re-injuring the fractured bone.

Full spastic flexion of my more spastic left arm at the elbow (my "chicken wing spasms") caused pain and made the arm virtually useless for moving around with a rollator walker. When my paretic left arm goes into a chicken wing spasm, the paretic left side of my trunk can join in the spasm, bending me over at the waist until my head is right beside the chicken wing. The first time it happened, I thought I was done for.

Spastic stiffness can be frustrating, as mentioned above. Nonvolitional motions can be similarly frustrating. For example, when I'm trying to remove my pajama shirt with my stronger right arm, the spastic left hand can grab hold of the sleeve that I'm trying to remove and hold on like this is a game of "tug-of-war" – a totally inane waste of my time.

A new spasm in my more spastic, left arm can cause it to retract so much that it loses its grip on the walker handle and cause me to fall. Spasticity can also cause myoclonus of my leg muscles that is so violent that it causes me to fall. This tends to happen when I am in a bout of increased spasticity triggered by severe pain from new fractures related to a recent fall. In this type situation, my legs can become so jumpy that myoclonic jerks seem to occur with a hair trigger.

Prevention and Control of Non-Volitional Spastic Movements

Sleep

As with spastic stiffness, sleep has a powerful restorative effect on spastic, non-volitional movements. Some may find this confusing since a number of the non-volitional movements occur at night during sleep, but, as mentioned above, this could be as much due to a recumbent position as it is to sleep. I believe that sleep has a calming influence on these movements and that is why I don't get chicken wing spasms or periodic limb movements in the morning even if I lie down in the recliner. If I lie down in the recliner in the evening (longer after my last sleep), periodic limb movements can start within 20 minutes in my more spastic left leg.

Stretches: active and passive

The first thing I actively tried to control periodic limb movements was stretching my more spastic left leg once daily by standing only on that leg for 1 to 2 minutes, which worked perfectly for months, allowing me to sleep the entire night without being wakened once by periodic limb movements or restless leg syndrome. As my spasticity continued to worsen, however, I had to progressively add more stretches per day, but this allowed the stretching alone to continue working to prevent periodic limb movements and restless leg syndrome from disturbing my sleep for six years.

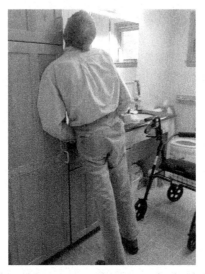

Figure 23-4 The author propped against the bathroom counter with his left hand propped on the flannel patch in front of the space heater, which provides necessary warmth on a chilly day, while he stretches his spastic left arm and spastic left leg. To do this, most of his weight is shifted to his left leg.

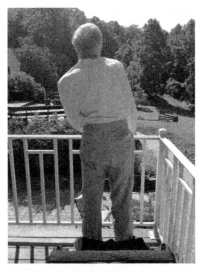

Figure 23-5 The author standing up leaning against a metal rail and stretching his spastic left leg while enjoying sunlight and fresh air.

But then I reached a point in the 20th year after my diagnosis with MS where stretching would neither prevent nor stop a very bad bout of periodic limb movements in my stronger, less spastic leg that started after I began standing propped against a desk several hours per day. At that point, I found a pharmacologic agent that helped control the problem (as discussed below). The stretching still helped, but only in an adjunctive fashion.

After years of increasing difficulty with periodic limb movements of my spastic left arm, I figured out that I could stretch the arm by trapping it between my two legs, and the periodic limb movements of that arm decreased after I started stretching it that way multiple times per day.

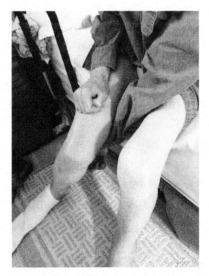

Figure 23-6 The author stretching his spastic
left arm between his two legs.

As mentioned above, I also used the head of the bed for stretching my spastic left arm at night. Stretching my spastic left arm at night was helpful during the night, but did not prevent periodic limb movements from occurring the following day.

Two other ways of stretching my spastic left arm were

recommended to me by a physical therapist – one sitting at a table leaning forward onto the spastic arm and thereby forcing it into a stretched position and the other with a device suspended from the top of a doorway while sitting in a wheelchair positioned in the doorway. I'm sure that both of these approaches can work but both seemed harder for me to use and less secure than the two approaches described above. For example, a device suspended from a doorway can't stay there and allow the doorway to be used normally, which means that the device has to be removed after each use; this is difficult for a patient with hemiparesis to do. Using a contraption suspended from a doorway seems about 10-fold more cumbersome to me than using the head of the bed. Moreover, a patient with hemiparesis like me has trouble sitting in a chair without falling out of it, and trying to lean forward onto a table to stretch my more spastic arm made me feel unsteady and more likely to fall.

Using an Elastic Waistband to Prevent Periodic Arm Movements from Traumatizing Anterior Rib Fractures

As mentioned above, I had problems with non-volitional spastic movements as a complication of severely painful anterior rib fractures. Periodic limb movements of my spastic left arm repeatedly traumatized the rib fractures. After that happened more than once, I figured out a way of preventing it: I would trap my left hand inside the substantial elastic waistband of L.L. Bean pajamas. Once trapped, the left hand could not escape from the elastic band without help from my right hand. After I started doing that, this marked increase in pain at the site of the anterior rib fractures stopped occurring while I was asleep.

A Powerful Physiologic Response (orgasm)

When I first started having involuntary periodic limb movements of my less spastic, stronger leg in the 20th year after being diagnosed with MS, they would start as soon as I got into bed and would not respond to stretching. I felt desperate to have a powerful medicine, but had none available at the time.

So I tried orgasm, a powerful physiologic response known to be associated with profound relaxation. It worked! No more limb jerking the entire rest of the night! This was a more impressive therapeutic effect than I had observed with the bedtime dose of baclofen that I took. On the other hand, there was only a mild reduction in spastic rigidity as compared with the dramatic reduction in spastic rigidity that had occurred with the first dose of baclofen that was discussed above.

But, after orgasm worked perfectly 15 times to prevent and control periodic limb movements over six months, my spasticity continued to get worse and orgasm started working less perfectly (i.e., the periodic limb movements would recur six hours later). If asked to guess, I would say that this lessening effect probably was not due to development of tolerance (like with baclofen), but rather due to the spasticity just continuing to get worse and become harder to manage (as occurred with stretching). Orgasm was also less convenient than taking a pill. A medication that could replicate orgasm would undoubtedly become a drug of abuse, but might provide relief for spastic patients with muscles jerking due to involuntary periodic limb movements.

Three years later, after reading that GABAergic drugs promoted the growth and metastasis of cancers, I decided to try using orgasm again. I wanted to see if it still worked reliably to prevent periodic limb movements (i.e., without taking zolpidem tartrate or baclofen at bedtime). I was able to go to sleep without developing periodic limb movements, but woke up one hour later due to periodic limb movements. What had worked well three years earlier didn't seem to work so well anymore.

Baclofen

The third thing I tried was baclofen, which had a dramatic effect on my chronic, spastic stiffness (as described above) but no effect at all on my periodic limb movements and did not prevent clonus or decerebrate rigidity. Baclofen reportedly makes spasms less frequent, but I was having them infrequently enough that it was hard to be sure whether there was a difference.

Zolpidem

The fourth thing I tried was zolpidem tartrate. When I first started trying zolpidem tartrate, I was just trying to sleep despite the movements, but found that the drug also had an inhibitory effect on my periodic limb movements. And, as the periodic limb movements got worse over time, the zolpidem tartrate was the only thing that reliably would calm the problem once it started. I continued to use lots of stretching during the day and at night when I got up for nocturia, which helped but only in an adjunctive fashion.

What happened was as follows. I started regularly taking zolpidem tartrate at night to sleep because restless leg syndrome and periodic limb movements were regularly preventing sleep. I found that 2-2.5 mg was usually sufficient to induce sleep for a person with my weight of 130 pounds.

Soon after that, I realized that I could take a slightly larger dose (e.g. an extra quarter to half milligram) and this larger dose would not only induce sleep but prevent development of periodic limb movements and restless leg syndrome during the time that I was asleep. In addition, I stopped having clonus, cramps in my calf or the arch of my foot, and decorticate posturing during the night (but it had no effect on episodes of sudden decerebrate rigidity accompanying dire urinary urgency). When I woke for nocturia, I would take a smaller dose of zolpidem tartrate to get back to sleep and to keep the concentration in my blood high enough to prevent the non-volitional movements from starting up again. To decide what small dose to use, I assumed that a 2.5 mg zolpidem tartrate fragment would work for five hours. The reason for the assumption was my first experience with the drug was during high-dose methylprednisolone courses prescribed for MS relapses. During that time, a 10 mg tablet would keep me asleep for five hours. To sleep more than five hours, I had to take more zolpidem after waking. So, assuming that two hours would use up 40% of my initial 2.5 mg dose at bedtime, I would need to take about 1 mg to go back to sleep after nocturia. That assumption seemed to work for me.

When I told my neurologist that zolpidem tartrate calmed my periodic limb movements and other non-volitional movements, she said that was not something neurologists recognized, but noted that it did bind to the benzodiazepine receptor like some other drugs that were used to treat spasticity.

After regularly using a larger dose for several months, I noticed that the frequency of periodic limb movements and other non-volitional spastic movements had also decreased during the following day as well. That continued for more than a year with me suspecting that the change in dosage was perhaps responsible but doing nothing to confirm that.

I was then forced to reduce my nighttime dosage of zolpidem tartrate because of a slight shortage of pills. The shortage was probably caused by multiple factors (e.g., cutting pills with a pill cutter into smaller fragments inevitably wastes part of the pill as unusable powder, spastic hands can cause pill bottles to fall over and pills to be lost, my slight increase in dosage had used pills faster than the previously used lower dose). After I reduced the dosage to the minimally effective hypnotic dose for putting me to sleep, I started getting periodic limb movements during the night waking me up again. After that happened, I also started having periodic limb movements the following day as well, usually commencing around supper or after supper. One night I was unable to use zolpidem tartrate at all and had very bad periodic limb movements through the night and periodic limb movements commencing before noon the next day. This was very unusual.

I raised the dose back to the slightly higher dose that I had used to suppress periodic limb movements at night, which worked, and the periodic limb movements occurring the following day disappeared again. After raising and lowering the zolpidem tartrate dose five times and having this pattern occur each time, it seemed obvious that zolpidem tartrate had powerful effects on spastic non-volitional movements that could extend for much of the following day despite taking the last dose at night.

I checked the medical literature again and found an uncontrolled case series of eight patients with restless leg syndrome unresponsive to other medications; all eight patients responded completely to therapy with 10 mg of zolpidem at bedtime without side effects. [Bezerra MLS, Martinez JVL. Zolpidem in restless legs syndrome. *European Neurology* 2002; 48:180-181.DOI: 10.1 159/000065514] Stopping the drug after a year without symptoms in two patients led to prompt recurrence of RLS in both; both responded again when zolpidem tartrate therapy resumed. Several case reports also reported that zolpidem had a powerful effect on spasticity in MS and other diseases. [Park IS, Kim JS, An JY, Kim YI, Lee KS. Excellent response to oral zolpidem in a sporadic case of the myoclonus dystonia syndrome. Mov Disord. 2009 Oct 30;24(14):2172-3. doi: 10.1002/mds.22745.] [Damm J, et al. Severe dependency on zolpidem in a patient with multiple sclerosis suffering from paraspasticity. World Journal of Biological Psychiatry. 2010; 11:516-8.] [Shadan FF, et al. Zolpidem for post-anoxic spasticity. South Med J 2004; 97:791-2.] There was also one study in laboratory mice suggesting that it reduced seizure activity.[Vlainic J, et al. Zolpidem is a potent anticonvulsant in adult and aged mice. Brain Res. 2010; 1310:181-8.]

How do these results compare with those of FDA approved treatments for RLS (dopamine agonists like ropinirole and the anticonvulsant gabapentin) or the old standby clonazepam? It's clear that not all patients respond to ropinirole or gabapentin because there have been plenty of studies. For example, a meta-analysis of randomized controlled trials including 1,679 adult patients taking ropinirole or placebo for moderate to severe restless leg syndrome reported the following: "At baseline, study patients slept an average of 5.8 hours per night. At the end of 12 weeks, ropinirole-treated patients slept a mean of 2.5 hours per week more and had a 21% greater improvement from baseline in sleep adequacy scores compared with patients receiving placebo. Ropinirole-treated patients also had 14% less sleep disturbance and 8% less daytime somnolence than patients receiving placebo. Clinicians rated 63% of ropinirole-treated patients and 47% of patients receiving placebo as responders based on the CGI-I scale."[Hansen RA, song L, Moore CG, et al. effect of ropinirole on sleep outcomes in patients with restless legs syndrome: meta-analysis of pooled individual data from randomized controlled trials. Pharmacotherapy. 2009;29:255-62. doi: 10. 1592/phco.29.3.255.] Translation of these data into everyday English: there was significant improvement, but it was modest (e.g., only sleeping 21 minutes more per night on ropinirole as compared with placebo). A meta-analysis by the Agency for Healthcare Related Quality (AHRQ) reported that the rate of response to gabapentin therapy was similar to that of dopamine agonists like ropinirole: (a relative risk of improvement with dopamine agonists of 1.6 and with gabapentin 1.66) .[Wilt TJ, et al. Pharmacologic therapy for primary restless legs syndrome: a systematic review and meta-analysis. JAMA Intern Med. 2013; 173:496-505. doi: 10.1001/jamainternmed.2013.3733.]

How about side effects? The review of gabapentin side effects mentioned in Chapter 13 said this, "Persons taking gabapentin can expect to have at least one adverse event (66%), withdraw because of an adverse event (12%), suffer dizziness (21%), somnolence (16%), peripheral edema (8%), and gait disturbance (9%)." [Moore RA, et al. Gabapentin for chronic neuropathic pain and fibromyalgia in adults. Cochrane Database Syst Rev. 2011 Mar 16; (3):CD007938. doi: spell 10. 1002/14651858.CD007938.pub2.] The meta-analysis by AHRQ reported that patients taking gabapentin or a similar drug had significantly more short-term adverse effects than those taking placebo: "somnolence (19% vs. 3%, RR=5.37 [95% CI, 2.38 to 12.12], k=5), unsteadiness or dizziness (17% vs. 4%, RR=4.11 [95% CI, 2.19 to 7.71], k=4), and dry mouth (6% vs. 1%; RR=3.31 [95% CI, 1.09 to 10.05], k=4) (overall high-strength evidence for these outcomes)." Patients treated short-term with ropinirole have complained of nausea, dizziness, orthostatic hypotension, hallucinations, and sudden sleep attacks; long-term use has been associated with augmentation (i.e., significant worsening) of the restless leg syndrome), compulsive behavior, and hypersexuality. The meta-analysis by AHRQ reported "short-term adverse effects from treatment with dopamine agonists compared with placebo were nausea (23% vs. 7%, RR=3.31 [95% CI, 2.53 to 4.33], k=15), vomiting (7% vs. 2%, RR=4.48 [95% CI, 2.68 to 7.48], k=8), and somnolence (12% vs. 6%, RR=2.04; [95% CI, 1.50 to 2.76], k=8) (overall high-strength evidence for these outcomes).

Reviewing two large open label studies of ropinirole, Cushida said that "the most commonly reported adverse events (≥10%) were nausea, headache, and arthralgia, and the majority of the adverse events were mild to moderate in intensity, with the first occurrence largely in the initial 12 weeks of therapy. There were few reports of augmentation (3.9%) ... a paradoxical increase in RLS symptom severity despite increased dose..., spread of symptoms to other limbs, and/ or symptom occurrence earlier in the day." [Cushida CA. Ropinirole for the treatment of restless legs syndrome. Neuropsychiatr Dis Treat. 2006 Dec; 2(4): 407–419.] The meta-analysis by AHRQ referred to above reviewed data from 18 observational studies (including open-label extensions of RCTs) that reported at least 6 months of follow-up to assess the percentage of individuals withdrawing from pharmacologic treatments and reasons for withdrawal (e.g., lack of efficacy, adverse events, and augmentation). Withdrawal from treatment was common, occurring in 13 percent to 57 percent of subjects. The highest withdrawals were in studies of levodopa (withdrawal greater than 40%). Withdrawal from gabapentin and the dopamine agonists was typically greater than 20 percent. About half of withdrawals were due to adverse events, including augmentation; 20 percent to 30 percent of withdrawals were due to lack of efficacy."

What are the data for the old standby clonazepam? There are studies suggesting that it works, but not quite as well as ropinirole or gabapentin. That's why it's no longer a drug of first choice for the problem. Its side effects are also a concern because they are numerous and some serious. The three most frequent are drowsiness, ataxia (clumsiness) and behavioral changes. Others include dizziness and confusion. There are also numerous potential drug interactions with a variety of other drugs. Clonazepam is a benzodiazepine, which can cause addiction. In my view, a drug with all of this baggage should be used as a last resort.

So, there are relatively clear data for the other drugs used for restless leg syndrome. How does zolpidem tartrate stack up against the competition? The proportion of patients whose restless leg syndrome will respond to zolpidem tartrate is less clear. In the uncontrolled case series mentioned above, eight of eight patients (100%) responded completely to zolpidem tartrate without side effects. But the sample size was too small to provide certainty (this was discussed in Chapter 1). The 95% confidence interval of 100% of eight patients is 63% to 100%, meaning that the response rate in a larger study could be as low as 63%; more data are needed for clarity. The lack of side effects in the small case series doesn't mean that zolpidem never causes side effects. As mentioned in Chapter 16, taking too much zolpidem is associated with a significantly higher rate of falls and fractures. It makes me weaker and more wobbly, so I have to avoid overdosing and get in bed quick after a dose before getting too weak or wobbly.

Bottom line: each of these drugs has advantages and disadvantages and each patient must balance such things and select what's best for her. My own approach has been to keep using zolpidem tartrate because I'd already been using it for several years successfully before my neurologist mentioned that we should consider the other drugs. The side effects of the other two drugs and of clonazepam seem worse to me (e.g., nausea, vomiting and dizziness would be very unpleasant for a debilitated patient like me already struggling to get up repeatedly at night for nocturia). The reason the other drugs seem worse is partly explained by the old adage "better the devil you know than the devil you don't know." After more than five years of use, zolpidem tartrate has not been associated with development of tolerance or augmentation of side effects for me. This seems to support the results of Bezerra described above, but certainty about performance will depend upon the results of larger, confirmatory studies.

Stretching To Control Chicken Wing Spasms

When I go into a spasm of spastic flexing of my paretic left arm, I have found that I can usually control the problem by doing several things. The first is assuring that my spastic, paretic left hand is attached to the walker handle, using my stronger right hand to place it there if necessary. I then twirl the hand around the handle advancing the fingers until I can get my palm securely around the handle. This usually works like a key in a lock for me, causing the spasm to abate enough that I can stretch that arm more easily and start stretching it several times until the pain and spasm are further reduced. I then stand straight up, stretching my spine, which seems to further reduce the spasm. After doing these two things, I can usually safely proceed across the room using the walker. What hasn't worked for me is 1) trying to directly arm wrestle the spasm, which is usually more difficult and more painful (this is a special problem if I am having back pain due to fractures or spasms at the time because struggling against the spastic flexion puts great tension on my back, which increases the pain of either) and 2) tripling my baclofen dose. The more I keep using the walker to navigate around the house, the fewer chicken wing spasms I have. If I have to reduce my ambulation (e.g., because of one or more fractures in my leg), the chicken wing spasms become worse and more frequent.

Chapter 24

What Is a Contracture and Are MS Patients at Risk for Getting This?

A contracture is usually a permanent change in a non-bony tissue (e.g., skin, muscle, ligament, tendon) resulting in tightening, limitation of motion and pain. The change is due to fibrosis. MS patients are at increased risk because of immobility. It occurs with flaccid paralysis, but many believe that it occurs more frequently with spasticity. For example, an NYU website said this, "Contracture is different from spasticity, but they are often related. Spasticity is an abnormal increase in muscle tone, which can worsen the development of contractures. " And a Wikipedia website said this, "A muscle contracture is a permanent shortening of a muscle or joint. It is usually in response to prolonged hypertonic spasticity in a concentrated muscle area, such as is seen in the tightest muscles of people with conditions like spastic cerebral palsy." I couldn't find controlled studies showing that, but the initial contracture in my left foot involved the second toe, which always seemed to have worse spasticity than the other toes in that foot (e.g., actually curling under in spastic response to stepping on a cold floor so that I sometimes had to walk on the dorsum of that toe).

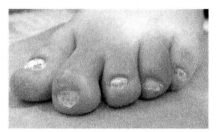

Figure 24-1 This photo shows a permanent, painful flexion contracture of the joint closest to the toenail of the second toe. Contractures occur more frequently with spasticity.

Can contracture be prevented? Yes, by moving the limb at risk as much as possible by active exercise or by passive stretching after the limb becomes too weak to cooperate.

Two of the four books by physicians for MS patients mentioned that contracture can be prevented by stretching, but there were problems with the way this was said. For example, Dr. Lechtenberg's book implied that the stretching needed to be done by a physical therapist. Not so. In its attempt to be encyclopedic, so many things were said that the very important recommendation to see a physical therapist also could get missed.

Dr. Giesser's book recommended that an MS patient set up care by a team of 15 different healthcare professionals, one of which was a physical therapist. This makes it unclear that seeing a physical therapist is vitally important while seeing most of the other 14 isn't as important. It also said that a neurologist or physical therapist can recommend a regimen of stretching to prevent contracture, which is true, but I wasn't told this by my neurologist or physical therapist and developed incipient contractures in both second toes (much worse in the weaker, more spastic left foot) before I figured out that regular stretching of the toes (every time I took off my shoes) stopped progression of the process. Stretching didn't cure the spasticity, just stopped the contractures from getting worse (sort of like the 1953 truce halting hostilities of the Korean War at a demilitarized zone along the 38th parallel).

The reason I believe that this brief chapter is important is so that the readers will have clear knowledge of how to prevent contractures -- by regular stretching.

Chapter 25
What Is a Frozen Shoulder and Are Patients with MS at Increased Risk?

Pathologic studies of a frozen shoulder (also called adhesive capsulitis) show inflammation and fibrosis. Does this mean a frozen shoulder is a contracture? They have similarities but aren't identical. Both are stiff and painful, but the type of fibrosis is different and a frozen shoulder is usually more reversible. [Uhthoff HK, Boileau P. Primary frozen shoulder: global capsular stiffness versus localized contracture.. Clin Orthop Relat Res. 2007; 456:79-84.] A frozen shoulder can occur in a patient with restricted motion following an injury or surgery but can also occur in an MS patient with a weakening arm that causes decreased mobility of the arm.

Can a patient with MS related hemiparesis avoid getting one? Yes, getting a frozen shoulder can be prevented. But nobody told me that until after I got one.

How can it be prevented? By using that arm as much as possible for as long as possible. My arm was weakening, but as long as I kept using it to do things like putting on a sport coat, shooting a bow and arrow, swimming, etc., there was no way a frozen shoulder could start. When the arm becomes too weak to actively exercise using normal shoulder motions, passive stretching of the arm is necessary to prevent a frozen shoulder. The passive stretches I have used were 1) lying prone and stretching my paretic left arm with the stronger right arm and then lying for several minutes with it in a stretched position and 2) lying supine and lifting my paretic left arm with my stronger right arm until the arm was fully extended and I could place my left hand against the head of the bed and then leave the arm hanging there for a couple minutes of stretching. Both of these approaches worked well for years and neither required a special device or a second person to do the stretching. I switched from the first approach the second after advancing hemiparesis made it impossible for me to roll over prone in bed without assistance.

Chapter 26
Preventing Falling

"Something there is that doesn't love a wall, that wants it down."
Robert Frost, "Mending Wall"
"Something there is that doesn't love an MS patient, that wants him down too." – Barry Farr, corollary to Frost's observation
"Humpty Dumpty sat on a wall. Humpty Dumpty had a great fall. All the King's horses and all the King's men couldn't put Humpty back together again." – English nursery rhyme
"Roll me over on the right side 'Cause the left side hurts me so" – "Frankie and Johnny"

Three of the biggest challenges to physically disabled MS patients are gravity, entropy, and microbes. This chapter will discuss falls – an important problem caused in part by gravity and entropy –and Chapter 28 will begin discussing the many threats posed by microbes.

Gravity, wonderful playmate of our youth (i.e., essential for playing with a pogo stick, a bicycle, a trampoline, etc.), seems to turn vicious toward MS patients. During many rude encounters with Mother Earth, I began to feel as if gravity was hurling the full weight of the planet at my increasingly frail body.

Like gravity, entropy is a force of nature, and thus hard to resist. It results in "everything evolving toward maximum disorder," according to Wikipedia. An MS patient falling over and breaking bones represents disorder – departure from a normal, healthy life.

Trauma from falling is a well-recognized cause of death dating back to antiquity. For example, Genghis Khan, Geronimo, and William the Conqueror all died from injuries sustained while falling off a horse. History tends to repeat itself, and this trend has continued. The actor Christopher Reeve (famous for his movie portrayal of Superman) died in 2004 because of injuries from falling off a horse in 1995.

For MS patients, things can go very bad after a fall, as they did for Humpty. Falls are an important source of both morbidity and mortality for MS patients. The pain of fractured ribs, clavicles, vertebrae, etc., can't be treated with a first line analgesic because of an MS patient's propensity for severe constipation and inability to tolerate the increased constipation due to a narcotic analgesic. Moreover, immobilizing a fractured bone for months may allow healing, but the immobility prevents exercise and stretching, allowing weakness and spasticity to get worse. After fracturing my clavicle, I lost the ability to do multiple things (e.g., wash my left foot in the shower, tie a tie, don or remove a sport coat, etc.). Fracturing a hip can make rehabilitation difficult for a debilitated MS patient. The required immobility can also make deep venous thrombosis (blood clot) more likely, and chronic anticoagulant therapy is more risky in patients who are continually falling.

Can an MS patient prevent falling by exercising? I have seen this recommended, and it seems true that a weak, debilitated patient is more likely to fall than a patient in better condition with greater strength. But it's important to understand that the reason an MS patient falls is not just weakness. An MS patient getting weaker usually also simultaneously becomes more spastic and loses her sense of balance. For these reasons, an MS patient can be optimally conditioned with as much strength as possible and still fall.

My first fall, in the ninth year after onset of MS, may serve as a good example because I was still working and still in good enough shape that I could get up off the floor relatively easily after falling. But I fell, nevertheless.

The cerebellum is a part of the brain that often gets attacked by MS. Because the cerebellum acts like the body's gyroscope, damage to it can cause a strong MS patient still able to walk without a cane to fall on the floor. I know. I did it. It was a surprise, being my first fall.

For most of my subsequent falls, weakness and spasticity were often important contributors like imbalance. All three tend to increase over time, and, as they do, a patient falls more frequently. But for me, there was often one particular wrinkle that differed with each fall. Paul Simon said there are "50 ways to leave your lover," and there are probably at least 50 ways for an MS patient to fall.

Regardless of the exact cause, patients with a weaker side tend to fall on that side. I fall on my left side about 98% of the time. In the song "Frankie and Johnny," Johnny gets shot and says, "Roll me over on the right side 'cause the left side hurts me so." That's what I usually say after a fall.

An important exception seemed to be falls caused by getting up when my blood level of zolpidem tartrate was too high for this to be safe. In that circumstance, I fell on the strong side as well as the weak.

The exact way my falls occurred was usually unexpected. Sometimes I tried to "hurry" and took a step too fast with my paretic leg, which didn't quite make a full step onto the floor, and this "foot drop" tripped me. Because MS symptoms often change, it becomes hard to rely on previous experience. You can do something a certain way thousands of times, but then weakness or spasticity can worsen and make it impossible to do it that way again.

A baseball pitcher only has a few pitches (e.g., a fastball, a curveball, a changeup, a slider, etc.), but the batter never knows which one is coming and whether it will be inside, outside, high, or low. So the batter is always guessing. An MS patient is always kept guessing as well even though the disease has only a limited number of manifestations because these symptoms often change. My weakness never seemed to hit a plateau and stay there. It was always changing, usually getting worse from one year to the next. Ditto for my spasticity. My imbalance also got worse over time.

One time, I was standing in the kitchen before I had to use a cane or walker and my spastic left leg just buckled. I assume this was "negative myoclonus" as referred to in the chapter on spasticity. Other times I fell due to "positive myoclonus," where the same spastic leg would suddenly react violently to something (e.g., being touched by something cold) seemingly with a hair trigger.

People joke about someone unable to "talk and chew gum" at the same time. As I became more impaired, it became risky for me to divert my attention from walking to listening to what someone else said. A visitor said something as I was walking down the hall, and I looked up and immediately fell.

An MS patient's gait can be so precarious that a spastic sneeze or a sudden, intense, unreachable itch in my spastic leg can cause me to fall.

I often fell in clusters (e.g., eight times over nine days); I believe that this is another example of positive feedback as referred to in Chapter 38 on the relatedness of MS problems. A first fall can cause a fracture, which can cause severe pain, which can immediately cause increased spasticity, which can cause increased difficulty maneuvering with a walker, making falling more likely. The increased spasticity could make my spastic arm retract so much that it lost its grip on the walker handle or cause an increase in sudden myoclonic jerks. For me, one fall seems to cause more.

When a patient is already struggling mightily just to get from the bed to the bathroom and back, having to endure significant pain while doing that makes this seem more arduous. In addition, there is a reflex that causes one to immediately withdraw a hand when it touches something painfully hot without time to think about it. I think such a reflex may be involved in my increased tendency to fall after a first fall because when I stand up grabbing hold of the walker handles and suddenly have a sharp pain, my body tends to want to withdraw from the effort just like the hand jerks away from a hot stove. It's only by conscious determination that I can force my unwilling body to go forward through the pain. The increased pain and accompanying increase in spasticity impede progress toward the bathroom, which can serve as a Pavlovian, conditioned stimulus that can cause a sudden spike in urinary urgency; this can in turn trigger incontinence and divert attention from walking. Walking on a tightrope requires confidence, and, to an MS patient struggling to walk at all, walking with a walker can be like walking on a tightrope. After having multiple clusters of falls, the patient having a first fall doubts himself and his ability, which doesn't inspire confidence.

I have fallen more than 200 times, and I believe that awareness is very important for preventing falls. Understanding that I can fall anytime, anywhere keeps me on the qui vive (i.e., being very careful). Although I'm much weaker, more spastic, and more unbalanced than on the day of my first fall, I can, by being very careful, avoid falling for eight consecutive months.

Early on, my falls were innocuous, resulting in no serious injury. This was because I was still sufficiently strong and coordinated that when I knew I was falling, my body would react to make the fall have little impact. As the disease progressed and I became more feeble, I began to fall more as dead weight – the way a tree falls. And once that happens, kersmash! Then I began to have serious injuries. An MS patient living in my town fell over in that way smashing his face into the floor and breaking out both front teeth. I have fallen over in almost an identical way but, by chance, luckily avoided breaking out my teeth. Instead, my teeth cut my lip, which bled all over the floor. An MS patient falling in that way generates more force for a blow against the head than Mohammed Ali's boxing glove did.

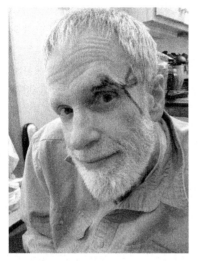 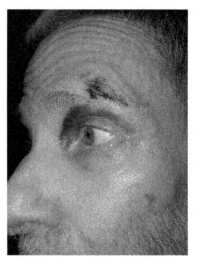

Figure 26-1 The author's face after a midnight fall was followed by re-bleeding during the night with blood congealing on the face.

Figure 26-2 The author's face two days after the midnight fall still showing a gory gash in his brow and a black eye caused by bruising from the fall.

I heard someone say that a patient predisposed to falling should "learn how to fall safely." But, as mentioned above, my body seemed to do this automatically without my thinking about it. And after imbalance, spasticity and weakness became severe, it seemed unlikely to me that knowledge of how to fall could have had much impact on how my body fell (other than avoiding hazardous places like a staircase). I will say, however, that I began trying to use the padded seat of my rollator walker as an intermediate landing site when I started to fall; this had the advantage of breaking the fall into two steps and falling off the walker pad onto the floor was usually associated with less likelihood of fracture.

After falling many times, it becomes clear that **EVERYWHERE** is a dangerous place, requiring great care.

Despite taking great care, some falls still occur for other reasons. Some of these are iatrogenic (i.e., caused by a physician, such as an adverse effect of a prescribed medication). The sleeping medication zolpidem tartrate is clearly a risk factor for falling, so its use requires careful balancing of risk versus benefit. [Finkle WD, et al. Risk of fractures requiring hospitalization after an initial prescription for zolpidem, alprazolam, lorazepam, or diazepam in older adults. Journal American Geriatric Society. 2011; 59:1883-90. doi: 10. 1111/j.1532-5415. 2011.03591.x. Epub 2011 Sep 21.] This study reported that nonvertebral fractures and hip fractures increased 2.55-fold with zolpidem therapy.

One thing that a patient using a sleeping pill should never do is take a pill, lie in bed for 20 minutes not feeling the least bit sleepy and get up to do something. The pill can unpredictably and instantaneously switch from seeming to have no effect at all to "lights out," which can cause a patient to suddenly black out and hit the floor. A constant problem for MS patients is that their nocturnal bladder capacity can be only a couple of hours, but a dose of zolpidem tartrate will usually last for five hours; this means that the patient will have to get up to pee while under the influence of the sleeping medication. A couple of hours after taking an appropriate dose, I am usually able to get up and safely navigate to the toilet with a rollator walker. One of the things that helps offset the negative influence of the sleeping medication is that sleep itself is restorative, making me stronger and less spastic.

The laxative polyethylene glycol 3350 (MiraLAX) isn't thought of as a risk factor for falling but has been instrumental in more than one fall for me. "Rushing" to the toilet for MiraLAX induced fecal urgency, an MS patient can fall because of the perceived need to rush. Trying to get up from the kitchen table after a gross MiraLAX spill onto the floor is a clear invitation to fall, but the design of the MiraLAX bottle has caused me to fall for a different reason. The MiraLAX cap is used to measure a dose and then replaced on the bottle, but the powder in the cap is hard to completely remove, which means that some powder often falls out of the cap when replacing it on the bottle or when removing the cap the next time.

A third way MiraLAX can end up on the floor can be visualized by thinking of a dump truck dumping a load of dirt. Most of the dirt is pulled straight down onto the ground by gravity, but some of it rises as a cloud of dust, which then settles onto the pile and around the pile of dirt. When a dose of MiraLAX is poured, something similar occurs: most of the dose just falls by gravity into the glass, but with the right lighting conditions, one can see a puff of powder that rises like a dump truck's cloud of dust and then re-settles. This fine cloud of powder can accumulate over time and cause the table and floor next to it to become slippery and pose a risk for falling. Tiny, invisible amounts of powder may end up on the table and eventually the floor where a shoe bottom may get contaminated with MiraLAX and become slippery. That happened to me and the slippery shoe lost traction with the bathroom floor WHILE I WAS HOLDING ONTO A GRAB BAR! The slippery shoe started spinning like a dancer's foot doing a pirouette and spun to the point of no return where a fall became obligatory. This shows how important traction is and how important it is for an MS patient to avoid getting slippery stuff underfoot. A pill cutter has been useful to an MS patient like me for cutting zolpidem tartrate or baclofen tablets to a smaller, more useful size, [see photo] but little bits of powder produced by the pill cutter can end up on the table and eventually the floor, again making the floor slippery. Similarly, a dirty floor becomes slippery. Sweeping MiraLAX powder, crushed fragments of zolpidem tartrate or baclofen tablets, or dirt with a broom can remove large, visible amounts of each, but still leave the floor slippery. These situations require wet mopping for optimal cleaning to restore good traction.

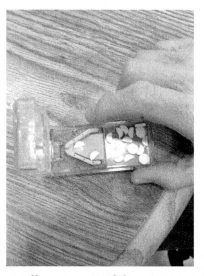

Figure 26-3 A pill cutter is useful to an MS patient when
certain medications are too large to be taken as marketed,
but a pill cutter invariably produces powder, which can spill
on the floor and cause a shoe to slip resulting in a fall.

MiraLAX powder is usually less expensive when buying larger
containers but large containers can be harder to hold and can result
in more spills or MiraLAX coming out in clumps. The 26.9 ounce
bottle is too large for me to use conveniently. The 17.9 ounce bottle
is cheaper than the smaller bottles, but when it's full, the powder
tends to come out too frequently as clumps, which can cause spills.
For that reason, I have used an inexpensive, 4-ounce funnel made by
Oxo to pour powder from a full 17.9 ounce bottle into an empty 17.9
ounce bottle. This results in my starting pouring doses from each
bottle when it is only half full. This means that there is less weight
in the bottle and the powder comes out easier with less clumping
and fewer spills. When pouring a dose into a glass, I also get fewer
rising puffs of powder if I pour it slowly (e.g., in 10 small increments
rather than just dumping the full load at once)

MS patients can have trouble accessing light switches, which can
be double trouble because cerebellar disease makes the MS patient

more likely to fall in the dark. A well-lit room is always safer for the patient to maneuver with a cane or walker. Because of the need for light, at all times, an emergency generator is a wise investment. If the patient is maneuvering with a walker and then plunged into darkness by a power outage at night, this could result in a fall with fractures, pain, etc. For that reason, we have an emergency generator that clicks on whenever the power goes off and I have an LED flashlight permanently mounted on my walker where I can reach it. It glows in the dark, making this easier if the power does flip off and the generator fails. When I get up at night for nocturia, I always carry an additional LED flashlight to the bathroom, resting it on the walker seat, where it sits securely. This way, if one of the LED flashlights fails, I have a backup and am not plunged into darkness.

When I get up from the toilet in a well-lit room, I have found that staring at something with a definite image (e.g., the toilet handle) is safer than staring at something with an amorphous pattern (like the floor), because I tend to be more stable with the former than the latter. The same is true when I stand up beside the bed at night for nocturia. Staring at the numbers on the digital clock seems to be safer than looking at something dimly lit. Similarly, when I pull a shirt over my head, I try to do so sitting down, making a fall less likely.

After falling many times, I have tended to wear more substantial clothes (e.g. L.L. Bean thicker cotton ["canvas"] shirts in the summer and flannel shirts in the winter), which seem more protective against abrasions. Wearing flannel and corduroy may be more protective against abrasions during falls, but it's too warm to wear with comfort during the warm half of the year -- not warm enough to cause Uhthoff's phenomenon, but uncomfortable.

Patients prone to falling are at risk for serious problems other than fractures, abrasions, infection, and pain. For example, falling on the floor with a hard blow to the head can cause significant bleeding both externally and internally. The external wounds are obvious and pressure can be applied to stop the bleeding before dressing the wound. But internal bleeding is not obvious and can become very serious. Blood can collect beneath the lining of the brain – the dura mater. The blood collection, called a subdural hematoma, can keep enlarging if blood keeps oozing from the injured site. The enlarging hematoma can apply pressure to the brain that is confined inside the skull, and this can cause herniation of the brain stem and death.

This is important to know because many people take aspirin to minimize their risk of atherosclerosis and ischemic heart disease. Aspirin makes bleeding more likely, and MS increases the chance of a subdural hematoma in a patient prone to falling. For this reason, patients prone to falling should avoid taking aspirin and other drugs that increase bleeding. Are there any other drugs such patients could take to counter an increased risk of ischemic heart disease (e.g. positive family history, increased cholesterol, sedentary life-style [due to MS related paresis])? A statin.

Should an MS patient's toilet seat be left up or down?

Some readers may think this is a joke, but it's not. Having fallen onto the toilet about 30 times and into the toilet once (where I got stuck like Winnie the Pooh in Rabbit's hole), I believe that the toilet seat should be left down for safety. Falling onto the toilet seat isn't comfortable, but falling into the toilet is worse.

Should an MS Patient's Bathroom Door Be Closed for Privacy?

For the first 20 years of MS, I routinely closed my bathroom door for privacy. But after falling multiple times while trying to close the door, I came to view this differently. During the day, the only problem with leaving the door open was my wife or my nurse coming into the bedroom when I was in there. Because both had had to rescue me in the bathroom because of desperate situations involving urinary incontinence, fecal incontinence or both, I figured that seeing me in the bathroom with the door open was probably no longer such a big deal. There also was little if any odor coming out of the open bathroom door to worry about (see Chapter 37). This made things easier and faster when approaching the bathroom using a walker or a motorized wheelchair. I continued to close the door when approaching the bathroom for nocturia to avoid disturbing my wife's sleep. Maneuvering at night after sleep was usually easier and safer because sleep always reduces my weakness and spasticity.

Chapter 27

Would a Rubber Coated Flashlight Be Helpful to MS Patients? If so, Why?

I believe it may. A rubber coated flashlight has been very helpful to me. MS patients need a flashlight handy more than healthy people do when they become prone to falling because cerebellar involvement makes falling in the dark more likely.

MS patients also have to get up at night repeatedly for nocturia. To avoid waking a spouse, a small flashlight can be used to help allow safe ambulation with a rollator walker from the bed to the bathroom. To do this, I turn on the flashlight, which rests on my bedside chest of drawers through the night. I then stand up using a bed rail for support, grab the flashlight and reach for the handles of my walker. After I have hold of the walker handle with my paretic hand, I place the flashlight on the vinyl seat of the walker and leave it there as a "headlight." The rubberized surface has plenty of friction, keeping it stable on the seat. Before I found a rubber coated flashlight, I tried many others. Metal and plastic surfaces have little friction, which causes a flashlight to slide off the pad onto the floor where

I have had flashlights break, damage the lightbulb, or burst open, spilling batteries on the floor. These are each relative disasters to a patient in urgent need of getting to the toilet because of nocturia. It's a disaster because lack of light means that the patient can't keep walking. It's also a disaster because anything untoward can serve as a conditioned, Pavlovian stimulus causing an immediate spike in urinary urgency, which can result in wet pajamas, wet slippers, a wet floor, etc. The latter disaster also requires cleanup and changing into a different pair of pajamas, which, in turn, means that the bladder will likely fill dangerously full before the next time to wake up again, which can result in repetition of the same disaster. My rubberized flashlight stays stable on the walker seat, never causing me such problems.

Another reason that a rubber coated flashlight is preferable is that my paretic hand can hold onto the rubbery surface better, allowing more independence with unscrewing and re-screwing flashlight parts together for battery changes. Yet another reason that a rubber coated flashlight is preferable is that touching cold surfaces is very uncomfortable for my spastic limbs and causes in-creased spasticity. A metal coated flashlight can become very cold.

A solar powered flashlight available at Amazon and at L.L. Bean is mostly plastic but has rubber on the front and back ends (made by Hybrid Light). It has a number of the same virtues and does not require battery change. This can be better for a patient with hemi-paresis having difficulty changing batteries. It's also inexpensive and friendly to the environment.

Chapter 28
Preventing Pressure-
Related Illness

Gravity contributes to another important problem for MS patients: pressure-related illness in the buttock of a paretic or paralyzed leg. Politicians use the phrase "press the flesh" to refer to shaking hands with their adoring public, but the phrase has an ominous meaning for MS patients.

The tissue of a leg being paralyzed becomes flaccid. Unrelenting pressure on this unmoving flesh can cause a variety of problems. One of these, for a patient with intact sensation, is ischemic pain. Another is necrosis of the skin (i.e., a pressure ulcer). A third is infection of the tissue undergoing sustained pressure. Infection usually occurs when the skin is no longer intact and microbes invade the pressure ulcer – a breach in the body's system of host defenses. But infection can also occur in skin under pressure before necrosis happens (i.e., recurrent pressure-related *Staphylococcus aureus* furuncles [boils]).

I started having pressure-related problems in the 11th year after my diagnosis of MS. At that time, I started getting recurrent, painful, *Staphylococcus aureus* furuncles in the buttock of my increasingly paretic left leg. The first furuncle occurred after a course of high dose methylprednisolone therapy administered for an MS relapse. The same dose of the same medication had been prescribed for treating relapses of MS for the preceding seven years with no infectious complications. After that first episode, a new furuncle followed every subsequent course of methylprednisolone.

As mentioned in Chapter 1, causation in epidemiology is usually multifactorial. *Staphylococcus aureus* is the main cause of furuncles, so one might say that the cause was *Staphylococcus aureus*. But the onset of a new furuncle following each course of methylprednisolone implies that immunosuppression was another important cause of these infections. And the occurrence of every furuncle in the buttock of my paretic left leg (and none in the healthier, right leg) shows that paresis was yet another important cause, due to unrelenting pressure on the weakening leg. If gravity wasn't pulling the paretic leg down against a seat (imagine the weightless astronauts in the International Space Station), there would be no pressure on the paretic leg, so gravity is a fourth cause.

Six years later, in the 17th year after my diagnosis of MS, I had my last attack of MS and stopped receiving courses of methylprednisolone. But the following year, I started having new pressure-related problems – ischemic pain in the buttock from sitting too long or on too firm a surface and development of new, pressur- related *Staphylococcus aureus* furuncles in that setting. The rate of infection kept rising and the pain of sitting on furuncles made it difficult for me to sit down and do anything. Hemiparesis made it difficult to lie in bed and do anything. I tried standing up, propped against the front of a desk, to see if I could work with a computer that way, but that was associated with a marked increase in periodic limb movements, and for the first time these involved my stronger, healthier right leg.

The pain of sitting on a new furuncle seemed sharp in quality, began immediately, and continued unchanged as long as I continued sitting: the larger a furuncle was allowed to get before applying effective therapy, the more it hurt. By contrast, the pain of sitting on a sufficiently paretic buttock was delayed (i.e., there was no pain when I first sat down); it usually began within an hour and increased in intensity as long as I continued sitting. Its quality reminded me of the pain described by patients with angina having impaired blood flow to the myocardium.

I asked my neurologist at each clinic visit for years what could be done about the infections in the paretic buttock and was repeatedly told that there were "no data."

Feeling desperate, I searched on the Internet and found testimonials reporting prevention and healing of pressure related necrosis of skin on the buttock of paretic or paralyzed legs using alternating air cushions. The two companies with the most testimonials claiming efficacy had both been marketing alternating air cushions for over a decade at that point, but neither company's products had been the subject of research and publication in the medical literature. I invited both of those companies to provide me with their products so that I could compare how they performed in preventing my pressure-related problems. Both agreed to participate.

The similar ratings of the two companies on that website did not prepare me for what the study would show. Use of one company's cushions was rapidly followed by onset of seven new furuncles during 18 patient-days of use, while the other company's cushion was followed by no infections during six months of use. The probability that this huge difference was due to chance (random error) was extremely small ($p = 1.47 \times 10^{-7}$), suggesting a relative risk greater than 66. [Farr BM. Preventing recurrent pressure-related furuncles using an alternating air cushion. *Infect Dis Clin Pract.* 2013; 21:21-24.] After the study ended, I sat on an Aquila cushion for the next six months with no new furuncles. It worked so well that it reminded me of Arthur C. Clarke's "Third Law": "Technology sufficiently developed is indistinguishable from magic."

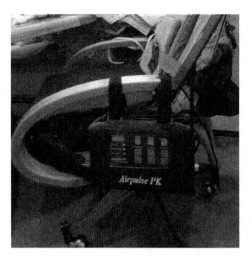

Figure 28-1 Pressure related illnesses (e.g., painful furuncles, pressure sores, etc.) can be prevented by using an effectively functioning alternating air cushion like the one shown. The cushion is lying on a kitchen chair and the box containing its pump and control buttons hangs on the arm of the chair from Velcro straps.

It's also unlikely that this study's result was false positive due to bias (systematic error) because a staphylococcal furuncle that is painful, visible, palpable, tender, and responsive to warm compresses is an objective endpoint. Subjective endpoints are more susceptible to biased interpretation (e.g., feeling less cold symptoms after sucking zinc lozenges).

One shouldn't conclude from the results of this study that all patients with paresis require an alternating air cushion for comfort or for prevention of infection. I had paresis of the left leg due to MS for 19 1/2 years before the study began, but problems with discomfort from sitting on a static cushion and painful furuncles developing merely from sitting too long on a static cushion didn't begin until the 18th year of MS (before that, recurrent, pressure-related furuncles had affected the paretic left buttock but only following courses of methylprednisolone).

For MS patients with severe paresis or paralysis, an alternating air cushion that works is important for preventing ischemic pain, infection, and necrosis of the skin on the buttock. For this reason, having at least one functioning system (i.e., pump, cushion, connecting tubes, etc.) is essential to me. Because such devices develop problems over time and require repair, there should be a plan of how to deal with unavailability of one or more parts of the system when something has to be shipped back to the company, repaired and then returned, which can take 2 to 7 days. Getting the system back within two days requires getting it there quickly enough with overnight delivery that there is time for both repair and shipping the following day. Trying to do this will obviously cost more because of overnight delivery in both directions. The patient can "pay his money and take his choice" about how best to do this. My preference was to have more than one operating system available in my house so that downtime of one system could be dealt with by substituting a part from the other system. As I write this paragraph, I have been sitting on Aquila alternating air cushions for five years. During that time, I have had to ship back the cushions of two different systems three different times and a pump once for repair. Each time, having a spare cushion available allowed me to insert it and confirm that a pressure loss was due to a problem with the cushion or pump. This meant that I only had to send back the part with the problem, lowering postage fees, while ensuring that that part was indeed being sent for repair.

Another conclusion of this study was that not all alternating air cushions are equally effective. Prior studies of the utility of alternating air cushions that I was able to find using Medline searching only used one type of alternating air cushion, apparently assuming that any alternating air cushion was as good as any other alternating air cushion (à la Gertrude Stein's assertion that "a rose is a rose is a rose.").

A recent Cochrane review said that it was unclear that alternating air cushions worked to prevent pressure ulcers, but that review included no studies evaluating the Aquila cushion that worked well in this study. [McInnes E, Jammali-Blasi A, Bell-Syer S, Dumville J, Cullum N. Preventing pressure ulcers -- are pressure redistributing support surfaces effective? A Cochrane systematic review and meta-analysis. Int J Nurs Stud. 2011 click file. [Epub ahead of print]]

_____

After I had had 14 medial furuncles temporally associated with clamping my buttocks shut to prevent fecal incontinence, I was feeling desperate. At that point, healing an individual furuncle was requiring a couple of months of warm moist compresses applied seven times per day. What happened then was I went into a particularly bad bout of constipation that kept me on the toilet for extra hours per day. That was associated with my getting four simultaneous furuncles [I had never had more than two simultaneous furuncles in the past and almost always had only a single furuncle]. These furuncles were also in a different distribution from those usually due to sitting on a chair and from those due to clamping my buttocks shut. The four simultaneous furuncles were all in the area that turns red after sitting on the toilet seat, suggesting that they were due to the extra time spent sitting on the toilet seat because of the bout of constipation; they also hurt immediately when I sat down on the toilet giving a clue as to their location and would pop discharging pus and blood onto the toilet seat. Four simultaneous furuncles would require so much time heating water and making warm moist compresses and applying each one to each of the 4 furuncles, that I initially felt hopeless. That was the first time I tried using an alternate heat source to apply enough heat to turn the skin pink without burning it, which would cause an even worse problem. I tried using a small Gillette, compact hairdryer – an old, no longer used one that had belonged to my wife, who had gotten a newer, niftier model. It worked well for treating the four simultaneous furuncles. They responded well to the heat, just as they had always done to the warm moist compresses, and it was much easier and quicker to apply the heat than it was using warm moist compresses. After that, I found that applying heat to the involved portion of my left buttock seemed to work to prevent development of such pressure-related furuncles (e.g., after a long session on the toilet seat or after crimping my buttocks closed to prevent fecal incontinence). Having had 14 medial furuncles and a half dozen more lateral "toilet seat distribution" furuncles before trying prophylactic application of heat, I was pleased to find that such prophylaxis was followed by no further development of such pressure-related furuncles. Another thing that I started doing later was rocking from side to side to lift my paretic buttock up off of the toilet seat about once every minute or two whenever I was constrained to sit there longer than usual. That also may have helped prevent further development of furuncles in the toilet seat distribution.

Before ending this chapter about pressure-related furuncles, I should mention one more possible source. As a leg being paralyzed by MS atrophies, bony prominences such as the hip become more prominent. This can become so extreme that lying on one's side while sleeping can cause too much pressure on skin beneath the hip, which may foster pressure-related furuncles at that site. This pressure under the hip becomes worse when weakness and paresis make it hard to move in bed (i.e., prolonged pressure is worse than brief pressure). Sleeping pills also may add to the problem because they can make a patient less likely to move.

Chapter 29

Microbes and MS:
Are Infections Important?

Chapter 22 said that microbes and gravity are two of the biggest threats to MS patients. This chapter will discuss risks posed by microbes.

Healthy people generally aren't troubled much by microbes. Most microbes are not especially pathogenic, and some are actually symbiotic (mutually beneficial) – aiding digestion, producing vitamins, turning undigested food into feces in the colon, completing the biblical cycle of "dust to dust" after death, etc. Those that are pathogenic are usually easily fended off by a healthy person's normal host defenses. Death rates due to infection have declined with modern medicine, sanitation, vaccinations, etc., and some believe that this means that concerns about infection are passé.

This isn't quite right. Infection has remained the leading killer of humans worldwide and continues to cause important morbidity and mortality for compromised hosts in the 21st century.

What is a compromised host? A compromised host is a patient with impaired host defenses who thus gets more frequent or more severe infections. MS patients are compromised hosts and should be more concerned about microbes and the risk of infection than a normal healthy person.

Some laymen think that a compromised host is a germaphobe (i.e., someone excessively and inappropriately concerned about infection like Howard Hughes was portrayed in the movie *The Aviator*). A compromised host and a germaphobe may both be concerned about infection, but for different reasons. Howard Hughes was not a compromised host. He wasn't predisposed to more frequent or more severe infections.

What makes MS patients compromised hosts? This can range from normal, age-related senescence of the immune system to a number of complications and therapies of MS. Like the old gray mare, who ain't what she used to be, geriatric patients are more susceptible to a variety of infections. Various treatments and sequelae of MS are also known to impair host defenses. For example, drugs used to halt or prevent relapses may suppress the immune system (e.g., methylprednisolone). Immunosuppression can make a variety of infections more likely. A good illustration is the recurrence of staphylococcal furuncles after every course of methylprednisolone for seven years mentioned in Chapter 28. The gastric acid suppression required during each course of methylprednisolone also predisposed me to food poisoning. MS patients also often take nonsteroidal anti-inflammatory drugs for pain from fractures caused by falling. Nonsteroidal anti-inflammatory drugs cause ulcers, which can also require gastric acid suppression with proton pump inhibitors (e.g., omeprazole).

Some studies suggest that hypnotic drugs like zolpidem also predispose patients to increased risk of infection. [Joya FL, Kripke DF, Loving RT, Dawson A, Kline LE. Meta-analyses of hypnotics and infections:eszopiclone, ramelteon, zaleplon, and zolpidem. J Clin Sleep Med. 2009;5(4):377-83. Review.] [Huang CY, Chou FH, Huang YS, Yang CJ, Su YC, Juang SY, Chen PF, Chou P, Lee CA, Lee CC. The association between zolpidem and infection in patients with sleep disturbance. J Psychiatr Res.2014;54:116-20.doi:10.1016/j.jpsychires.2014.03.017.].

The data suggested that the risk was not confined to a particular type of infection but extended to infections in general (e.g., some might have suspected an increased aspiration pneumonia risk because of the hypnotic drugs causing a reduced level of consciousness, since this seems to be so for alcoholics on a binge). Is this correct? I can't say. The publications suggesting an increased risk of infection are recent and will require confirmation as noted by Joya et al. For immunosuppressive drugs, the mechanism of enhancing infection is known. For zolpidem, it's not known.

Receiving methylprednisolone therapy as an infusion through an intravenous catheter can increase risk of a couple of other types of infection. Having a catheter in place creates risk for catheter related infection. Intravenous infusion of methylprednisolone can also sometimes cause bloodstream infection due to contamination of the medication due to an error in the pharmacy compounding it. Contaminated methylprednisolone was linked to 751 cases of fungal infection resulting in 64 deaths during an investigation in 2012. The contaminated methylprednisolone came from the New England Compounding Center.

Impaired glottic reflexes during one of my early attacks increased my risk of aspiration of saliva, food and drink, which also increased my risk of pneumonia. Impaired emptying of urine from my urinary tract after my first attack resulted in post void dribbling and wetting of underclothes, but also increased my risk of urinary tract infection. Increased weakness of my left leg after multiple attacks made it more susceptible to *Staphylococcus aureus* infections and to pressure sores, which also increase risk of infection.

Other MS problems can also make infection more likely. For example, MS patients often require hands-on care because of paresis or paralysis. Such frequent touching by healthcare workers can result in transmission of microbes from one patient to another via the healthcare worker because of unwashed hands, unwashed white coats, contaminated equipment not disinfected between patients, etc. Such transmission can result in colonization by various antibiotic-resistant bacteria that cause more serious infections because initial antibiotic therapy often fails due to antibiotic resistance; in some cases, antibiotic resistant bacteria have been resistant to all known antibiotics, further increasing the gravity of this problem.

Some believe that homebound MS patients avoid the risk of infection by not going out into the public or to their physician's office. In some ways, this is true (e.g., less exposure to casually contagious microbes like the common cold, influenza, tuberculosis, etc.). But in other ways, it may not be true. For example, MS patients can get pneumonia by aspirating microbes living in their upper respiratory tract or stomach, they can get urinary tract infection by contamination of their urinary tract with microbes from their own colon, and they can get serious skin infection from microbes already colonizing their skin.

MS patients have problems with infection from the beginning of their illness until the end. At the beginning, when relapses of autoimmunity are striking the central nervous system, a viral respiratory infection can reportedly stimulate the immune system and trigger a relapse. Near the end of the disease, more serious infections can cause death; a recent national study of causes of death among MS patients reported that acute respiratory infection was the most frequently reported cause of death on death certificates that didn't just list MS as the cause of death. [Redelings MD, McCoy L, Sorvillo F. Multiple sclerosis mortality and patterns of comorbidity in the United States from 1990 to 2001 *Neuroepidemiology*. 2006; 26:102-7.] When physicians didn't attribute death to MS and recorded what else contributed, the 5 most frequent causes were pneumonia and/or influenza (19.7%), ischemic heart disease (10.9%), septicemia [bloodstream infection] (10.1%), cancer (8.5%), and urinary tract infection (8.4%). Another study confirmed that infections were the most frequent cause of death for MS patients. [Sumelahti ML, Hakama M, Elovaara I, Pukkala E. Causes of death among patients with multiple sclerosis. *Multiple Sclerosis*. 2010; 16:1437-42.]

There are many different manifestations of infection, in part because there are numerous types of infection. Fever can be an especially bad problem for MS patients, because it can make them very weak. When I was still able to walk without a cane, I developed a mild temperature elevation twice (once as a complication of a new MS therapy and once due to gastroenteritis caused by food poisoning at a restaurant). Both times I became so weak that I could barely walk or sit without danger of falling. Both times my oral temperature did not quite reach 38°C, the usual threshold for defining fever. If I had had high fever, the problem would have been worse. A patient already suffering with a weak, ineffectual cough will have a weaker, more ineffectual cough.

As stated in the introduction, this book won't attempt comprehensive coverage of MS, and that is true of this chapter regarding infectious complications of MS. There are so many different infectious diseases that could cause so many different problems that complete coverage would require an entire book. A few brief examples of infections to which I had potential exposure inside my house after becoming homebound due to MS may help illustrate the diversity of this problem.

A nursing aide assisting me with activities of daily living poured me a glass of tomato juice that looked discolored. If I had not been paying attention, I might have sipped it without noticing, because she said nothing to draw my attention to it, just put it beside me at the table. When I glanced up and said that it looked abnormal, she tried to convince me that it was okay, saying, "it smells fine." An MS patient who can barely ambulate with a walker doesn't need weakness caused by botulism, a disease that can be fatal after swallowing tiny doses.

A nursing aide also left an exterior door ajar, which allowed a bat to get inside unobserved. I woke up for nocturia at 2 AM and, while navigating to the bathroom with my walker, saw a bat fly into the bathroom in front of the flashlight I was using. Bats can sometimes transmit rabies, which can be fatal.

Somebody left at least two doors open long enough for mosquitoes to fly into the kitchen and then migrate through the rest of the house to my bathroom (like the bat). A slow moving MS patient repeatedly disrobing for nocturia is an easy target for a hungry mosquito. Mosquito borne West Nile virus infections are unpleasant and sometimes fatal. Mosquito borne chikungunya fever rarely causes death in healthy patients, but in MS patients could pose serious problems (e.g., weakness from Uhthoff phenomenon due to the high fever, and significant problems with mobility from the musculoskeletal pain that can become chronic). It recently spread from Africa to the Western Hemisphere. In 2014, it reportedly caused more than 750 cases in the southeastern United States. Chikungunya infection results in high fever, joint and muscle pain, and headache.

Family members coming down with new respiratory viral infection during the annual winter epidemic of influenza could have influenza. Some patients infected with influenza virus experience milder symptoms, perhaps because of pre-existing, partial immunity, leading them to believe they have a common cold, but the virus they transmit can cause lethal infection in other patients. Getting too close to someone with a virus that can spread across the dinner table could lead to transmission. Influenza is a special problem because it routinely causes excess mortality each winter and its high fever can make MS patients weaker and less able to cope.

Chapter 30
Preventing Infections

D ifferent infections occur at different sites for different reasons and therefore often require different measures for prevention.

For example, the alternating air cushion mentioned in Chapter 28 prevented recurrent pressure-related furuncles but would do nothing to prevent influenza.

An MS patient with impaired glottic reflexes (which are supposed to protect the trachea and lungs from aspiration of food, drink, saliva, etc.) is at increased risk for aspiration pneumonia, but daily oral hygiene may reduce the amount of microbes being aspirated and lower the risk of pulmonary infection (see Chapter 31).

Oral hygiene does nothing to protect the same MS patient from risk for urinary tract infection, which requires preventing fecal contamination of the hands (I did this by carefully cleaning with soap, water and toilet paper after a bowel movement) and keeping the urethra as clean and dry as possible (by avoiding fecal contamination of the urethral meatus and carefully blotting the urethra after voiding). Other books for MS patients recommend cleaning the urethral meatus regularly, but I believe it is safer and more effective to avoid fecal contamination of the urethra in the first place.

One can prevent acquiring a common cold by avoiding people

with symptoms of a common cold (e.g., sniffles, cough, etc.), and by regular hand hygiene. One can avoid acquiring influenza by getting the annual flu vaccine and by having others coming in contact with an MS patient also get the annual flu vaccine. Importantly, the patient should also avoid contact with anyone with symptoms of a respiratory virus during the flu season.

I ask the aides assisting me with activities of daily living to avoid coming on days when they have symptoms of infection and allow a backup to cover that day. During the first 2 ½ years of aides caring for me in this way, four of them came down with a flulike illness (i.e., fever, cough and other flu symptoms during the winter flu season), six came down with a cold (i.e., nasal congestion, a runny nose, sore throat, etc. without fever) and there were 14 reported episodes of nausea and vomiting (but 12 of those 14 episodes were reported by a single individual).

Insect vectors of disease (e.g., ticks, mosquitoes) may be unimportant for many housebound MS patients, but risk can be increased by well-meaning friends and family who insist on the patient getting out into the great outdoors. The great outdoors is admittedly wonderful, but the insect vectors are there. Infections transmitted by such insects can be severe and cause considerable problems for a compromised host. Wearing clothes that cover the skin and applying insect repellents containing DEET are reasonable precautions. Keeping mosquitoes out of the house by keeping doors shut and opening only windows covered by screens is also reasonable.

Chapter 31
Preventing Pneumonia

Is pneumonia a big deal for MS patients?

It's important in a variety of ways. Pneumonia and influenza were frequently reported causes of death for MS patients in a recent national study.[Redelings M, et al. Multiple sclerosis mortality and patterns of comorbidity in the United States from 1990 to 2001. *Neuroepidemiology.* 2006; 26:102-107.] Another study of the same topic confirmed that influenza and pneumonia caused death significantly more frequently for MS patients than for the general population. [Sumelahti ML, Hakama M, Elovaara I, Pukkala E. Causes of death among patients with multiple sclerosis. Multiple sclerosis. 2010; 16:1437-42.]

In addition to mortality, pneumonia causes patients to suffer significant morbidity, including a vigorous cough, which itself can cause multiple problems for MS patients. A sudden vigorous cough can cause an MS patient teetering about with tenuous balance to fall. Vigorous coughing in a patient already suffering severe pain from rib fractures, vertebral fractures, or clavicular fractures (from previous falls) also makes the pain much worse with each cough. And, worse pain can cause worse spasticity, which can also make falling more likely.

As compromised hosts, MS patients have an increased incidence of a variety of infections including pneumonia and also have more frequent hospital admissions for care of infections including pneumonia. [Marrie RA, Elliott L, Marriott J, Cossoy M, Blanchard Temakoon A, Yu N. Dramatically changing rates and reasons for hospitalization in multiple sclerosis. Neurology. 2014; 83:929-37. doi: 10.1212/ WNL.0000000000000753. Epub 2014 Aug 1.] Several studies have reported that MS patients with difficulty swallowing (dysphagia) get more pneumonia. Overall, 24% to 43% of MS patients reported dysphagia which was a permanent symptom starting early in the disease for some.[De Pauw A. Dejaeger E. D'hooghe B. Carton H. Dysphagia in multiple sclerosis. *Clin Neurol Neurosurg* 2(X)2;104:345-51.] [Calcagno P. Ruopptilo G. Grasso MG. De Vincentüs M, Paoiucci S. Dysphagia in multiple sclerosis — prevalence and prognostic factors. *Acta Neurol Scand* 2002:105:40-3.] [Abraham S, Scheinberg LC, Smith CR, LaRocca NG. Neurologic impairment and disability status in outpatients with multiple sclerosis reporting dysphagia symptomatology. *Neruorehabil Neural Repair.* 1997; 11:7-13. doi:10.1177/1545 9683 9701100102.] Dysphagia increased in frequency and in degree as time passed and MS disability progressed from mild to severe. .[De Pauw A. Dejaeger E. D'hooghe B. Carton H. Dysphagia in multiple sclerosis. *Clin Neurol Neurosurg* 2(X)2;104:345-51.]

What is pneumonia?

It is a lower respiratory tract infection of the lung itself often associated with fever and cough productive of sputum, which can be purulent, blood tinged, grossly bloody, etc. There may be chest pain, shortness of breath, and rapid breathing (tachypnea). Chest x-ray usually shows an infiltrate (opacity) that can involve a segment, an entire lobe, or an entire lung, but this opacity may lag a day or so behind initial symptoms.

What microbes infect the lung?

The microbes causing pneumonia are usually bacteria, but occasionally viruses and other microbes such as protozoa.

Where do these microbes come from that infect the lung?

Most episodes of pneumonia occur because of aspiration (i.e., liquids or solids "going down the wrong way" into the trachea and lungs instead of the esophagus and stomach), but these pneumonias are usually caused by small bits of aspiration, and they are not called "aspiration pneumonia." About half of normal, healthy people have been found to aspirate small amounts of saliva into the lungs when asleep. Normal healthy people can also occasionally regurgitate stomach contents (this is related to the ability to burp up swallowed air from the stomach) and they can rarely aspirate small bits of these regurgitated stomach contents into the lung.

The microbes aspirated into the lungs that cause most pneumonias come from the upper airway (e.g., mouth or throat), where they may be transient or chronic colonizing flora. The microbes that cause pneumonia for people with a normal healthy nervous system are usually aerobic bacteria like *Streptococcus pneumoniae*; this streptococcal pneumonia is usually the most frequent cause of community acquired pneumonia.

A small proportion of pneumonia cases are due to inhalation (e.g., those due to *Mycobacterium tuberculosis*). And an even smaller proportion is due to spread from infections in other parts of the body through the bloodstream to the lung.

Influenza is often acquired by inhalation. It routinely causes lower respiratory tract infection with fever and cough. There can be sputum, but it's not purulent, and a chest x-ray is usually clear (i.e., it's not pneumonia). *Staphylococcus aureus* can colonize the upper respiratory tract and be aspirated into the lung to cause pneumonia but also can spread from other infection sites to a lung through the bloodstream and cause expanding pneumatoceles – round opacities with central necrosis and cavitation (i.e., a different pattern on chest x-ray).

The term "aspiration pneumonia" is reserved for particular episodes of pneumonia in patients aspirating larger amounts. Impairment of the nervous system can result in more frequent aspiration and aspiration of larger volumes. This impairment can be temporary (e.g., decreased level of consciousness due to general anesthesia for surgery or acute alcohol intoxication) or chronic (e.g., glottic reflexes absent due to MS). A patient with a neurologically impaired lower esophageal sphincter causing gastroesophageal reflux disease is also more likely to regurgitate stomach contents. Lying in bed supine makes regurgitation and aspiration of stomach contents more likely [Torres A, Serra-Batlles J, ros E, Piera C, puig de la bellascasa J, cobos A, lomeña F. Pulmonary aspiration of gastric contents in patients receiving mechanical ventilation: the effect of body position. *Ann Intern Med.* 1992; 116:540-3.] . Tube feedings also make regurgitation and aspiration of stomach contents more likely.

Such aspiration can include saliva, food, drink, and regurgitated stomach contents – a suspension of macerated food (chime) and hydrochloric acid and sometimes bile and/or blood. Foreign bodies (e.g., food particles) at the site of an aspiration make infection more likely and harder to treat; they make it harder for the immune system (macrophages and white blood cells) to devour and dispose of microbes. The more foreign bodies there are, the likelier an aspiration will result in pneumonia. Regurgitated hydrochloric acid can cause a chemical pneumonia (Mendelson's syndrome) that is often fatal; symptoms resemble those of pneumonia.

When aspiration occurs, many different microbes can be aspirated into the lungs, but some are more likely to cause pneumonia than others. One reason is that some microbes are more virulent (powerful) than others (e.g., *Streptococcus pneumoniae* and *Staphylococcus aureus* are more virulent than *Staphylococcus epidermidis,* which colonizes virtually all human beings but is relatively wimpy and almost never causes pneumonia even when aspirated). Another reason is numbers (i.e., some microbes are far more numerous than others in the fluid being aspirated; for example, patients with poor oral hygiene can have very high concentrations of bacteria in saliva and patients requiring gastric acid suppression because of gastroesophageal reflux disease or because of mechanical ventilation in an intensive care unit can develop very high concentrations of bacteria in the stomach).

"Aspiration pneumonia" caused by larger volume aspiration tends to be associated with a different set of microbes—aerobic bacteria transiently colonizing the throat or stomach or anaerobic bacteria chronically inhabiting the gingival crevices between teeth. Aerobic bacteria are those that can live happily in the presence of oxygen while anaerobic bacteria are those that prefer an absence of oxygen (e.g., there is a low concentration of oxygen in the crevices between teeth and anaerobes living in those crevices typically metabolize food particles left on the teeth and produce foul-smelling metabolites [the source of "morning breath"]).. Aerobic and anaerobic bacteria live in the other end of the gastrointestinal tract (the colon) as well, metabolizing undigested foodstuffs flowing downstream where the anaerobes produce foul-smelling metabolites that impart the characteristic feculent odor of feces

Methods of Prevention

Can patients who aspirate larger amounts do anything to prevent aspiration pneumonia, the type of pneumonia for which MS patients are a special setup? Only one of the other 8 books about MS mentioned above discusses prevention of pneumonia. It says that MS patients prone to aspirating larger amounts can reduce their risk with swallowing exercises prescribed by a speech pathologist. I'm a great fan of exercise, which can strengthen muscles weakened by deconditioning, but I'm somewhat doubtful that actual paresis or paralysis due to MS-related destruction of the central nervous system can be corrected by exercise. And I'm doubtful that swallowing exercises do much to prevent aspiration pneumonia.

Why am I doubtful? There doesn't yet seem to be consistent evidence from randomized trials documenting significantly lower pneumonia rates after swallowing exercises. One recent review of exercise-based dysphagia rehabilitation concluded that there were "more questions than answers" about this topic and that more research was needed.[Burkhead LM, Sapienza CM, Rosenbek JC. Strength-training exercise in dysphagia rehabilitation: principles, procedures, and directions for future research. Dysphagia. 2007; 22:251-65.] Another recent review said that "reduction in post swallow residues [was] uncommon after such swallowing exercises."[Steele CM. Exercise-based approaches to dysphagia rehabilitation. Nestlé Nutr Inst Workshop Ser. 2012; 72:109-117. doi. 10.1159/000339999.]

Another reason I'm skeptical is that my choking often happens when I'm not trying to swallow (i.e., saliva or drink just slides down at the wrong time). This can happen during the day or during the night when asleep. After fracturing a metatarsal bone in my foot once and another bone in my left hip (femur) 3 different times, I slept in a recliner for a cumulative total of 78 days and had markedly increased aspiration of saliva each time. I woke many times in the recliner choking and coughing. I believe this increased aspiration was due to the back of the recliner being up 10° to 20° above horizontal and that gravity made saliva slide "downhill." Because this can happen when I'm not swallowing, it seems unlikely that swallowing exercises would prevent that.

As stated above, pneumonia due to *Streptococcus pneumoniae* is not the type of pneumonia MS patients are specially predisposed to get, but there is a very effective vaccine for preventing it and its complications, and I believe MS patients should get that vaccine – because they do poorly with respiratory infections in general. [Centers for Disease Control and Prevention. Updated recommendations for prevention of invasive pneumococcal disease among adults using the 23-valent pneumococcal polysaccharide vaccine (PPSV23).

Morbidity and Mortality Weekly Report. 2010; 59:1102-1106.] This ounce of prevention will usually be worth more than a pound of cure for a pneumococcal infection.

So is there another way that works to prevent aspiration pneumonia? I believe there may be multiple things a patient can do to make regurgitation and aspiration less likely.

Being chronically slumped over with poor posture due to weakness and spasticity makes regurgitation more likely. I have noticed that my episodes of regurgitation tend to occur after meals when the stomach is full and I feel the need to burp. Burping is a normal way that the stomach can remove air swallowed with food, but tends to bring up liquid gastric contents in a patient with GERD (gastroesophageal reflux disease due to impairment of the lower esophageal sphincter). When I feel a burp coming on, I therefore try to brace myself (whether sitting or standing) and straighten my spine as best I can and try to burp (twice or three times is better than once). Sitting up straighter during the burp uses gravity to help reduce the risk of regurgitation. Since I started doing this, I have had no regurgitation of stomach contents. So, taking such precautions may help prevent aspiration of stomach contents during the day. Preventing regurgitation of stomach contents can also be done by avoiding lying down while eating and during the time required for gastric emptying (about five hours seems to work for me). For patients unable to do these things, lying down in a semi recumbent position (e.g., raising the head of the bed 30° to 45° from horizontal) uses gravity to make regurgitation of stomach contents less likely. [Draculovic MB, Torres A, Bauer TT, Nicolas JM, Nogue s, Ferrer M. Supine body position as a risk factor for nosocomial pneumonia in mechanically ventilated patients: a randomized trial. *Lancet.* 1999; 354:1851-8."]

Choking on food obviously occurs only when the patient is eating, so being careful and taking smaller bites make sense. Socializing while eating – telling jokes, boisterous laughing, etc. – becomes more risky once the MS patient starts choking. I still socialize at dinner, but less often than before and I try to be especially careful (e.g., I try not to become overly engaged in the conversation while chewing food).

Another strategy that might be more important for preventing aspiration pneumonia is reducing the inoculum of bacteria that gets aspirated by improving oral hygiene. In studies of hospital patients, use of chlorhexidine mouthwash or gel was associated with a 40% reduction in ventilator associated pneumonia. [Shi Z, xie H, Wang P, zhang Q, Wu Y, Chen E, ng L, Worthington HV Needleman I, Furness S. Oral hygiene care for critically ill patients to prevent ventilator associated pneumonia. Cochrane Database Syst Rev. 2013;8CD008367. doi: 10. 1002/14651858.CD008367.pub2:] This suggests that the microbes causing ventilator associated pneumonia often come from the mouth and oral hygiene may help prevent such episodes. But there was no added benefit from tooth brushing. The benefit of other oral mouthwashes was not documented in this meta-analysis. Microbes coming from regurgitated stomach contents would be unlikely to respond to oral hygiene.

Something else that may help is daily flossing of the teeth. I say that not because I found studies documenting efficacy (I actually couldn't find any evaluating use of dental floss), but because it seemed to help me prevent aspiration pneumonia.

Here's what happened to me: I had for years used dental floss daily for dental hygiene at the recommendation of my dentist and dental hygienist (for clarity, their recommendation had nothing to do with my diagnosis of MS). As my left arm became increasingly paralyzed, in the 17th year after diagnosis, I lost the ability to floss my teeth because using dental floss the conventional way requires two hands. After I became unable to floss my teeth, my daily oral hygiene consisted of brushing my teeth with Crest toothpaste after breakfast, supper and sometimes lunch.

Months after I lost the ability to floss my teeth, I had a series of three episodes of vigorous cough associated with purulent, blood tinged sputum, each lasting a couple of weeks. I was sure that these episodes of cough and purulent sputum must be related to my in-creasing inability to control saliva, food and fluids in my throat. I also knew that the vigorous cough and purulent blood tinged spu-tum had to be coming from my lungs-- most likely mild aspiration pneumonias. At the time, I didn't think about the recent cessation of dental flossing and assumed like most everybody else would have that this was just due to aspiration from continuing progression of my long-standing MS-related dysphagia.

Some months later, I went to visit my dentist for regular care and was informed that dental floss picks could be used with one hand. I ordered some (Oral-B Glide Floss Picks), started using them, and never had another episode of cough with purulent blood tinged sputum. My approach to oral hygiene at that point was as follows: After breakfast, I would rinse my mouth with water until no more flecks of food were visible. Then I would floss between my teeth, starting with the upper and lower incisors, and then, switching to a different, older, Oral-B Glide Floss Pick, I would floss the rest of my teeth. Switching to a different, older, Oral-B Glide Floss Pick was done because the floss of a new pick was thicker, stiffer and more likely to break than an older, previously used Oral-B Glide Floss Pick when forced between my molars and premolars. When flossing my teeth, I would routinely gently force the floss between two teeth and then gently force the floss down below the gum line twice beside each of the two teeth. After flossing, I would rinse the pick free of food particles and let it air dry, discarding a pick only when the floss broke—usually after about a week of use. After finishing, I would rinse my mouth with water again until no more flecks of food were visible. Then I would brush my teeth with Crest toothpaste. After that, I would rinse my mouth with water again until no more flecks of food were visible. After lunch and supper, I would follow the same procedure, except that I didn't repeat the floss picking. To do this much tooth brushing, I found that it was more comfortable for me with a very soft toothbrush. My dental hygienist said that the softest toothbrushes available were "postsurgical" toothbrushes intended for patients to use after oral surgery (ordered online from Gum).

As mentioned above, aspiration pneumonias are often caused by bacteria that inhabit the gingival crevices. Putting my observations together with what was already known led me to believe that worsening aspiration due to MS and my losing the ability to floss had caused the 3 mild aspiration pneumonias. I didn't reach this conclusion until several more years had passed with worsening dysphagia and choking but without any more episodes of vigorous cough with purulent sputum.

The probability that this sequence (i.e., three months [25%] with new, mild aspiration pneumonia during 12 months of not flossing as compared with none [0%] in the next 84 months after resuming daily flossing using the dental floss pick) happened by chance was 0.0019, Fisher's exact test, 2-tailed. This means that this change in rate was unlikely to have been due to chance (i.e., daily flossing probably prevented recurrent aspiration pneumonia).

My career in internal medicine with sub-specialization in infectious diseases and epidemiology helped me recognize what had happened. Pasteur said, "Chance favors the prepared mind."

So, if oral hygiene with daily flossing prevented recurrent aspiration pneumonia for me, does that mean that it will work for all MS patients? That will depend upon the results of follow-up studies. If an MS patient suffering recurrent aspiration pneumonia understands and is able to do what I did, it seems likely that it should work. But, if someone doesn't understand or lacks the manual dexterity to do it, it probably won't work for that individual. A relatively small study (e.g., 10 patients randomly assigned to use the same oral hygiene that I used with daily flossing and regular tooth brushing and 10 more randomized to just use regular tooth brushing) would probably give a good idea whether and how well the approach might work. For the study to have meaningful results, the 20 patients would have to have impairment of glottic reflexes severe enough that they were already experiencing episodes of aspiration pneumonia like I was.

In the meantime, what should an MS patient at risk for aspiration pneumonia be doing? My recommendation would be to use daily flossing and regular tooth brushing. Your dentist will be pleased whether this works to prevent aspiration pneumonia or not.

Postscript: I suffered a really bad aspiration while awake 6 years after I resumed flossing my teeth – so bad that I assumed that another episode of aspiration pneumonia probably would occur. The aspiration happened just after supper (a bowl of pea soup, a piece of blackberry and blueberry pie and a 12 ounce glass of orange juice). The volume aspirated was apparently larger than usual for me because I immediately became dyspneic (short of breath) and started coughing vigorously and repeatedly. The dyspnea and coughing lasted most of an hour. These symptoms were much worse than those of any aspiration I'd ever had. The French have a phrase "*grand mal*" ("great ailment") that is often used to denote a particularly bad form of epilepsy. I think of that instance as my "*grand mal*" aspiration.

It also seemed that this event might pose another rigorous test of my hypothesis that daily flossing of my teeth was protecting me from aspiration pneumonia. No symptoms of pneumonia developed. This implies that the microbial inoculum is a key determinant of whether aspiration leads to pneumonia even when there is regurgitation of enough gastric contents to cause significant respiratory embarrassment (hard coughing and difficulty breathing for an hour).

Chapter 32
My Approach to Preventing Urinary Tract Infection

"Will all great Neptune's ocean wash clean this my hand? Nay, this my hand will rather the multitudinous seas incarnadine." – William Shakespeare, *Macbeth*

Pretty much all publications addressing the issue seem to agree that urinary tract infections are a big problem for MS patients. They are right.

But two thirds of MS patients are women, and women are anatomically more predisposed to urinary tract infection anyway (up to half getting a bladder infection at some point) because of a shorter urethra and the urethral meatus being closer to the anus (bacteria from the colon like *Escherichia coli* being the usual cause of urinary tract infection). Women are so used to urinary tract infections that they often regard it as more a nuisance than an important problem.

So, what's the big deal with UTIs in MS patients? They are worse for MS patients partly because they occur more frequently due to neurophysiology scrambled by MS damage to the central nervous system, which makes urine stay in the urethra after voiding. Fluid in the urethra facilitates transmission of microbes to the bladder by capillarity after contamination of the urethral meatus.

They are also worse because MS patients already struggling with urinary urgency, nocturia and incontinence have these problems accentuated during cystitis.

In addition to this increased suffering, urinary tract infection can be lethal for MS patients. In a recent national study of causes of death in MS patients, urinary tract infection was one of the leading proximate causes of death (MS itself was the most frequent "underlying" cause of death).[Redelings MD, McCoy L, Sorvillo F. Multiple sclerosis mortality and patterns of comorbidity in the United States from 1990 to 2001 *Neuroepidemiology*. 2006; 26:102-7.]

As mentioned in Chapter 2, my approach to preventing urinary tract infections differed from what other books for MS patients recommended. And the other books' recommendations didn't always jibe with one another either. For example, the books by Drs. Lechtenberg and Giesser each made 4 recommendations for preventing urinary tract infection but only agreed about two: the need to acidify urine by consuming products such as cranberry juice and avoiding orange juice and tomato juice and, if all of their recommendations failed and the patient had frequent urinary tract infections anyway, taking chronic antibiotics such as trimethoprim sulfamethoxazole. Their approaches to preventing UTIs in MS patients seemed to accept fecal contamination of the urethral meatus as inevitable.

The reason that Drs.Lechtenberg and Giesser disagree about this is that their recommendations are mostly not evidence-based and thus subject to opinion.

Acidifying the urine with cranberry juice is an old time nostrum that, as mentioned above, was recently reported by a Cochrane meta-analysis to be ineffective. If patients are going to be having frequent infections and have to take chronic antibiotics, this would seem to be an admission that their other prophylactic measures don't work very well. Reasons for disagreeing with their other four recommendations were listed in Chapter 2.

My approach to preventing urinary tract infections also involved four preventive measures, but focused more on preventing a) fecal contamination of the urethral meatus and b) retrograde transmission of any contaminating microbes from the urethral meatus to the bladder:

1) trying to minimize urine left in the urethra after voiding by blotting the urethral meatus with toilet paper using hands cleaned with soap and water washing, alcohol hand gel, or both [this blotting was done in three stages after voiding –i) holding a sufficient stack of toilet paper over the urethral meatus while massaging pelvic floor muscles in the perineum, ii) next wringing urine remaining in the urethra by holding the same stack of toilet paper over the meatus while clasping the penis between the thumb and index finger of my paretic left hand, and iii) a final more bibulous blot with a single new sheet of toilet paper] (it has been said that "necessity is the mother of invention," and I discovered as my hemiparesis worsened that I could do steps i and ii almost as well with one hand by holding the toilet paper stack over the urethral meatus with thumb and index finger while the third finger massages pelvic floor muscles and my hand tries wringing out urine remaining in the urethra);

2) trying to minimize the risk of fecal contamination after a bowel movement by using soap and water on toilet paper to clean the anus;

3) trying to minimize the risk of fecal contamination after an episode of fecal incontinence by immediately removing the contaminated clothes and cleansing myself with soap and water in the shower; and

4) trying to minimize the risk of fecal contamination of the urethral meatus during bathing by finishing all washing of the genitalia before washing of the buttocks.

Like the 4 measures recommended by Dr. Lechtenberg and the 4 measures recommended by Dr. Giesser, my 4 preventive measures were not based on data from epidemiologic studies, but their measures were routinely associated with high rates of UTI among MS patients and my 4 measures were associated with no UTIs during my first 20 years and 8 months of MS. During that time, I was at high risk for developing a UTI the whole time, but got none while giving myself more than 7,500 showers and having fecal incontinence more than 30 times. The reason that I didn't use their preventive measures was that I couldn't find supportive data (i.e., none of the measures seemed to be evidence-based).

Could the observed difference (i.e., a high rate of UTI with conventional measures and a low rate of UTI with the four measures that I was using) be due to chance alone? Yes, but, as explained in the Introduction, the probability of such a large difference being due to chance would be low. A recent review said that most MS patients got bladder infection (cystitis). I had none over 20.6 years. If one assumes that half of 200 MS patients would get cystitis over 20 years (i.e., 4,000 patient-years), then my getting none over 20 patient-years was unlikely due to chance ($p < 0.0001$).

When my neurologist referred me to another neurologist specializing in care of MS patients to see if a second opinion about possible therapeutic approaches would prove useful, the MS specialist expressed skepticism that I could have gone so long without urinary tract infection and insisted that I submit a urine specimen for urinalysis and urine culture. I was told that she believed this would document acute and/or chronic urinary tract infection. She was wrong. The urine showed no evidence of infection. My specialty before retirement due to MS was infectious disease epidemiology (i.e., the study of the causes and prevention of infectious diseases).

After 20 years and eight months of having no UTIs, I stopped being able to bathe myself in the shower when I fell eight times during nine days, which caused multiple fractures. One of the falls occurred as I exited the shower, which made me lose confidence in my ability to walk in and out of the shower safely. This development made it harder for me to adhere to my third and fourth preventive measures (showering immediately after fecal incontinence and always washing the genitalia before the anus when showering). During the first week of being bathed by nursing aides, one of the aides violated my fourth preventive measure. Instead of proceeding from front to back with a washcloth, she washed the anus and then reached around front and grabbed my genitalia with the now contaminated washcloth and started scrubbing the glans penis. I said, "No, stop!" But it was too late.

Exactly 7 hours later I began to have dramatic symptoms of a urinary tract infection: pain over the urinary bladder, urgency to urinate, increased frequency of urination, burning painful dysuria when I voided, and burning pain following voiding; an additional confirmation that this was a urinary tract infection due to an aerobic gram-negative bacillus was rapid response of all of the symptoms to starting ciprofloxacin therapy (i.e., within hours).

Unfortunately, the rapid response was no guarantee that there would be no more problems for the urinary tract. Because the urinary tract in an MS patient is so impaired, I decided to treat for a week to be sure that the last microbe was indeed dead in the urinary tract. That duration of therapy resulted in prominent overgrowth of *Candida* (a fungus that is commonly present inside the gastrointestinal tract) with redness and irritation around the anus.

I was well aware when that happened that a ricochet urinary tract infection due to *Candida* was an important risk because the urinary tract was so impaired by MS and because I had to do blotting of the urethral meatus every time I voided to avoid dribbling urine on my underwear, pants and shoes. This posed a risk for contaminating the urethral meatus with the abundant *Candida* that was overgrowing due to the ciprofloxacin.

I decided to stop the ciprofloxacin after the sixth day because of the *Candida* infection. The symptoms of the urinary tract infection had ended four days earlier. The same day, a new urinary infection due to *Candida* started (same symptoms as before). This time I started an antifungal drug, fluconazole, and the symptoms immediately began responding like before, but took longer to completely disappear. The recommended duration of treating a *Candida* bladder

UTI (cystitis) is two weeks, and when that was finished, I remained asymptomatic with no more ricochet urinary tract infections.

After that, I continued to receive daily care from the nursing aides including help with bathing, which after a couple of months started being a shower using a shower chair, but I always insisted on using my only good hand to do the washing of my own genitalia and buttocks. I stopped having urinary tract infections after I started doing that again. I also did the drying of those private parts while the nurse aides helped to make sure that I didn't fall while doing that and helped me dry other anatomic parts that I couldn't reach such as my back, underarms, elbows, etc..

I had a third bacterial urinary tract infection six months later following an episode of fecal incontinence in my pants (i.e., the day after), again confirming the importance of fecal contamination from incontinence as a cause of urinary tract infection. This occurred six months after I stopped being able to shower myself immediately after fecal incontinence. Losing the ability to bathe oneself makes showering immediately after fecal incontinence difficult to do. I still tried to wash the contaminated buttocks with soap and water while sitting on the toilet and then change clothes, but that's not as thorough as bathing the area under running water in the shower.

I believe that these three UTIs after I stopped being able to bathe myself serve to confirm the importance of fecal contamination of the urethral meatus in causing UTIs in MS patients and of preventing this contamination by bathing immediately after fecal incontinence.

It's important to understand that any visible fecal staining represents unacceptable contamination that could make urinary tract infection considerably more likely. This means that a "wet fart" can require as much time and trouble for cleanup as a full bowel movement does. This may seem much more than normal, healthy people might do, but an MS patient isn't healthy. If the "wet fart" stained the underwear, I would immediately remove them and put on a new pair after cleaning up as for a bowel movement).

Chapter 33
Preventing Other Types of Skin Infections

"What an agony it is to cut the fingernails of my right hand."
  – Anton Chekhov
"Chekhov had no idea about the difficulty of cutting fingernails."
  – Barry Farr

M S patients are predisposed to skin infections for a variety of reasons. Preventing skin infections requires different measures from those mentioned above for pneumonia and urinary tract infection.

Chapter 28 discussed how MS-related paresis and gravity collaborate to cause pressure-related infections of skin and how this might be prevented.

Gravity also causes fluid to pool in a paretic extremity (i.e., edema), which causes multiple problems for MS patients including an increased risk of infection. Cellulitis (a common bacterial infection of the skin usually due to *Staphylococcus aureus* or *Streptococcus pyogenes*) is more frequent in an edematous leg. This has happened in my paretic leg multiple times.

Untreated cellulitis can cause important problems for MS patients (pain, fever [which can make MS patients weak], nausea and vomiting [which can lead to aspiration that can result in trouble breathing and pneumonia], or bloodstream infection, which can be lethal).

Cellulitis often begins where there is a defect in the skin. One of my family members got infected from getting a splinter in her finger while lighting a fire. She was a fully healthy 54-year-old woman who died of bloodstream infection. Infection can kill an MS patient more easily.

Fatal infections can start off appearing trivial (e.g., an ingrown toenail on a toe that had never before caused any problem, an abrasion that didn't get fully covered by antibiotic ointment and bandaged etc.) and advance rapidly if not promptly treated. In a study referenced above, bloodstream infection was the third leading cause of death in MS patients, most often from infection at the site of a pressure sore. [Redelings MD, McCoy L, Sorvillo F. Multiple sclerosis mortality and patterns of comorbidity in the United States from 1990 to 2001 *Neuroepidemiology*. 2006; 26:102-7.]

Any defect in the skin can become infected. In my paretic left leg, an ulcer started forming two separate times over the malleolus at the ankle. I found that applying Vaseline lotion to it made these small ulcers better. After that I applied lotion to my legs daily, and the ulcers stopped forming.

MS patients fall frequently, which can result in many abrasions, each of which needs to be carefully cleaned with soap and water, dried, and then bandaged after application of antibiotic ointment to the abrasion (I used polymyxin, neomycin, bacitracin ointment).. But all of the effort and assistance required for repeatedly applying ointments and Band-Aids can pose considerable difficulty for a profoundly disabled patient.

Band-Aids help heal abrasions when placed correctly over an abrasion, but are counterproductive when placed incorrectly; for example, placing the Band-Aid pad on the abrasion reduces pain and speeds healing, but placing the sticky tape directly on the abrasion does the opposite. Tape applied across an abrasion causes considerable pain and tears the healing skin when the bandage is removed. I mention this because I have had nurse aide helpers do the latter six times despite my pleading to avoid that. Because a disabled MS patient is often unable to see abrasions after a fall, it's important to have clear communications with those applying bandages because some bandages work better than others. The nonstick pad of a Band-Aid keeps antibiotic ointment on the abrasion; plain, sterile cotton gauze absorbs the ointment, so it doesn't work as well. Cotton gauze also causes pain (i.e., as compared with a nonstick pad) when I'm trying to get into bed, which puts pressure on the bandage.

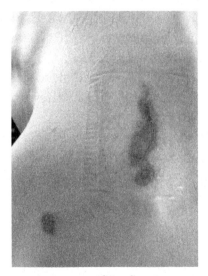 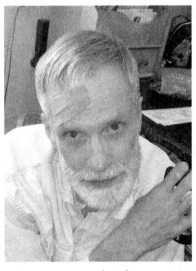

Figure 33-1 Skin abrasions like this occur frequently and require careful application of antibiotic ointment and bandages to promote healing and prevent infection.

Figure 33-2 Band-Aids covering an abrasion on the forehead.

Another type of infection also got worse in my paretic, edematous leg – athlete's foot (tinea pedis). After having athlete's foot involving both feet for decades with good control with tolnaftate cream therapy each day after a bath, the athlete's foot got worse in the paretic, edematous foot despite continuation of that therapy in both feet.

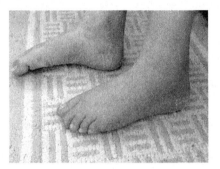

Figure 33-3 The swollen, paretic left leg has worse fungal infection due to *Trichophyton rubrum* (athlete's foot), visible as redness and scaling.

Athlete's foot causes cracks and fissures which can predispose to repeated cellulitis. Regular bathing of the feet with soap and water, towel drying, and then application of antifungal cream (tolnaftate or clotrimazole) can help control athlete's foot.

MS patients often lose the ability to clip their own nails. This is important because untrimmed nails are more than just unattractive. Overly long nails, especially on spastic extremities, can dig into the skin like claws or the talons of raptors, which can cause a bloody mess, a problem for cleanup and also for possible potentiation of falling (e.g., from a slippery floor). The damaged skin can get infected, an important problem for MS patients in more than one way. Moreover, untrimmed nails can break, which can become an even larger problem than just gouging the skin.

Ingrowing toenails also can cause repeated cellulitis. Ingrowing toenails can be prevented by stuffing cotton under the edge of the toenail before it can grow into the flesh. This is a conventional approach, which a surgeon taught me to do. After a toenail biopsy, I started putting 4% chlorhexidine gluconate on that same toenail every day before a bath and the toenail stopped growing. The toe had been injured in a compulsory woodshop class when I was 13 years old in the ninth grade and, after falling off, the toenail repeatedly grew back for 45 years causing many infections as it grew into the flesh of the toe. I started putting the chlorhexidine gluconate on the toenail daily for a different reason, but noted the fortuitous result mentioned above – the toenail stopped growing. For the next five years, it required no clipping and didn't grow into the flesh of the toe. I then clipped several other (rams horn) toenails short and treated them with daily application of the same antiseptic, but they didn't stop growing. It may only work for toenails that fall off and repeatedly grow back. An answer will require trial on other such toenails.

Toenail management is a difficult problem for many elderly patients, but especially so for a patient with hemiparesis (i.e. a very weak leg and arm) due to MS because sitting anywhere becomes a risk for falling, and leaning over to cut toenails increases this risk. MS related spasticity also causes the toes tend to curl under like claws, which makes reaching a toenail with the one good arm more difficult.

The WE Bassett company in Shelton, Connecticut makes barrel spring toenail nippers for cutting thick toenails (Neat Feet Pedicure by Trim). I have found these to be handy for clipping toenails with onychogryphosis (i.e., Ram's horn toenails). Would such special toenail clippers be helpful for MS patients, and if so, why? I believe they would because they have helped me. As one proceeds further into disability everything gets harder to do including cutting toenails. With increasing age, toenails can become thicker and harder to cut for various reasons. Such nippers are very helpful for cutting such toenails that can be impossible to cut with regular toenail clippers.

Patients with cognitive deficits or with insufficient strength or dexterity to cut their own toenails need regular help from someone to do this. In some cases a podiatrist might be required, but maneuvering a homebound, wheelchair patient to and from regular clinic visits for any purpose becomes increasingly difficult as the disability increases and other problems emerge (e.g., urinary frequency and urgency).

To help prevent cellulitis in the foot, the MS patient also should regularly stretch spastic toes to prevent their turning into claw toes or mallet toes because these evolving deformities put unnatural pressure on the toe, which can cause such infection. During my 24th year of MS, my fourth right toe started turning into a mallet toe, which put so much pressure on the nail that an ingrown toenail and cellulitis resulted. After therapy with dicloxacillin, I started stretching the toe regularly and the toe turned back into a regular fourth toe, which caused no further trouble.

Avoiding high salt intake can help minimize edema. My biggest problem with salt intake was processed, commercial food products, which often include more sodium than optimal. One of the reasons for this was that I had stopped adding salt to food with a salt shaker at the table decades earlier when I was a freshman medical student. An example of a processed food with high sodium content that would reliably be followed by increased edema of my paretic leg was Amy's Asian Noodles (610 mg sodium). Two more examples were Amy's Teriyaki Bowl (780 mg sodium) and Amy's Brown Rice with vegetables (550 mg sodium). Amy's Light in Sodium Brown Rice with Vegetables (270 mg sodium) did not cause as much swelling.

I've seen no data from studies addressing this, but I seem to get worse abrasions when I fall wearing thin summer pajamas than when I wear thicker flannel pajamas.

Pressure sores usually occur on the bottom (buttock or sacrum) of a patient with paralysis or advancing paresis. Preventing pressure sores requires keeping the paralyzed patient from lying or sitting too long in one position (because the pressure impedes blood flow in the paralyzed flesh, eventually resulting in necrosis [death] of the skin and thus giving microbes the upper hand). I got two pressure sores after lying on the floor all night when my helpers were unable to hear me and I was unable to move enough.

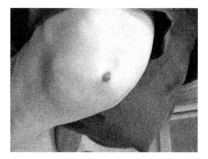

Figure 33-5 A pressure sore over the right knee three days after lying on the floor all night.

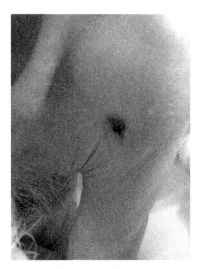

Figure 33-4 A pressure sore over the left shoulder three days after lying on the floor all night.

Before the paresis gets bad enough to cause a pressure sore, it can result in pressure-related furuncles (boils) on the buttock of the leg being paralyzed (as discussed in Chapter 28). If nothing is done, the furuncle can keep growing and turn into a carbuncle, a larger infection from which bloodstream infection is more likely.

The proper, medically accepted therapy of a furuncle is repeated application of a warm moist compress. The risk of not applying heat is that the infection will keep getting worse and result in bloodstream infection. The risk of using hot water on a washcloth to apply a warm moist compress to a furuncle on the buttock is that too much heat can be applied, scalding the skin. For that reason, the patient should only apply warm moist compresses herself if she still has intact sensation at that site. If the skin is numb, the only safe way to apply warm moist compresses would be to have an assistant do it with direct visualization of the skin. The assistant would need to understand that a burn injury could be much worse than a furuncle and therefore avoid applying too much heat.

Applying warm moist compresses is difficult for a patient with hemiparesis, requiring use of a hand mirror to confirm that the compress applied heat to the correct site. An easier approach for me has been using a handheld hair dryer. I turn it on and blow warm air over the likely site, trying to include generous margins so I don't miss. By using a continual, circular motion, I am able to avoid applying too much heat to any square centimeter of skin. After applying heat this way for several minutes, my mirror has always confirmed success (not true with the warm moist compress). In addition to making application to the correct site easier, using the hairdryer is quicker than heating and pouring water for warm moist compresses. A down side of using a hairdryer is that it still could be used incorrectly and scald the skin. It also can heat up the bathroom 2° to 3° within those few minutes. Either way, an MS patient with hemiparesis has to be careful to avoid scalding skin or falling while applying heat to the buttock.

Can antibiotics be used to treat *Staphylococcus aureus* furuncles? In a pinch, they may be useful, but in a patient with furuncles due to unrelenting pressure, the pressure impedes blood flow, which makes delivery of the antibiotic to the site of infection unreliable. This made antibiotic therapy less effective for me when I tried it in a desperate situation.

Pressure-related furuncles on the buttock from sitting too long on a chair or on too firm a surface can be prevented with an alternating air cushion, as discussed in Chapter 28. But an alternating air cushion can't prevent furuncles related to other types of pressure (e.g., from pinching the butt cheeks closed [i.e., to prevent fecal incontinence] or from sitting too long on the toilet without moving). The location of a furuncle will usually give a clue as to which type of pressure was responsible. For example, pinching the butt cheeks closed will result in more medial furuncles, closer to the anus. And sitting too long on the toilet without moving results in a furuncle on part of the buttock, sacrum or leg that would correspond to where the toilet seat supports flesh. If the patient has any question, the area of toilet seat pressure often can be easily confirmed with a hand-held mirror after getting up from the toilet.

If an alternating air cushion can't be used to affect risk from pinching the butt cheeks or from sitting on the toilet, are any alternative measures available for preventing those types of pressure-related infection? I believe the former can be prevented by applying heat (e.g., with warm moist compresses or a hairdryer in the area of the butt that was pinched) and the latter can be prevented by raising up off of the toilet seat every minute or two when stuck with prolonged waiting for an "imminent" bowel movement. Heat can also be applied in the distribution of the toilet seat after being stuck on the toilet seat and unable to move for too long (e.g., because of the need to clean up after fecal incontinence). Using these three measures, I have been able to go more than a year without getting a new furuncle on the buttock of my paretic leg.

Folliculitis is another red bump that is not the same as a furuncle. It's smaller, doesn't cause pain and occurs in the setting of dry skin. Furuncles require warm moist compress therapy, while for folliculitis, moisturizing lotion usually does the trick for me.

Chapter 34
Food Poisoning

Food poisoning caused me difficulties throughout the time that I had MS – during high-dose steroid therapy for an MS relapse early in the disease and also late in the disease (perhaps due to senescence of the immune system, immunomodulatory drugs, proton pump inhibitor therapy, etc.). How I dealt with these problems varied at different times with different particular problems. During the early phase of the disease, the problem almost always occurred when I ate food at a restaurant that was not fully cooked (e.g., eating a fast food sandwich with raw lettuce, tomatoes, etc). That was addressed by avoiding such fast food sandwiches and asking that any food ordered at a restaurant be cooked well done and delivered to the table "sizzling hot" with no raw foods or flowers added as a garnish. In the tropics where *tourista* is frequent, travelers are advised to eat only food that is recently cooked and still steaming hot unless it's fruit that they clean and peel themselves.

Later on, as the problem changed somewhat, the way I had to deal with it also changed. After I began taking a proton pump inhibitor daily, I started having problems with foods stored in the refrigerator (i.e., using the system of refrigerator storage that my wife had learned from her mother), which had not previously caused me any problem. For that, we had to change the method of refrigerator management so that foods were refrigerated promptly after being cooked and stored in the refrigerator for a much shorter period (especially foods more prone to cause food poisoning such as potato salad or mashed potatoes [as opposed to a baked potato or hashbrowns]). I also had to stop eating fresh fruit because I got food poisoning multiple times after eating raw fresh fruit (e.g., strawberries). After doing without fresh fruit for an extended period, I decided to try using heat to make food poisoning less likely (e.g., pouring boiling water into a cup containing blueberries or an apple or grapes and letting them sit in the hot water for a couple of minutes). It worked. This approach cannot be applied to all fruit (e.g., strawberries), since some fruits like strawberries are more fragile and will become a macerated mush in the hot water.

A modification of this also had to be used after I developed food poisoning from trying to eat guacamole. Heating the guacamole in a microwave didn't work (i.e., still caused food poisoning), but putting the guacamole in a saucepan and adding some water so that it could be boiled for a full five minutes while continually stirring to avoid burning. This did the trick. After boiling off the excess water, the guacamole returns to its original consistency with no alteration in taste and does not cause food poisoning in a compromised host.

On the other hand, I was able to eat tomatoes that had been washed with soap and water, sliced and then "nuked" for a few minutes in a microwave. Aesthetically compromised tomato slices are much better than no tomato slices at all.

Because an MS patient becomes klutzy due to the combination of weakness and spasticity, an episode of food poisoning with diarrhea can make it hard for the patient to make it to the toilet and get his pants down in time. Diarrhea all over one's clothes, one's shoes, and the floor will make an MS patient begin to think that maybe retirement isn't such a bad idea – especially when this happens repeatedly. Cleaning up the mess is also much harder for an MS patient, who is more likely to fall if he steps in something slippery like a pool of diarrhea. Getting his clothes and shoes off can become a tricky proposition. Then the clothes and shoes have to be washed and the patient has to change clothes. All of this can take hours, which can become an extreme problem for someone still trying to work, and be available at the office answering everyone's questions. Some gastrointestinal infections don't just affect the lower gastrointestinal tract, but can cause both nausea and emesis. Nausea and emesis are special problems for an MS patient in more than one way. If the patient has to suddenly vomit, just like with diarrhea, it may be impossible to reach the toilet in time, meaning that the emesis may end up on the floor, in the patient's bed, on the rug, all over the patient's clothes and shoes. These are nightmare scenarios for an MS patient who has not yet begun having a nursing aide provide assistance with activities of daily living. If the MS patient were to make it to the toilet, it's not clear that the patient could bend forward and vomit vigorously into the toilet without falling into the toilet himself and getting stuck. The author has fallen into a toilet and gotten stuck and had to be pulled out by someone else. Emesis can also result in aspiration causing pneumonia and death. Anorexia making the patient unable to eat and drink normally can result in constipation after the first illness subsides.

The grim prospect of such possibilities convinced me to stop eating raw salads or any other raw food sold commercially or in a restaurant.

Chapter 35
Treating Infection

The gold standard for treating infection for the past half-century has been use of an antibiotic or a synthesized antimicrobial drug (e.g., a sulfonamide). But this can be difficult for an MS patient, I found, due to rapid development of abdominal pain and diarrhea after starting a course. I asked my neurologist and infectious disease specialists focusing on gastrointestinal infections why they thought I had lost the ability to tolerate antibiotics. They said they had no idea.

During the time that I felt unable to take an antibiotic, I found several abrasions with early infection already starting. When this happened, I began a course of dicloxacillin while applying generous amounts of PNB (triple antibiotic) ointment to the abrasion and bandaging it. By doing this, I was able to cure several early infections despite continuing the dicloxacillin for only a couple of days at most and continuing once daily application of the PNB ointment until the lesion healed.

As mentioned above, the problem causing my intolerance of antibiotics was MS-related, but complicated. Because I had MS related constipation, I had to eat a special diet and take a laxative just to have a normal bowel movement. During a desperate situation in which cellulitis in my foot did not respond rapidly to dicloxacillin, I determined that I would have to keep taking the drug despite the abdominal pain and diarrhea, but tried reducing the doses of both dicloxacillin and the laxative I was taking (polyethylene glycol 3350 [MiraLAX]). This intuitive decision based on desperation rather than knowledge allowed me to figure out what had been making antibiotic therapy impossible for years: antibiotics and laxative both tend to loosen stools and combined, cause abdominal pain and diarrhea. By reducing the dose of one or both, I found that I was able to tolerate antibiotic therapy again. The problem was not specific to MS per se, but to a common treatment of MS (laxatives for constipation).

I used dicloxacillin to treat cellulitis at the site of a recurring ingrown toenail, to treat pre-popliteal bursitis, and to treat an occasional incipient infection at the site of an inadequately bandaged abrasion. It's very difficult for a patient with hemiparesis to see all of the abrasions occurring due to a fall and even harder for such a patient to apply antibiotic ointment and Band-Aids. If helping hands fail to apply ointment to all of the abraded skin, infection can start rapidly and things can go downhill in a hurry. Some doses of dicloxacillin in such situations can come to the rescue like the cavalry in an old western movie.

For an *Escherichia coli* urinary tract infection, ciprofloxacin for three days worked great, but if I tried treating longer, I got a very sore bottom by the sixth day due to overgrowth of yeast (*Candida*), which also resulted in an immediate ricochet urinary tract infection due to *Candida*. Of interest, ciprofloxacin therapy caused me less loose stools and no abdominal pain (unlike the dicloxacillin). The response to ciprofloxacin was immediate improvement of burning bladder pain, dysuria, urinary urgency and frequency. The *Candida* cystitis (bladder infection) responded well to fluconazole (two week course) but more slowly than the response to ciprofloxacin for treating bacterial cystitis.

Conventional, accepted therapy of *Staphylococcus aureus* furuncles is warm moist compresses. I found that a small hairdryer could provide the same heat and cure furuncles more easily with less time expended per application. Another important measure for treating a furuncle is getting weight off of it (e.g., standing, lying down in bed or in a recliner, etc.) for as little as a half hour during the morning and afternoon. After struggling for months using warm moist compresses alone, I found that lying down this much greatly enhanced the effect of the warm moist compresses.

Candida infection of the buttock (the same as a baby's diaper rash) may seem a trivial infection but can be an important and difficult complication to control. This is made more likely by increasing paralysis, which leads to staying on the buttock too much of the day. Incontinence adds to the problem because damp clothes increase the risk. Wearing incontinence pads or adult diapers also increase the risk because the bottom gets less air inside occlusive covers. Wearing a condom catheter to deal with incontinence also increases the risk. And if the infection occurs, all of these factors make it harder to treat. A diaper rash usually isn't fatal, but can be very uncomfortable to someone unable to get off of the bottom. Therapy usually requires a nystatin (antifungal) cream, often concocted with hydrocortisone and zinc oxide and applied three times per day. A similar product using nystatin cream with triamcinolone would give similar results initially, but the triamcinolone is far more potent and should not be used for days (because of the steroid's own side effects [e.g., too much steroids can cause a new problem called "red bag syndrome," in which the scrotum can become chronically red and painful]).

This may seem counterintuitive, but bathing with soap and water can make a *Candida* infection feel worse because of difficulty getting the bottom thoroughly dry before putting a paralyzed bottom back on the wheelchair seat. Spending more time drying the bottom is worthwhile and blowing cool air over it also seems to help. The Vidal Sassoon 1875 hairdryer mentioned above has a button for blowing cool air that seems useful for that purpose.

Chapter 36
Would Urine Dipsticks Be Helpful to MS Patients?

U rine dipsticks can be useful to MS patients when questions arise that they might help answer. For example, MS patients are at high risk for urinary tract infections. When urinary tract infection occurs, urine gets hazy, which the patient can see easily, but crystals in the urine (e.g., calcium oxalate) can also make urine hazy. A urine dipstick showing white blood cells and positive nitrite suggests a bacterial urinary tract infection. Urinary tract infection due to yeast (*Candida albicans*) is associated with pyuria (white blood cells in the urine) but a negative nitrite test. Sometimes the urine dipstick will also show red blood cells in the urine with urinary tract infection, but not as often as white blood cells. By contrast, when the patient has colicky pain from a kidney stone passing from the kidney into the ureter and thence into the bladder, red blood cells are almost always seen in the urine dipstick and white blood cells would be unusual. Nitrite would also be negative with most kidney stones (unless the kidney stone was associated with urinary tract infection, which can sometimes happen). If the patient develops hepatitis with pain in the right upper quadrant of the abdomen, the urine dipstick can show increased bilirubin and urobilinogen. Dipsticks allow patients to check urine pH, which may help patients attempting to acidify the urine.

As mentioned above, MS patients tend to be overweight. Being overweight predisposes a patient to diabetes mellitus ("sugar diabetes"). When diabetes is poorly controlled, sugar (glucose) spills into the urine. A dipstick can tell whether sugar is spilling into the urine and how much.

Chapter 37

How to Prevent Feculent Odor Due to a Rectal Sphincter Incontinent for Flatus?

In the 16th year after my diagnosis with MS, my rectal sphincter became incontinent for flatus. As revealed in Chapter 6, I had been mortified when flatus leaked out one time in a social situation in the third year after onset of my MS. That initial problem of losing control of flatus was dealt with by never leaving home before a morning bowel movement at the recommendation of my neurologist. This approach worked to prevent recurrence of the problem for 12 years.

But the new development was much worse. Instead of happening a single time, flatus floated out willy-nilly and frequently – sometimes five times per minute. This resulted in my being surrounded by a cloud of feculent odor over and over again throughout every day.

People often make fun of and laugh at the physical failings of others. A consummate comedian of the silent movie era, Charlie Chaplin practically made a career out of imitating physical failures (e.g., falling flat on his face, falling over backwards, etc). In the novel *The Old Man and the Boy*, Robert Ruark observed that, "Old dogs and old men smell bad." Likewise, the novel *Empire Falls* by Richard Russo humorously depicted a grandfather as senile and flatulent.

Actually, most old men don't smell bad. The reason some do is often that they lose control of their bowels because of various diseases (e.g., a stroke). The unpleasant smells of the human gastrointestinal tract from mouth to anus come from byproducts of microbial metabolism (mostly by anaerobic bacteria). And it's not just old men or old people in general that have such byproducts in their gastrointestinal tract. The same byproducts are usually present in the gastrointestinal tract of a toddler. Anybody who's visited a day care center or a nursing home probably knows what dirty diapers smell like.

To people losing control of their bowels, there's nothing funny about it.[Williams J. Flatus, odor, and the ostomist: coping strategies and interventions. *Br J Nurs*. 2008;17:S10,S12-S14.] This new loss of control seemed too embarrassing for me to want to be around people – even my family.

This unpleasant situation and the fact that my cumulative neurologic deficits had increased every year since onset of the disease made me believe that these changes would probably persist. This view convinced me that I needed to find something to control the problem as soon as possible.

As of that time, researchers had tried for many years without success to figure out what foods served as the substrate metabolized by colonic bacteria to produce the odoriferous gases that make flatus feculent. [Levitt MD. Intestinal gas production -- recent advances in flatology. *N Engl J Med*. 1980; 302: 1474-5.]

But I had a theory – based on three chance observations of my own:

1) I had been trying to eat very little animal fat over the previous year because routine blood work had shown a progressively rising cholesterol over the preceding decade. I had noted no change in odor from this attempted dietary change, but had to undergo colonoscopy and, because of the few "low fiber" food items I was

allowed to eat during preparation for the colonoscopy, I chose to take a holiday from the diet and eat fried eggs with toasted white bread. There was a surprising increase in the feculent odor of my flatus the following day.

2) I had been invited 32 years earlier to a gourmet dinner very rich in animal fat that was followed the next day by a similarly surprising increase in feculent odor despite an omnivorous diet at the time.

3) I had started drinking skim milk when my sons were young to show them that it was a healthy beverage to drink and I was still drinking it until just before I ate the eggs that were followed by a dramatic increase in odor, suggesting that the copious animal protein in fat free, skim milk must not get metabolized to cause feculent odor.

These three observations suggested to me that animal fat might be a principal substrate for producing the feculent odor of flatus. To see if this was right, I conducted a study similar to the one described above that evaluated different alternating air cushions.

The study began in late 2007 with open trial of avoiding ingestion of animal fat. After my flatus became odorless with this approach, an n-of-1 trial was used to prospectively test 201 food items during 1,826 patient-days, usually one item at a time though some foods contained multiple items (e.g., vegetable soup).[Guyatt G, Sackett D, Taylor DW, Chong J, Roberts R, Pugsley S. Determining optimal therapy -- randomized trials in individual patients. *N Engl J Med.* 1986;314(14):889-92.]

When a food test was positive, feculent odor typically returned the next day, but I waited 72 hours before declaring a test negative and testing a different food item. Foods with a negative test were often retested the next day with leftovers from the first test meal. Food products identified as odor-producing could only be retested after waiting until the flatus became odorless again. The numbers of tests of food items that were followed by odor are noted in Table 37-1 and Table 37-6.

When feculent odor became barely detectable, it wasn't present in every emission of flatus during a day. If faint feculent odor was detectable at any time during the day, this was defined as a low level positive. Flatus was called odorless only when I was unable to detect feculent odor at any time during a day.

Fisher's exact test (2-tailed) was used to calculate the probability that different frequencies of odor developed by chance with different diets. A probability (P value) < 0.05 was considered statistically significant

Here's the main result: after more than five decades of eating an omnivorous diet, I stopped ingesting any animal fat at all, and for the first time my flatus became odorless after a few weeks.

After that, animal products containing animal fat were ingested 26 times (Table 37-1) and followed the next day by recurrence of feculent odor in flatus (usually lasting 10 to 14 days). Switching back to a diet avoiding animal fat and limited to foods already documented to result in no odor was followed by a return to odorless flatus 26 times ($p < 1 \times 10^{-10}$). This low p value means that these changes were very unlikely due to chance.

Swallowing human blood after dental extraction or trauma to the tongue or gums was followed by feculent odor lasting 8-14 days (Table 37-1).

Ingesting animal products from which animal fat had been removed was never followed by feculent odor (e.g., drinking 2 gallons of nonfat, skim milk per week for over four years and eating nonfat Egg Beaters egg substitute made with egg whites multiple times); by contrast, ingesting foods containing bacon, milk, milk products, or eggs each resulted in easily detectable, feculent odor (Table 37-1).

186 different food items lacking animal fat were followed by no feculent odor (Tables 37-2-37-5). No fruit, vegetable, nut, seed, mushroom, vegetable oil, margarine, cereal, grain or pasta was followed by odor. Multiple products made from soybeans (four different brands of soy milk and over 30 other commercial soy products) were followed by no odor.

Five different food items lacking animal fat but containing hydrogenated vegetable oil (Table 37-6) were followed by less intense feculent odor. These included servings of five Mrs. Smith's fruit pies (3 apple, 1 blueberry, and 1 cherry), a homemade vegan pumpkin pie, and a loaf of homemade cornbread. Multiple servings of an apple pie and of a strawberry rhubarb pie made with palm oil (but not with animal fat or hydrogenated vegetable oil) and of 2 homemade peach pies using olive oil as shortening were followed by no odor. Odor followed all ten different items with animal fat (Table 37-1) versus 5 (2.6%) of the 191 lacking it (RR=38.2, 95% CI: 16.1-90.7).

Having noted the regular occurrence of odor after eating pies made with hydrogenated vegetable oil, I experimented with a sixth (homemade vegan pumpkin) pie made with hydrogenated vegetable oil (Crisco). I ate a thin sliver of pumpkin pie on two consecutive days. On the day following each of those two days there was faint feculent odor. On the third day, I ate a large piece of the same pumpkin pie, and the next day there was easily detectable feculent odor.

Several other foods made with hydrogenated vegetable oil weren't followed by feculent odor (e.g., generous helpings of Jif peanut butter filling two sandwiches, servings of two Duncan Hines cakes, servings of a batch of oatmeal-chocolate chip cookies, servings of multiple different brands of margarine, and Ritz crackers). Homemade apple and pecan pies made using Smart Balance margarine and a pumpkin pie using Willow Run margarine as shortening contained hydrogenated vegetable oil but were followed by no odor

Various types of beans (including soybeans) were followed by a marked increase in odorless gas production (starting within a few hours and continuing as long as 24 hours after ingestion) but never by feculent odor.

After drinking skim milk every day for more than four years, I took a break from drinking it. After a three month hiatus, I resumed drinking skim milk, which, like beans, was promptly followed by a marked increase in odorless gas production but no feculent odor. On the second and third consecutive days after resuming drinking skim milk, there was more odorless gas than usual but less than the day before. On the fourth day, gas volume returned to normal.

Limited to one patient, this study will require confirmation. The colonizing bacteria in some patients' colons produce 10 million-fold more methane than in others.[Levitt MD. Intestinal gas production -- recent advances in flatology. *N Engl J Med.* 1980; 302: 1474-5.] And people could differ in ability to smell odoriferous gases in flatus (some people can smell a stinkbug and others can't).

Nevertheless, the results of this study – the largest yet regarding flatus odor substrates and the first to avoid ingestion of a hypothesized substrate until flatus became odorless before re-challenge – suggest that the familiar, foul odors emanating from the human colon may derive from eating animal products. More specifically, the data suggest that animal fat is likely the principal substrate metabolized by colonic bacteria producing the trace odoriferous gases that give rise to these odors. My flatus became feculent 26 times on the day after swallowing animal fat and then odorless again 26 times after switching back to a diet excluding animal fat. The calculated probability that this pattern occurred by chance (< 1×10^{-10}) was lower than in prior studies of flatus odor substrates.

Previous studies found that strongly odoriferous compounds were lipid soluble,[Schiffman SS. Characterization of odor quality utilizing multidimensional sealing techniques. In: Moskowitz HR, Warren CB, eds. Odor quality and chemical structure. Washington DC: American chemical Society, 1981:1-21.] supporting the notion that animal fat might be the principal substrate.

The results of this study make it seem unlikely that most other foods (including animal protein) could be the principal substrate. Ingesting the proteins in nonfat skim milk, in nonfat Egg Beaters, and lesser amounts of animal protein in multiple processed foods weren't followed by odor. Markedly increased flatus after resuming drinking skim milk likely was due to transient lactase deficiency and metabolism of lactose by colonic bacteria; absence of odor suggests that lactose is not a substrate that produces flatus odor.

Animal fat and animal protein could both be required for colonic bacteria to produce odoriferous gases, but this seems unlikely because of Occam's Razor, which suggests that a simple hypothesis is more often correct than a complicated one.

This study's most certain results were that eating animal products that included animal fat was always followed by feculent odor while eating plant products was never followed by odor. Less intense feculent odor was observed after eating seven baked products containing hydrogenated vegetable oils, but other food products containing hydrogenated vegetable oils weren't followed by odor. If hydrogenated vegetable oil is another substrate, these variable results could be due to qualitative or quantitative differences between such foods (e.g., Mrs. Smith's apple pie contained more hydrogenated vegetable oil per serving than did Jif Peanut Butter, which wasn't followed by odor, and Jif was made using different vegetable oils). Commercial products often change (intentionally or inadvertently), which might result in different results with the same product during consecutive years.

Human blood isn't food, but swallowing it was reliably followed by feculent odor even when little was swallowed (e.g., a slight pink tinge of saliva while flossing teeth), but the level of odor after swallowing blood wasn't enough to be noticed in an omnivorous patient because more intense feculent odor is an everyday occurrence in omnivores. When I was a resident physician, a patient with gastrointestinal bleeding was admitted with a foul odor so pungent it could be smelled throughout half a medical ward. This study's findings suggest that the bleeding might have caused the pungent odor. Blood usually has no feculent odor, but could after metabolism by colonic bacteria (probably requiring a bleed with slow enough transit for this to occur) and might be greater in patients with hyperlipidemia. Medline searching found only one report of foul odor in a patient with gastrointestinal bleeding, the authors hypothesizing this to be due to metabolism by colonic bacteria.[Walker V, Mills GA, Fortune PM, Wheeler R. Neonatal encephalopathy with a pungent body odor. *Arch Dis Child Fetal Neonatal Ed.* 1997; 77: F65-F66.]

Some might question a study using an instrument as simple as the human nose, but the nose can be as sensitive as (or more sensitive than) gas chromatography and mass spectroscopy for detecting trace odoriferous gases and is said to be the only instrument that can both detect and interpret odors due to such gases.[Levitt MD. Only the nose knows. *Gastroenterology.* 1987;93(6):1437-8.]. Olfactory ability can wane with age, but I could still smell bread toasting or popcorn popping 70 feet away through the house at the end of the study (unaided by a fan) and never lost the ability to detect the stronger feculent odors issuing from a bathroom after use by an omnivore.

Earlier research demonstrated that "organic molecules containing sulfur or nitrogen at reactive sites often have very powerful, offensive odors,"[Levitt MD. Only the nose knows. *Gastroenterology.* 1987;93(6):1437-8.] and two studies of the odoriferous gases in human flatus suggested that the responsible molecules contained sulfur.[Moore JG, Jessop LD, Osborne DN. Gas-chromatographic and mass-spectrometric analysis of the odor of human feces. *Gastroenterology.* 1987;93(6):1321-9.][Suarez FL, Springfield J, Levitt MD. Identification of gases responsible for the odor of human flatus and evaluation of a device purported to reduce this odor. *Gut.* 1998;43(1):100-4.] They disagreed about which molecules caused the odor, but both speculated that vegetables might be the substrate metabolized by colonic bacteria to produce the odor, noting that 15 vegetables contained sulfur-bearing compounds and that some of these vegetables contained the same molecules identified in flatus. It seems likely that sulfur-bearing compounds might contribute to the odor of human flatus, and it was reasonable to speculate that vegetables might serve as the substrate. Eating asparagus had been known for three centuries to cause unpleasant odor in the urine of a portion of the population (though too quickly to involve colonic bacteria),[Mitchell, SC. Food idiosyncrasies: beetroot and asparagus. *Drug Metabolism and Disposition.* 2001; 29: 539-543.] and eating garlic had been known to cause halitosis, but the present study's findings suggest that vegetables probably don't serve as the substrate for feculent odor in flatus.

Implicating vegetables would have been more convincing if volunteers avoiding ingestion of vegetables developed odorless flatus and odor recurred when re-challenged with vegetables. The only vegetables followed by feculent odor in flatus in the present study were coated with melted butter or cooked with bacon or a fatty piece of ham in the pot as flavoring at a restaurant. The same vegetables eaten at home many times and in large quantity without butter or animal fat as flavoring were never followed by feculent odor. It remains possible that vegetables could be the principal substrate in one subset of patients and animal fat the principal substrate in another subset, but this seems unlikely because this hypothesis would be more convoluted than the idea that both animal protein and animal fat are required to produce odoriferous gases. Occam's razor would again favor the simpler alternative.

One study [Moore JG, Jessop LD, Osborne DN. Gas-chromatographic and mass-spectrometric analysis of the odor of human feces. *Gastroenterology*. 1987;93(6):1321-9.] also mentioned coffee, beer and cocoa as potential substrates (of which cocoa was ingested in the present study and followed by no odor). It seems unlikely that they would be a principal cause of colonic odor, since pediatricians agree that all infants develop stinky diapers (i.e., long before most babies would consume those products).

A third study focusing on infants[Jiang T, Suarez FL, Levitt MD, Nelson SE, Ziegler EE. Gas production by feces of infants. *J Pediatr Gastroenterol Nutr*. 2001;32(5):534-41.] suggested that the stools of soy formula fed infants produced more hydrogen sulfide when incubated anaerobically than did stools of infants drinking breast milk or cows' milk formula and hypothesized that soy might be a substrate. But a study of canine diets concluded that a diet emphasizing soy was associated with significantly less fecal odor metabolites and a trend toward less hydrogen sulfide in flatus than was the other diet (poultry byproduct meal, which contained more fat and more animal fat). [Yamka RM, Harmon DL, Schoenherr WD, Khoo C, Gross KL, Davidson SJ, Joshi DK. In vivo measurement of flatulence and nutrient digestibility in dogs fed poultry byproduct meal, conventional soybean meal, and low-oligosaccharides low-phytate soybean meal. *Am J Vet Res.* 2006;67(1):88-94.]

The patient in the present study didn't drink infant formula, but drank four different brands of soy milk and ate more than 30 different food items containing soy that weren't followed by feculent odor. Nevertheless, it's known that different cultivars of soybeans can have different biological properties, so the infant formula could have contained a different cultivar from what was used in the many soy products consumed in the present study or the difference could be due to other things added to the infant formula (if not dietary treats given to infants by relatives).

A dog's nose is 1,000- to 10,000-fold more sensitive than a human's, suggesting that some foods could produce odoriferous gases in a quantity undetectable by the human nose.[Levitt MD. Intestinal gas production -- recent advances in flatology. *N Engl J Med.* 1980; 302: 1474-5.] A dose-gradient was demonstrated for two items in this study (i.e., a thin sliver of pumpkin pie was followed by faint odor and a large slice by more odor; likewise, a slight tinge of blood in saliva resulted in less odor than copious bleeding). A large gourmet meal rich in animal fat was also followed by more intense feculent odor than was a single bite of bacon, but that small bite of bacon was followed by considerably more odor than the (much larger) sliver of pumpkin pie. If some foods produced subliminal amounts of odoriferous gas, larger servings could possibly reach the threshold of detection.

A small, short-term study (10 healthy adults for three to seven days) showed 95% reduction in hydrogen sulfide in flatus in volunteers taking bismuth subsalicylate tablets.[Suarez FL, Furne JK, Springfield J, Levitt MD. Bismuth subsalicylate markedly decreases hydrogen sulfide release in the human colon. *Gastroenterology.* 1998;114(5):923-9.] This doesn't mean taking an antimicrobial drug long-term to reduce odor is necessarily good. The results of long-term studies doing that aren't available. Taking antimicrobial drugs permanently can have unintended consequences. Prolonged courses of bismuth had adverse neurologic effects in one report, spurring some to recommend drug-free holidays lasting months.[Gorbach SL. Bismuth therapy in gastrointestinal diseases. *Gastroenterology.* 1990;99(3):863-75. Review.]

A small laboratory efficacy study (6 healthy adults with a tube releasing artificial flatus [hydrogen sulfide, methylmercaptan, and hydrogen] at the anus) reported that activated charcoal-impregnated briefs captured almost all of the two sulfide gases,[Ohge H, Furne JK, Springfield J, Ringwala S, Levitt MD. Effectiveness of devices purported to reduce flatus odor. *Am J Gastroenterol.* 2005;100(2):397-400.] but a laboratory efficacy study is not the same as an epidemiologic effectiveness study of patients in their home environment. The undergarments of patients with hemiparesis often go awry shortly after being donned correctly. Patients with rectal incontinence for flatus often have urinary incontinence requiring a pad inside the briefs. The only activated charcoal briefs I have seen were too skimpy to accommodate such a pad. Activated charcoal briefs also cost more than regular underwear and wear out (all fabric does) with repeated laundering.

Other reasons to consider not eating animal products include the following:

1) Carefully selected vegan diets cost less because growing plants costs less than raising animals.
2) A vegan diet results in a much smaller "carbon footprint" (e.g., raising cows reportedly resulted in release of 57-fold more greenhouse gases than did growing an equivalent amount of potatoes).[Nathan Fiala. Producing beef for the table has a surprising environmental cost: it releases prodigious amounts of heat-trapping greenhouse gases. *Scientific American.* February 4, 2009.] The Chairman of the UN

Intergovernmental Panel on Climate Change said the single most effective thing an individual could do to prevent global warming was to eat less meat.[Bryan Walsh. Meat: making global warming worse. *Time.* September 10, 2008.]

3) If most American grain wasn't fed to livestock, it's been estimated that it could feed all Americans plus 500 million hungry people in the Third World. Many are trying to use less fossil fuels by eating locally produced food ("locavores"), but eating locally raised animals remains a problem because raising animals requires much more fossil fuels than growing plants.

4) Eating animal fat creates risk for atherosclerotic cardiovascular disease, the leading cause of death in the United States, and eating animal protein may increase one's risk for cancer, the second leading cause.[Pan A, Sun Q, Bernstein AM, Schulze MB, Manson JE, Stampfer MJ, Willett WC, Hu FB. Red meat consumption and mortality: results from 2 prospective cohort studies. *Arch Intern Med.* 2012;172(7):555-63.] [Key TJ, Appleby PN, Spencer EA, Travis RC, Allen NE, Thorogood M, Mann JI. Cancer incidence in British vegetarians. Br J Cancer. 2009 Jul 7;101(1):192-7. *Br J Cancer.* 2009;101(1):192-7.] [Campbell TC, Parpia B, Chen J. Diet, lifestyle, and the etiology of coronary artery disease: the Cornell China study. Am J Cardiol. 1998; 92:18T-21T.] [Appleton BS, Campbell TC. Dietary protein intervention during the post-dosing phase of aflatoxin B1-induced hepatic preneoplastic lesion development. *J Natl Cancer Inst.* 1983; 70: 547-9.]

Those seeking to confirm this study's results will have advantages (e.g., being able to draw measured amounts of blood and have volunteers swallow their own blood [to determine a dose response] and to fractionate the blood [or other test items] to determine the effects of lipids versus proteins), but they need to be aware of some potential confounders (e.g., dried smudges of animal fat persisting on silverware or dishes through the dishwasher, waiters occasionally bringing the wrong food, and blood getting in one's mouth).

How big does a dried smudge of animal fat on a plate have to be to cause odor? Not very big. When one of our sons got married, the house filled up with relatives and the dishwasher filled up with lots of plates with dried smudges of food. Our KitchenAid dishwasher was never able to remove such smudges. Two days after the wedding, I had a recurrence of odor (luckily this was after the guests departed). At that point, I happened to notice a plate coming out of the cabinet with dried smudges of food that had persisted through the dishwasher cycle. I checked 10 more plates sitting in a stack in the cabinet and found six more with dried smudges of food. What do I conclude from this? It can be difficult to avoid swallowing animal fat in a house where animal fat is regularly consumed unless someone is fastidious about wiping food off plates before they go in the dishwasher.

Postscript

As mentioned above, I was very upset when my anal sphincter first became incontinent for flatus, but after the feculent odor disappeared, this incontinence stopped bothering me. It almost never resulted in an embarrassing noise (the exception being during a bout of constipation), and silent passage of odorless flatus during the afternoon and evening eventually became a reassuring comfort because it indicated that no bout of constipation was looming ahead to make my night miserable.

Table 37-1. Animal products containing animal fat → feculent odor (usual onset within 1 day & duration about 2 weeks)

Food item	Frequency*
blueberry muffin made with milk	1
yogurt	1
cheese (in soup, in quiche, in pizza, and in Lance Toastchee --cheese cracker peanut butter sandwiches--"Nabs")	1 each
butter melted on vegetables	3
butter as a faint glaze on a roll of French bread	1
Alfredo sauce containing butter, cheese and cream	1
eggs	1
pig fat used to season turnip greens and green beans at a restaurant	3
salmon, baked with no visible sauce	3
bacon (accidentally ingested one bite followed by feculent odor the next day that persisted for 13 days)	1
human blood	7 (following tooth extraction, inadvertent biting of tongue (twice), accidentally harsh flossing of gums (twice), brushing teeth with a toothbrush with hard bristles, and intentionally causing bleeding with dental floss at the end of the study as a positive control)

* number of times ingested on different days when flatus was odorless

Table 37-2. Animal products containing animal protein but no animal fat → no feculent odor

Food item	Frequency*
nonfat skim milk—several brands	2 gallons per week for 4 years
nonfat Egg Beaters egg substitute (eaten as scrambled eggs and in baked products)	> 3

* number of times ingested on different days when flatus was odorless

Table 37-3. Plant products containing no animal fat → no feculent odor

Food item	Frequency*
vegetables: artichoke, asparagus, basil, beans (navy beans, black beans, red beans, Pinto beans, soybeans), beets, broccoli, brussels sprouts, cabbage, carrots, cauliflower, celery, chick peas, corn (as corn on the cob[up to 4 large ears at a meal], in succotash, in soup, sautéed with squash and onions, in shepherd's pie, and as grits, etc.), cucumber, eggplant, garlic, green beans, green peppers, kale, lentils, lettuce, lima beans, mustard greens, okra, onions, peas, potatoes [baked, French fried, roasted, mashed, pieces cooked in soup, sautéed, and boiled new potatoes], pumpkin, rhubarb, spinach, squash (yellow squash, acorn squash, spaghetti squash), sweet potatoes, turnip greens, tomatoes, zucchini	each > 3

fruits: apples (Red Delicious, Golden Delicious, Rome, green Granny Smith), avocados, bananas, blackberries, blueberries, cantaloupe, cherries, clementines, grapefruits, grapes (red, green, black), honeydew, kiwis, lemons, melons, olives (green, black), oranges, peaches, plums, pomegranates, raisins, raspberries, strawberries, tangerines, watermelons	each > 3
nuts: almonds, peanuts, pecans, pistachios, walnuts	each > 3
seeds: sunflower seeds (raw or roasted),sesame	each > 3
mushrooms: button, portobello, shiitake	each > 3
vegetable oils: canola, corn, olive, palm, safflower, soybean, sunflower	each > 3
margarines: Bluebonnet, Promise, Smart Balance, Willow Run, and multiple unspecified margarines used on bread and vegetables and for cooking at multiple restaurants from 2008-2011	each > 3

* number of times ingested on different days when flatus was odorless

Table 37-4. Bread, cereal, grains, and pasta containing no animal fat → no feculent odor

Food item	Frequency*
bread (bagels, French, dinner roll, hamburger buns, hot dog buns, Italian, rye, wheat)	each > 3
pasta (spaghetti, angel hair, lasagna, linguine, cannelloni, manicotti, couscous)	each > 3 except cannelloni and manicotti (1 each)
grains: rice, oats	each > 3
cereals: Cheerios, Raisin Bran, Life, Cracklin' Oat Bran, oatmeal	each > 3

* number of times ingested on different days when flatus was odorless

Table 37-5. Processed food products with no animal fat (most being vegan) → no feculent odor

Food item	Frequency*
Amy's Brown Rice with Vegetables (contains soy)	> 3
Amy's Asian noodles(contains soy)	> 3
Amy's Teriyaki(contains soy)	> 3
Amy's Nondairy Vegetable Pot Pie(contains soy)	> 3
Amy's Roasted Vegetable Pizza	> 3
Amy's Tofu Scrambler(contains soy)	> 3
Amy's Veggie Loaf [product contains olive oil, safflower and/or sunflower oil and soy milk]	> 3

Amy's Vegetable Lasagna [product contains coconut oil and safflower oil but no soy]	> 3
Amy's Ziti [product contains safflower or sunflower oil and soy]	> 3
Garden Protein's Tuscan ['chicken'] breasts(contains soy)	> 3
Garden Protein's "Chicken Scaloppini"(contains soy)	> 3
Garden Protein's Crispy Chicken fillets (contains soy)	> 3
Light Life's Smart Barbecue(contains soy)	> 3
Veggie Patch Portobello Mushroom Burger (apparently no longer available)	> 3
MorningStar Farms Soy "chicken" cooked with mushrooms and mustard sauce	> 3
MorningStar Farms soy "chicken" patty(contains soy	> 3
MorningStar Farms Griller(contains soy)	> 3
MorningStar Farms breakfast patty(contains soy)	> 3
MorningStar Farms hickory Barbecue Riblet(contains soy)	> 3
MorningStar Farms sweet-and-sour "chicken"(contains soy)	> 3
MorningStar Farms chicken cutlet(contains soy)	> 3

pizza made with Kroger Pizza Crust, Kroger Mozzarella Melt Topping [imitation], MorningStar Farms Crumbles(contains soy), and sliced olives and mushrooms	> 3
spaghetti sauce made with Prego tomato sauce and MorningStar Farms Crumbles(contains soy)	> 3
Talk o' Texas Pickled Okra	> 3
dill pickles	> 3
Jif peanut butter (contains fully hydrogenated rapeseed and soybean oils [< 2%]) (generous amounts for making two sandwiches)	> 3
Smuckers' Simply Fruit (strawberry, blueberry, blackberry, raspberry)	> 3
2 homemade peach pies using olive oil as shortening	> 3
apple pie made by the Willamette Valley Fruit Company using cold pressed (Spectrum) palm oil as shortening	> 3
homemade pumpkin pie using Willow Run margarine as shortening	1
homemade apple pie using Smart Balance margarine as shortening	> 3
strawberry-rhubarb pie made by the Willamette Valley Fruit Company using cold pressed (Spectrum) palm oil as shortening	> 3

rum cake cooked with Duncan Hines yellow cake mix [contains partially hydrogenated soybean oil], nonfat Eggbeaters (contains animal protein), olive oil, water, Pam with olive oil, rum, sugar, and walnuts	> 3
chocolate cake cooked with Duncan Hines devil's food cake mix [contains partially hydrogenated soybean oil], nonfat Egg Replacement by ENER CT, olive oil, water, and Pam with olive oil (using icing made with cocoa, powdered sugar and Willow Run margarine)	> 3
Turtle Island Tofurky roast (contains soy)	> 3
Turtle Island chocolate cake	> 3
oatmeal chocolate chip cookies (5 per serving) cooked with Crisco(contains fully and partially hydrogenated soybean and palm oils)	> 3
ketchup—multiple different brands	> 3
soy milk (brands: WestSoy, Soy Dream, Better Than Milk, and Silk)	each > 3
Good Seasons Italian Dressing (mixed with olive oil, vinegar and water)	> 3
Tostitos tortilla chips with guacamole	> 3
Fritos corn chips	> 3
Ritz crackers (contains partially hydrogenated cottonseed oil)	> 3
vegetable soup	> 3
homemade vegetable stew with cabbage, carrots, and mushrooms	> 3

semi-sweetened chocolate chips made by Enjoy Life	> 3
Tofutti Cuties soy vanilla ice cream sandwiches	> 3
So Delicious soy vanilla ice cream sandwiches	> 3
So Delicious soy vanilla ice cream	> 3
vegan pad Thai with tofu(contains soy)	> 3
Veganaise (a vegan version of mayonnaise made by Follow Your Heart) [contains canola oil and soy]	> 3
homemade vegan potato salad using Vegenaise	> 3
homemade vegan cole slaw using Vegenaise	> 3
homemade vegan soy "chicken" tetrazzini	> 3
homemade pesto sauce with pasta	> 3
homemade ratatouille	> 3
homemade vegan Reuben sandwiches using Garden Protein's Tuscan ['chicken'] breasts(contains soy) and Kraft's Light Thousand Island Dressing	> 3
Hershey's chocolate syrup (contains unspecified hydrogenated vegetable oil[s])	> 3

* number of times ingested on different days when flatus was odorless

Table 37-6. Processed vegan food products simulating animal fat → feculent odor (less intense than observed with animal fat)

Food item	Frequency*
homemade vegan pumpkin pie cooked with fully and partially hydrogenated soybean and palm oils (Crisco)	1
homemade cornbread cooked with fully and partially hydrogenated soybean and palm oils (Crisco)	1
Mrs. Smith's prebaked fruit pies cooked with hydrogenated palm and soybean oil shortenings and palm and soybean oil margarines	3 apple, 1 blueberry and 1 cherry

* number of times ingested on different days when flatus was odorless

Chapter 38

The Relatedness of
MS Problems

Albert Einstein received a PhD in physics in 1905 and immediately shocked the scientific community by publishing four ground-breaking articles. One reported the relativity of some phenomena in physics previously regarded as independent.

The complications of MS are often interrelated as well.

I didn't find that statement in any of the 8 books about MS mentioned above, but 4 didn't focus on complications, and the others generally included only previously published information (i.e., few if any original observations).

Interrelatedness of different MS complications can make discussing each only in separate chapters difficult, as mentioned in the Introduction. For example, it's hard to talk about an MS patient's pain without discussing spasticity, and conversely, it's hard to talk about spasticity without mentioning pain.

An example of interrelatedness of MS complications was mentioned in Chapter 7 regarding my experience with actively constipating foods – they repeatedly caused me constipation, urinary urgency, and urinary incontinence. Many publications about MS note that constipation, urinary urgency and urinary incontinence are common complications of MS, but none that I found linked these three problems together.

I'm not the first physician to figure out that constipation, urinary urgency, and urinary incontinence can be related, but the prior publications I saw about this involved patients with diseases other than MS,[Kim JH, Lee JH, Jung AY, Lee JW. The prevalence and therapeutic effect of constipation in pediatric overactive bladder. Int Neurourol J. 2011; 15:206-10. doi: 10.5213/inj.2011.15.4.206.] [Wesnes SL, Lose G. Preventing urinary incontinence during pregnancy and postpartum: a review. Int Urogynecol J. 2013; 24:889-99. doi: 10.1007/s00192-012-2017-3]. The website of the National Association For Continence (NAFC) says that constipation can cause urinary urgency and incontinence.

At the time I was writing this chapter, the Multiple Sclerosis Society website said that bowel problems could cause bladder problems. This is a bit vague and not the same as specifically stating that constipation causes urinary urgency and incontinence, but the latter is not incompatible with the former.

The other books written by physicians for MS patients didn't say that constipation causes urinary urgency, and the therapeutic approaches that they recommended for controlling urinary urgency and incontinence didn't mention the importance of controlling constipation. Instead of emphasizing optimal control of constipation for helping control urinary urgency, they seem to advise the opposite – that a bowel movement every three days is adequate. Dr. Giesser's book also noted that the anticholinergic medications usually recommended to control bladder problems frequently cause constipation.

The fact that constipation, urinary urgency, and urinary incontinence appear to be interrelated in me implies that they may be interrelated in other MS patients. I won't hazard a guess what proportion that is, but a relatively small study would be able to begin to find out.

What are some other relationships among MS complications?

Regarding fatigue, Dr. Lechtenberg says that MS patients can have it because of MS related CNS damage (demyelination) or any of five MS complications – sleep deprivation, infection, fractures, anemia, or kidney disease. He says that "daytime fatigue often proves to be from [an MS complication] sleeplessness associated with [another MS complication] depression, pain or drug reactions." Dr. Giesser says the same, but lists different MS complications as potential causes of fatigue (the extra effort required by everyday activities in patients with weakness, spastic stiffness, and impaired balance; side effects of medications frequently prescribed for MS patients [e.g., interferon, baclofen, tizanidine, diazepam, pregabalin, duloxetine, gabapentin, amitriptyline, sertraline, paroxetine, and venlafaxine]; sleep disturbances due to corticosteroids, nocturia, spasms, periodic limb movements, depression, or alcohol use; the effects of deconditioning; or the effects of reduced lung function).

So, from looking at fatigue, a single MS complication, one could gather that Drs. Lechtenberg and Giesser may agree with my statement that MS complications are often interrelated.

More interactions? The books by Dr. Lechtenberg and Dr. Giesser both note that bowel and bladder distention and pain can cause increased spasticity and that spasticity can cause pain. Dr. Giesser also notes that spasticity of the urinary sphincter can cause loss of bladder control.

Dr. Giesser says that constipation in MS patients is caused by CNS damage and worsened by 1) relative dehydration, 2) medication side effects (particularly for medications used to treat bladder symptoms) and 3) reduced mobility due in turn to a) weakness, b) fatigue, or c) stiffness.

Dr. Lechtenberg says that constipation in MS patients can be caused by "inactivity and medication side effects. Constipation often develops in people who, either because of pain or weakness, cannot be active. Fluid restrictions designed to improve bladder control may exacerbate constipation."

As paresis of a leg worsens, it becomes edematous. As it becomes edematous, urinary urgency worsens because edema fluid gets reabsorbed when the patient lies down, which increases the amount of fluid volume in the blood and thus urine volume that needs to be excreted through the urinary tract.

Physiologist Dr. Arthur Guyton said that in physiology there was no positive feedback but that in pathophysiology there was. Because of positive feedback, many of the problems in MS are circular. For example, an MS patient with a bout of increased constipation spends more time on the toilet and less time walking, which makes the patient weaker and more spastic; this increased spasticity and decreased activity can cause additional constipation. Waking one time for nocturia with severe urinary urgency and incontinence causes a hemiparetic patient to spend an hour taking off wet clothes and getting redressed, which makes incontinence more likely when waking the next time for nocturia because the bladder will inevitably be more full (i.e., delay getting back into bed after nocturia usually delays going back to sleep and waking for the next nocturia). Why does "nature's alarm clock," the bladder, not wake an MS patient at the appropriate time? The sensory nervous system can be damaged by MS and not be totally up to snuff. It still may be able to sense urine in the bladder, but not as well as a normal nervous system would.

If one episode of urinary incontinence at night can lead to a second, can one episode of urinary urgency be directly tied to another episode of urinary urgency? Yes. One way is for a spastic urinary sphincter to clamp shut soon after urination commences; this would guarantee that the bladder would become full (and overfull) quicker than usually expected.

Damage to the cerebellum, the body's "gyroscope," causes imbalance which causes MS patients to start falling. A fall can cause a fracture, which can cause severe pain, which can cause increased spasticity, which can cause increased difficulty maneuvering with a walker and an increase in sudden myoclonic jerks, which can make additional falls more likely. Increased pain and spasticity can spur increased urinary urgency and increased constipation, which can also cause increased urinary urgency. The increased pain, increased urinary urgency, and increased spasticity can each make the patient more likely to fall again, which, of course, can cause more pain, which can cause all of these things to increase again.

Spasticity and weakness cause different symptoms but are so intertwined in the dysfunctional limb of an MS patient that they almost seem like two heads of the same coin. Both are caused by MS destruction of the central nervous system (an upper motor neuron lesion). The weaker an MS patient gets, the harder it is to move. The harder it is to move, the less the patient moves. The less exercise the patient gets, the weaker the patient gets (positive feedback). Similarly, the less the patient moves, the more spasticity increases. Intertwined from the start, weakness and spasticity usually get worse together over decades. Occasionally, their effects can be separated. For example, after a fall, there may be an acute, dramatic increase in spasticity. The patient may not be able to tell which of the two got dramatically worse, but a neurological exam can show the increased rigidity and a dose of baclofen (if not already being taken regularly, which can make the body too tolerant to the effects of baclofen for use as a diagnostic tool) can lessen the increased rigidity and show that the recent worsening was more spasticity than weakness.

The other books note that if bowel and bladder are distended, this will increase spasticity, but don't talk about all of the implications. For example, my hand can become so spastic that it cannot grab hold of the walker handle. This impedes progress to the toilet, which causes an increase in urinary urgency and makes falling more likely.

The more weakness and spasticity you have, the more likely you are to fall. The more falls you have, the more likely you are to have fractures. The more fractures you have, the more likely you are to have to immobilize some to allow healing. The more you have to immobilize a limb, the less exercise and stretching you can do. The less exercise and stretching you can do, the more weakness and spasticity you will have.

Spasticity and weakness of my mostly paralyzed arm make it hard to use that arm for walking with my walker. When I get up at night for nocturia and reach for the walker, trying to grab the walker with my spastic left hand can require me to strain. Straining is like a modified Valsalva maneuver, which puts increased pressure on the bladder, making it feel more urgency to urinate. This increased urgency to urinate can in turn cause the spasticity of my mostly paralyzed left arm and left leg to increase acutely. This increased spasticity in turn causes me to strain still more to walk and to re-grab the walker handle when spasticity causes my hand to lose its grip. Straining more to walk and to re-grasp the handle are again like modified Valsalva maneuvers that further increase pressure on the bladder. So it goes, causing a crescendo of urgency that increases step by step as I approach the toilet. When my hand loses the grip on the walker, this is perceived as untoward because I have to stop and apply the brake, impeding progress toward the toilet. Anything untoward impeding progress toward the toilet acts as a Pavlovian conditioned stimulus causing an immediate increase in urinary urgency.

Spasticity can cause rigidity and periodic limb movements of skeletal muscle in a spastic limb and can cause hyperreflexia of the bladder urinary muscles, which can cause nocturia. Each of these things makes it harder to sleep, which results in sleeplessness, daytime somnolence and fatigue. Fatigue, spasticity, weakness and imbalance make an MS patient more likely to fall. Corticosteroid therapy for MS makes an MS patient more likely to have osteoporosis. Falling with osteoporosis makes fractures more likely. Fractures can cause severe pain. Pain causes increased spasticity. Bladder distention and urinary urgency can cause my spastic left leg to decerebrate, seemingly becoming as stiff and heavy as concrete. The dramatic increase in stiffness with decerebration impedes motion toward the toilet, which causes a conditioned Pavlovian reflex that in turn causes an immediate spike in urinary urgency. Such cycles of positive feedback due to the interrelatedness of different MS complications can cause continually increasing severity of symptoms.

I won't try to exhaustively list every possible interaction between different MS complications, but will conclude this chapter by reviewing some apparent interactions of complications mentioned in Chapter 23 that I suffered after a fall. After almost a year of not falling, I fell, causing two fractures. The fall was caused by spasticity of my left arm that had been increasing for 22 years. The fractures were associated with a marked increase in pain. The marked increase in pain was associated with a marked increase in spasticity. The increased spasticity seemed to affect my entire body (e.g., increased difficulty ambulating with my walker, increased nocturia, increased urinary urgency at lower volumes of urine than previously observed, etc.). Because I needed to immobilize the fractured metatarsal and because I was unable to function with a cast, I put on a tightly fastened shoe and left it on day and night. Because I was unable to go to bed with a shoe on, I had to sleep sitting in a recliner. Sleeping in the recliner was associated with increased aspiration of saliva clogging my throat, which woke me frequently with coughing fits. Reducing my ambulation to heal the fractures resulted in a further increase in spasticity. During this marked increase in spasticity, I experienced worse constipation that was different from what I had experienced before (i.e., rather than resulting in fecal incontinence, loose stools seemed to make the constipation worse), apparently involving spastic constriction of my rectal sphincter (the external anal sphincter). This spastic constriction was associated with spastic contractions of my left leg and sometimes simultaneous contractions of my left arm and right leg as well. Spastic adduction of my spastic left leg also increased. This new form of constipation was associated with increased urinary urgency even when the stool in the rectum was so loose because of antibiotic therapy that the stool was unformed. And the urinary urgency became so bad that

I started having urinary incontinence again for the first time in over a year. These were associated with incontinence occurring with nocturia and worse sleep deprivation followed by increased daytime fatigue and somnolence. The constipation was so bad and so prolonged that I started sitting on the toilet too long and had furuncles start forming on the buttock of my paretic leg for the first time in over a year. After having had trigeminal neuralgia about 200 times in the maxillary division of my trigeminal nerve, I got the worst episode of trigeminal neuralgia I'd ever had and it involved the mandibular branch of my left trigeminal nerve. I can't prove that it was interrelated with all of these other problems, but it occurred about four days after the two fractures, making at least a temporal association. Not only was the pain of this episode worse than any of my previous episodes, but it went on for a couple of days (all of the prior episodes had only lasted a few minutes). So, weakness, spasticity, falling, fractures, fracture pain, worse constipation, urinary urgency, increased aspiration of saliva, urinary incontinence, nocturia, insomnia, increased fatigue, daytime somnolence, pressure related furuncles, and renewed pain in the buttock added up to 15 MS complications all apparently interrelated (with trigeminal neuralgia being a 16th complication temporally associated with the simultaneous occurrence of all the others).

A doubting Thomas could say that the simultaneous occurrence of those 16 MS complications was mere coincidence due to chance, but the probability of joint occurrence and worsening of so many symptoms is very low.

Chapter 39
Do MS Patients Need Evaluation by a Physical Therapist

"Let's Get Physical" --Olivia Newton John

I highly recommend that MS patients see a physical therapist. For MS patients with a benign form of the disease, this may not be so important. For patients who receive an effective drug, converting aggressive MS to a benign form of the disease, this again may not be very important. But for patients like me who have to suffer through the horror of decades of increasing weakness and spasticity, I believe it is very important.

In Chapter 22, I said that the first physical therapist who evaluated me was not particularly knowledgeable about MS. She mainly just photocopied exercises and stretches said to be useful for MS patients.

If true, how could physical therapy be so important? The experience helped me understand that exercise and stretching were important tools for countering the weakness and spasticity of MS. My disease was worse than that of most MS patients and what mainly kept me going was exercise and stretching. Over time, my main exercise became walking with a walker. Nothing fancy, but exercise and stretching seemed to have more powerful effects than most of the drugs I took. Stretching spastic limbs proved to be helpful for combating spasticity in general and periodic limb movements in particular.

Having experienced the ravages of the disease during early attacks, an MS patient may assume that MS weakening is always irreversible and therefore do nothing about it. But for the weakening of deconditioning, the truth is the opposite – aggressive physical therapy exercises of the weakening limb may be able to extend its utility for years. By doing nothing, the weakening speeds along and the limb also becomes contractured (as discussed in Chapter 24).

Chapter 40
The Overuse Syndrome of the Remaining Functional Arm

"What's done cannot be undone." -- W. Shakespeare

What is "the overuse syndrome of the remaining functional arm"? When someone loses the function of one limb, there is a natural tendency to try to compensate by overusing another limb. This occurs in a variety of different patient populations in which the loss of function of one arm can be due to all sorts of problems (e.g., paresis, paralysis, amputation, etc.). With great effort, the patient may initially be able to come close to doing this, but with an important price.

Overuse of a remaining functional arm can cause serious problems. Together, these problems are referred to as "overuse syndrome of the remaining functional arm." [Sato Y, kaji M, tsuru T, oizumi K. Carpal tunnel syndrome involving unaffected limbs of stroke patients. Stroke. 1999; 30:414-8.] [Jones LE, Davidson JH. Save that arm: a study of problems in the remaining arm of unilateral upper limb amputees. Prosthetic orthot int. 1999; 23:55-8.] This also occurs in patients with paraplegia who have two functional arms. [Akbar M, et al. Prevalence of rotator cuff tear in paraplegic patients compared with controls. *J Bone Joint Surg Am.* 2010; 92:23-30. doi: 10. 2106/JBJS. H.01373.] [Sie IH, Waters RL, Adkins Rh, Gellman H. Upper extremity pain in the post rehabilitation spinal cord injured patient. *Archives Physical Medical Rehabilitation.* 1992;73:44-8.]

Are MS patients at increased risk of getting this overuse syndrome? I found no publications saying that, but I believe they are.

As MS related hemiparesis progresses, moving the weakened body about the house for activities of daily living begins to approach the physics of a beached whale. Repeated herculean efforts of the strong arm and leg to leverage the paretic half of the body out of the bed, off of the toilet, etc., wear out the strong limbs (e.g., torn rotator cuff in the shoulder, carpal tunnel syndrome in the wrist, repeated herniation of lumbar and cervical discs with radicular pain into the strong arm and leg, etc..).

Age and decades of high dose corticosteroid therapy take their toll on an MS patient's body, which becomes like the old gray mare (i.e., "ain't what she used to be"). Tissues become weakened and more susceptible to injury. For example, just standing only on my right leg to stretch it, without doing anything fancy, repeatedly resulted in herniation of an L5-S1 lumbosacral disc and sciatic pain for me; standing only on my left leg to stretch it never caused a problem. The only way I found I could stretch the right leg safely was by standing balancing my weight equally on both legs.

Similarly, merely lifting the hand of my paretic left arm passively to hold it in front of a space heater on a cold winter morning injured my left shoulder. Weeks of rest were required for recovery. This injury was probably due to weakening of tissues and also to spasticity of the paretic arm, which made lifting the paretic hand put unnatural stress on the paretic shoulder.

When I first started falling, it was very easy to get back up on my feet. As disability progressed, it got harder. But with considerable effort, I was able to continue getting back up on my feet. I did this because I figured that a little extra effort and a little extra time weren't that big a problem, and I valued staying as independent as possible. I also did not want to bother my helpers unnecessarily. When I fell on the floor and someone offered to help me up, I often said, "Let me try to get up first."

In 1999, Jones and Davidson concluded that patients with only one functional arm are not able and shouldn't try to resume their previous level of activity because this creates a high level of risk for developing overuse injuries. They recommended counseling these patients about recognition and prevention of overuse injuries. [Jones LE, Davidson JH. Save that arm: a study of problems in the remaining arm of unilateral upper limb amputees. Prosthetic orthot int. 1999; 23:55-8.] That recommendation was made 9 years before I began having symptoms of a torn rotator cuff in the shoulder of my stronger arm and 12 years before I began having symptoms of carpal tunnel syndrome in that arm.

Data on "overuse syndrome of the remaining functional arm" suggest that there is a high probability of permanent damage to the joints of that arm, (e.g., 50% to 60%) but the risk is not 100%. This is important, because it implies that this damage may be preventable by avoiding unnecessary stresses to the joints.

If I had known that there was a high risk that struggling to get up off of the floor would likely cause permanent, painful damage to my shoulder and wrist, I would have viewed this differently and accepted help getting up earlier. I often had considerable pain in my shoulder after struggling to get up from the floor. That pain would last for days. I assumed that this was just temporary pain from muscle overuse. But there was also serious joint damage. I didn't know that. I wasn't warned by the neurologist or two physical therapists caring for me that overuse syndrome of my more func-tional arm was likely or possibly could be prevented by avoiding unnecessary stress on that arm. I also was not warned by another neurologist who sub-specialized in the care of MS patients to whom I was referred in my 14th year of MS. And this wasn't because I was receiving care in Podunk; all of this occurred at a large, tertiary care, academic medical center. I don't believe that neurologists or physical therapists had focused upon this problem as of that time. I looked at the Multiple Sclerosis Society website in October 2014 and found nothing warning MS patients about the danger of overuse causing a torn rotator cuff or carpal tunnel syndrome. Similarly, the other books written by physicians for MS patients didn't warn about this.

The reason for this chapter is to make MS patients aware of this risk so they can try to prevent permanent damage to the joints of their more functional arm.

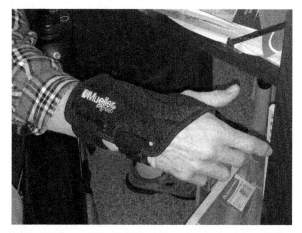

Figure 40-1 A wrist splint helps manage carpal tunnel syndrome due to overuse syndrome of the remaining functional arm.

Chapter 41

What is a peptic ulcer and are MS patients at increased risk?

A peptic ulcer is a defect in the protective lining (mucosa) of the stomach or first part of the small intestine (duodenum), which allows acidic stomach secretions to injure the wall of the bowel. This is painful and can lead to other complications. The most frequent cause of peptic ulcers is infection due to *Helicobacter pylori*. Once a defect in the mucosal lining of the stomach or duodenum forms, concentrated hydrochloric acid and digestive enzymes produced by the stomach can make the ulcer self-perpetuating and enlarging.

I never had an ulcer until my 17th year of MS, and I believe that MS patients may be at increased risk for getting an ulcer. Why do I say that if *H. pylori* infection is the most frequent cause? If an MS patient has already had an ulcer due to *H. pylori*, the patient is at increased risk for getting another ulcer, and MS patients often take medications that make that more likely. If an MS patient has *H. pylori* infection but has not yet had an ulcer, the patient will be at increased risk for getting a first ulcer because of the *H. pylori* infection and treatment with those same medications.

MS patients frequently have pain and can't take first line narcotic analgesics because this would further impair balance and cause additional constipation. This means that MS patients are frequently given other analgesics, one of which is acetaminophen, which provides only minimal relief for severe fracture pain. Orthopedists frequently prescribe nonsteroidal anti-inflammatory drugs (NSAIDs) for fracture pain when the patient cannot tolerate a narcotic. NSAIDs are frequent causes of peptic ulcer. I had been given NSAIDs several times for different musculoskeletal injuries complicating my MS and was never prescribed an accompanying drug for gastric acid suppression. I had always taken an accompanying drug for gastric acid suppression when I took many courses of methylprednisolone, which can also cause a peptic ulcer.[Chen KJ, et al. Risk factors for peptic ulcer disease in transplant patients – 11 years of experience from a single center. Clinical Nephrol. 2004; 62:14-20.][Rohrer CH,et al. Gastric hemorrhage in dogs given high doses of methylprednisolone sodium succinate. Am J Vet Res. 1999; 60:977-81.] I developed indigestion discomfort every time I took methylprednisolone, but never developed an ulcer while using the gastric acid suppression. 13 days after starting naproxen as treatment for a fracture of my clavicle without using gastric acid suppression, I developed pain due to an ulcer, which continued for months.

As mentioned above, MS patients often have osteopenia (less dense bones as seen by x-rays) due to low vitamin D levels, corticosteroid therapy, gastric acid suppression during corticosteroid therapy, gastric acid suppression for ulcers and/or gastroesophageal reflux disease, and increasingly frequent immobility and decreased weight bearing exercise, etc. When the MS patient develops significant osteopenia documented by bone densitometry, the patient is prescribed calcium, vitamin D, and bisphosphonate therapy (e.g. alendronate). Alendronate is another drug that can help cause or exacerbate a peptic ulcer.

An important reason for talking about gastric ulcers in this book is to recommend that MS patients ALWAYS take an accompanying drug for gastric acid suppression if prescribed high-dose steroids like methylprednisolone for an MS relapse or an NSAID for fracture pain. Will this always prevent an ulcer? Probably not, but the risk will be lower than if no gastric acid suppression is used.

Another way of protecting against peptic ulcer is using a drug called misoprostol, but it has a higher rate of side effects.[Rostom A, Dube C, Wells GA, Tugwell P, Welch V, Jolicoeur E, McGowan J, Lanas A. Prevention of NSAID-induced gastroduodenal ulcers. Cochrane Database of Systematic Reviews 2002, Issue 4. Art. No.: CD002296. DOI: 10.1002/14651858.CD002296.]

Chapter 42

What Is Nephrolithiasis (kidney stone disease) and Are MS Patients at Increased Risk?

In my ninth grade science class, we poured different amounts of a solute (e.g., sugar) into a beaker of water, suspended a string into the solution from a pencil lying across the top of the beaker and waited to see what would happen.

The beakers with more sugar started forming crystals along the string. This showed that a solution with a high enough concentration of solute can form crystals.

The same thing happens in the urinary tract when the concentration of a solute in urine (e.g. calcium oxalate) gets too high because of ingesting too much dietary oxalate or too little fluid or both (resulting in supersaturation of the solution). Calcium oxalate crystals are a relatively frequent finding in analysis of human urine, but the crystals can grow larger if the concentration rises and stays high. This is how a kidney stone forms. Calcium oxalate is the most frequent type of kidney stone among American patients (about 70% of stones).

When a stone gets large enough, it can cause colicky pain as it traverses the ureter, which conducts urine from the kidney to the bladder. In addition to pain, kidney stones can cause obstruction of the urinary tract, which can cause damage to the kidney and sometimes renal failure. They can also make treatment and cure of infection more difficult.

I saw no data from studies documenting a higher risk of kidney stones for MS patients, but I believe that MS patients are at higher risk. The other books written by physicians for MS patients said nothing about such an increased risk, but they noted that MS patients tend to drink less fluid as problems develop with urinary frequency, urgency and incontinence. Drinking less fluid causes increased concentration of urine, which makes crystal formation and development of stones more likely.

Patients with a positive family history of kidney stones are often at increased risk for developing stones. For example, in one family found to have excess calcium excretion and calcium oxalate stones, one man told me he had had 19 kidney stones by the age of 63 and his niece had had eight kidney stones by the age of 28.

MS patients with a positive family history have an increased risk for that reason. Drinking less fluid makes them have higher risk.

In my 22nd year of MS, I developed a kidney stone for the first time. There was no history of kidney stones on my father's or mother's side of the family. A recent study suggested that the prevalence of kidney stone disease among Americans was 8.8%. Roughly 15% of patients developing a stone have a positive family history and about 55% of patients developing more than one stone have a positive family history.

In addition to relative dehydration and supersaturation of urine predisposing to an increased risk for stone formation, there are other potential risk factors among MS patients that can increase the risk. One of these is diet. Many MS patients over the past several decades have chosen to reduce their consumption of animal fat (and animal products) and eat more vegetables and fruits; this change results in more consumption of oxalate (e.g., the Swank diet or the Jelinek diet that's mostly derived from the Swank diet, etc.). As mentioned above, MS patients are often advised to eat a wheat bran cereal such as Raisin Bran. Raisins are low in oxalate, but wheat bran is very high in oxalate. This alone may not cause MS patients to get a kidney stone, but combination with other high oxalate foods (e.g., spinach, chocolate, almonds, peanuts, peanut butter, etc.) could pose a risk.

Moreover, MS patients with nocturia can get treated with DDAVP (desmopressin), which concentrates the urine, making supersaturation and stone formation more likely. Treatment with DDAVP can result in hyponatremia and some important related side effects; to avoid these complications, the FDA advises patients taking DDAVP to stay NPO overnight (i.e., swallow nothing, including fluids). This additional fluid restriction makes the supersaturation of urine still worse and kidney stone development more likely. When I considered trying DDAVP, my neurologist warned that this treatment was a risk factor for developing kidney stones and that she had had a patient develop a stone after starting DDAVP.

So, an increased risk of kidney stones wasn't mentioned in the other books by physicians for MS patients, but I believe it exists and that patients should take precautions.

What precautions do I use? Dilution is the usual solution for kidney stone patients, but I can't increase fluid intake beyond the two liters I usually consume. It's recommended that a patient with a calcium oxalate kidney stone drink 3 to 4 L of water per day (101-135 ounces), but being an MS patient with a spastic bladder I am only able to drink about 53 ounces per day (39% to 52% of what is recommended to flush out the urinary tract, and keep new stones from forming). My water intake per day (including the water content of fruits and vegetables) is approximately 64 ounces (2 quarts). But that was my water intake per day when I developed a calcium oxalate kidney stone, so I have to be careful about ingesting large amounts of oxalate.

I carefully measure my fluid intake to be sure that I don't by chance drink less on one day than another.

The patient can avoid or eat only small to moderate portions of foods known to predispose to kidney stones (e.g., spinach, chocolate, peanuts, almonds, beets, and rhubarb are some foods that are very high in oxalate). After much thought, I chose the latter, feeling that life wouldn't be the same without an occasional taste of a special food. ("If we're treading on thin ice, then we might as well dance." – Jesse Winchester, "Third down, 110 to Go")

I also try to avoid ingesting too much oxalate during a short time span. Why should the time span matter? I found no data from studies of this question and saw nothing about this in the other books written by physicians for MS patients, but I believe this may matter for several reasons:

1) If I eat a food high in oxalate, my urine changes from clear to hazy because of crystals in the urine (the more oxalate I ingest, the hazier it gets).

2) The natural history of crystals in the urine is, in the vast majority of cases, to be peed out.

3) If I wait a day or two, my urine turns clear again and no symptoms develop.

4) When I got a kidney stone in my 22nd year after diagnosis of MS, relative dehydration due to limiting fluid intake was likely an important contributor, but the first symptom of a stone happened after I ate foods very high in oxalate two days in a row. The pain then abated and did not recur until I again ate foods very high in oxalate two days in a row.

5) Over the next 19 months, I spent a lot of time avoiding high oxalate foods, but then experimented with eating them one day but not eating the leftovers until several days later. So far, this approach has not resulted in another stone despite my inability to drink as much fluid as would normally be recommended for someone with a history of kidney stones (i.e., 3 to 4 liters per day).

How is one to know which foods are high in oxalate? There are a number of published tables available through Google that list a variety of foods and the concentration of soluble oxalate they contain. They don't always agree with one another. Be aware that such tables can change, sometimes adding or modifying information.

Another thing I do is to swallow a calcium citrate tablet (containing 630 mg of calcium) just before eating a food high in oxalate. The tablet dissolves in the stomach and the calcium binds with oxalate in the high oxalate food. The calcium oxalate formed by this chemical reaction in the stomach precipitates and doesn't get absorbed; it just flows downstream with undigested food and turns into feces.

As mentioned in Chapter 6 regarding incipient bowel problems, I began eating raisin bran soon after my MS started to deal with constipation. Bran cereals have high concentrations of oxalate, but I still depend upon the raisin bran to help control constipation 24 years later. To deal with the high oxalate, a calcium tablet just before eating the cereal may help (e.g., if I swallow the tablet but eating the cereal gets delayed, my urine becomes hazier than usual).

Does an MS patient have to get a urinalysis at the doctor's office to know when her urine starts having too many crystals?

That would help, but she might have a clue before that. Urine with lots of crystals is hazy, as mentioned above. It may thus be possible for her to do what I have done. The toilets in my house are water conserving, low flow Church brand toilets (about 1 gallon per flush). In such a toilet, the haziness mentioned above is obvious. In a toilet that uses twice as much water per flush, it might be more difficult to be certain. If so, urinating into a bedside commode or handheld urinal should allow the patient to see whether urine is clear or hazy. It can be poured into a clear plastic cup where haziness is obvious.

Can hazy urine be due to urinary tract infection rather than crystalluria? Yes, but crystals in the urine usually cause no symptoms at all while urinary tract infection causes pain over the bladder, burning pain in the urethra during and after voiding, increased nocturia, increased frequency of voiding, and/or increased urinary urgency. Infected urine may also have an unpleasant odor. With upper urinary tract (i.e., kidney) infection, there can be pain and tenderness over the flank, fever, shaking chills, nausea and vomiting.

Crystals don't change the odor of urine.

If crystals grow enough, they become kidney stones. Kidney stones cause colicky pain perceived in the abdomen or back over the kidney and ureter (the tubular structure that conducts urine from a kidney to the bladder) and sometimes change urine color to red or brown. When a stone is in a ureter, this can sometimes increase urinary frequency and urinary urgency, which may confuse some patients, but other symptoms don't overlap with those of a UTI (e.g., the colicky pain of a kidney stone and burning dysuria of urinary tract infection are not similar). One problem, however, is that some patients can have both stones and urinary tract infection.

In the absence of a centrifuge and microscope needed for performance of a urinalysis, one could use a dipstick to confirm or exclude the possibility of bacterial urinary tract infection. When there are no symptoms of urinary tract infection, it's very unlikely that new urine haziness would be due to subclinical, cryptic urinary tract infection. A urine dipstick with no white blood cells, red blood cells, or nitrite makes urinary tract infection still more unlikely. (Nitrite is produced by gram-negative bacilli like *Escherichia coli*, the most common cause of bacterial urinary tract infection.) When urinary tract infection is very unlikely, the most likely explanation for new urine haziness is crystals in the urine.

With a kidney stone, the urine dipstick will usually show red blood cells but no white blood cells or nitrite.

The more crystals one has in urine and the more frequently crystals are present, the higher the risk for stone formation. [Daudon M, Hennequin C, Bouielben G, Lacour B, Jungers P. Serial crystalluria determination and the risk of recurrence in calcium stone formers. *Kidney International.* 2005; 67:1934-43.] The nutrients absorbed from the diet most frequently resulting in supersaturation and crystal formation in urine are calcium and oxalate, which combine to form calcium oxalate. In people who are overweight or over 60, uric acid causes an increasing frequency of crystals and stones (i.e., with increasing weight and increasing age), but most stones in old and/or overweight patients are still composed of calcium oxalate, which, as mentioned above, accounts for about 70% of all kidney stones in American patients. [Daudon M, Lacour B, Jungers P. Influence of body size on urinary stone composition in men and women. Urol Res. 2006; 34:193-9.]

For completeness, I should mention that there is one other time that my urine predictably becomes hazy that is not due to dietary changes (or to urinary tract infection): whenever I have used a bit too much polyethylene glycol 3350 (MiraLAX) and my stools become so loose that the water in the toilet becomes too murky to see the feces and these loose stools are in the colon when I urinate. The same thing happens with other causes of loose stools. I have seen this at least 30 times and assume that this is due to better colonic absorption of oxalate from loose than from well formed stools. Anybody eating raisin bran can see that undigested insoluble bran fiber contributes greatly to stool appearance, and, as mentioned above, bran is very rich in oxalate, so I would guess that the high oxalate bran in unformed stools could be a source of increased oxalate being absorbed by the colon resulting in hazy urine in the absence of any change in diet. I was unable to find any studies evaluating this question, but did find studies showing that oxalate is absorbed from the rectum.

Chapter 43

What Is Osteoporosis and Are MS Patients at Increased Risk?

Osteoporosis is a bone disease characterized by a loss of bone mass and density, resulting in an increased risk of fracture. MS patients usually start off with a relative vitamin D deficiency as compared with a healthy population, which may result in reduced bone mass and density. Corticosteroid therapy for MS frequently causes more thinning of bones, resulting in osteoporosis.[Duzen O, et al. The course of hypercalciuria and related markers of bone metabolism parameters associated with corticosteroid treatment. Ren Fail. 2012;34(3):338-42. doi: 10.3109/0886022X.2011.648596. Epub 2012 Jan 20.][Li gw, et al. Marrow adiposity recovery after early zoledronic acid treatment of glucocorticoid induced bone loss in rabbits assessed by magnetic resonance spectroscopy. Bone. 2013;52:668-75.]

Gastric acid suppression with a proton pump inhibitor is frequently prescribed for MS patients during a course of high dose methylprednisolone therapy. MS patients can develop peptic ulcers as discussed above or gastroesophageal reflux disease, that both require gastric acid suppression. Gastric acid suppression is associated with decreased absorption of calcium and further thinning of bones.

Increasing MS related weakness and spasticity make a limb hard to move. These things result in reduction in the mass and density of bone (osteoporosis) and deposition of collagen (fibrosis) in non-bony tissues (skin, muscles, ligaments, tendons). Contracture makes a limb still harder to move, accelerating the process.

Osteoporosis is made more likely by hemiparesis reducing general muscular activity and weight bearing. A recent study suggested that the immobility of disability may be a more important risk factor for osteoporosis in MS patients than corticosteroid therapy. [Zorzon m, et al. Long-term effects of intravenous high dose methylprednisolone pulses on bone mineral density in patients with multiple sclerosis. Eur J neurol. 2005; 12:550-6.] A hemiparetic MS patient can try to increase exercise and weight bearing, but when the patient has a fractured bone in a leg or a torn rotator cuff in the shoulder, these things can make weight bearing exercise very difficult.

When the MS patient develops significant osteopenia as documented by bone densitometry, the patient is prescribed calcium, vitamin D, and bisphosphonate therapy (e.g. alendronate). Because it is difficult to increase bone density without using a bisphosphonate, it's important for the MS patient to try to avoid getting a peptic ulcer, which makes bisphosphonate therapy contraindicated because it can cause or exacerbate a peptic ulcer.

Chapter 44
Long-Term Healthcare Insurance

It's a good idea. Especially for a patient with MS for whom the average life expectancy has been about three decades, two of which usually occur after the patient is physically disabled and no longer able to work. The patient often receives disability insurance payments and Social Security disability payments until reaching a 65th birthday whereupon the patient is supposed to live on retirement savings. By that time, the patient is often more profoundly disabled than upon retirement after 10 years of the disease and often requires assistance with activities of daily living (e.g., mobility, eating, bathing, shaving, etc.) and long-term healthcare insurance would pay for a nursing aide to provide those services seven days per week. My own long-term healthcare insurance policy was obtained through my employer while I was still working at a cost of $43 per month. After my claim was accepted, the policy began paying $110.50 per day for care by nursing aides (i.e., a long-term healthcare insurance policy quickly reimburses the patient for all of his costs and continues paying nursing aides for a decade). In my own case, I applied for this benefit after 20.5 years of the disease, which means that care by nursing aides in the home will be available until I have had the disease for 30.5 years (if I should be so lucky to survive that long [vital statistics studies show that MS patients don't usually live to be 65 years of age even though the average longevity is three decades after diagnosis – partly because many of the diagnoses are made in early adulthood]). Paying my insurance premium for a decade cost $5,160. After my claim was approved, my investment of $5,160 was paid back to me (to pay my nursing aides) within the first month and a half. Over the ten-year life of my policy, it will pay $403,601.25 (i.e., at an annual rate of $40,360.12).

Chapter 45
Interacting with Caregivers

"As far as possible without surrender, be on good terms with all persons." – "Max Ehrmann", "Desiderata"
"I get by with a little help from my friends." –the Beatles, "With a Little Help from My Friends"

For the first 20 years of my MS I tried to remain as independent as possible. But there is a time "for every purpose under the heaven" (Ecclesiastes 3:2) and at 20 years and seven months, it became clear to me that new "handwriting was on the wall" (Daniel, 5:5-9). I fell 8 times over 9 days, once when I was walking out of the shower. I no longer felt comfortable walking on the slippery floor of the shower even when holding onto a grab bar. It was time for change. That was when my neurologist and I decided that it was time for me to have nursing aides assist me with activities of daily living, such as getting a shower using a shower chair.

How can a single nurse's aide get an MS patient up off of the floor after a fall? With a Hoyer lift. Such equipment is available through Medicare for MS patients who have frequent falls. It's well worth having. A 5'1" nurse's aide was able to lift me off of the floor within 10 minutes after a fall using a Hoyer lift. The floor was very uncomfortable, partly because of a large, new abrasion that was very painful.

I was fortunate to have many wonderful care providers over the next several years. That experience impels me to say several things about an MS patient's relationship with care providers.

A telephone interview may be good for starting the process of finding a nursing aide, but can never take the place of a face-to-face meeting, which should precede any final decision about hiring. For example, I told one applicant that the hardest physical task she would have to perform in caring for me was drying my feet after a shower. I asked if she was physically fit enough to squat down and do that. She assured me that she was, but in a face-to-face meeting, she wasn't. She struggled getting up out of a chair and walking across the kitchen due to age, weight, or both. Sometimes applicants are more guilty of wishful thinking than of downright dishonesty. She probably was one of those.

During a telephone interview, everything can seem compatible and appropriate, but the applicant may save other issues to raise only during the face-to-face meeting. For example, one applicant appeared to be very keen over the telephone to get the job, but informed me during our face-to-face meeting that she had already applied for a full-time job and thus would likely be available for backup care for only about one week. Another applicant sounded wonderful over the telephone but inquired during our face-to-face meeting whether the government would know that she was working for me. I told her that my wife and I had always been sticklers for following the law. She seemed disconcerted.

Infections are usually contagious and never helpful to an MS patient, so I ask each aide to let me know when she gets an infection so a backup can substitute until she's well. I ask each care provider to get an annual flu vaccine and to avoid people with viral infections when possible. Over the first three years, four of my aides came down with a flulike illness with fever and cough despite getting the annual flu vaccine and a fifth had fever and cough due to pertussis.

Six more took time off for colds with no fever, and there were 16 reported episodes of gastrointestinal infection (nausea, vomiting, diarrhea, etc.) requiring me to get a backup, but 12 of the 16 reported episodes of vomiting all occurred in the same individual (some aides may play hooky).

Communication is the lifeblood of a relationship and this is true of those between MS patients and their care providers. For this reason it's important to be open and direct. Max Ehrmann said that one should "be on good terms with all persons," as far as possible without surrender. Unlike the Dixie Chicks, MS patients probably should "make nice." Like the Beatles and most everybody else, we get by with a little help from our friends. So it's not good to alienate helpers. This can seem both straightforward and tricky depending upon the caregiver. Some are very easy to work with and others "a piece of work," as a friend of mine likes to say. As in dealings with everyone else, "honesty is [always] the best policy." Tact is also important, but keeping your preferences secret from caregivers is probably a mistake.

In the first week that I had nursing aides, two were alternating care and one seemed to do everything just right; the other didn't. When I tried to let the second one know what seemed to be working better for me, she took offense. She said that doing things differently was her style and resigned.

At that time, I was distressed because I only had the two workers and had not yet assembled a list of backups. After finding several backups, I was actually glad she had resigned. I started using that story for orienting future applicants. During an interview before hire, I asked each one whether they considered it appropriate for a patient to have and express preferences about the way things were done. Every applicant said it was appropriate. After that, I felt comfortable making my helpers aware of what I needed. Nobody objected.

There are a number of things that can interfere with this relationship. Many patients with late stage MS can develop cognitive deficits, which can make communication impossible. For those with intact mental status, other problems can interfere. One of those is the frequent use of medications like methylprednisolone which cause the patient to suffer and also sometimes the patient's caregivers to suffer. Methylprednisolone can cause the patient to say things she never would otherwise have said. This disinhibition can be countered by "biting one's tongue" (i.e., actively trying to avoid saying anything and specifically avoiding situations in which conversation will be emotionally challenging). The first important step in doing this is to recognize that methylprednisolone causes a change in what the patient says. In my case, I recognized this when my family attended a YMCA basketball game and, instead of just thinking that the referee had made a bad call, I immediately said so. The action surprised me because I realized immediately that the methylprednisolone was causing "loose lips." Later in the disease, dysarthria can become an important problem with communications. Spastic dysarthria can make it hard to articulate a sentence, and the patient straining to get the words out sometimes gets the tone "wrong" (i.e., sounding inappropriately harsh for what is being said). This can mislead caregivers into thinking that the patient is impatient or unappreciative or easily angered. After being told that my vocal tone had switched to an angry one many times and replying that I felt no anger but was merely trying to get words out, it finally dawned on me that people around me were constantly misinterpreting what I said because spastic dysarthria was causing the tone to be inappropriate. Wikipedia says that dysarthria can change the following 10 features of the patient's speech: range, tone, strength, steadiness, speed, breath control, volume, pitch, vocal quality, and timing.

Chapter 46

Do MS Patients Have a
Problem with Aerophagia?

"I never saw a moor,
I never saw the sea,
yet now I know how heather looks,
and what a wave must be."
    – Emily Dickinson, "Chartless"

What is aerophagia? It is a medical problem that literally means "swallowing air." But all human beings swallow air, so the medical problem is usually defined as "excessive air swallowing." I believe excessive amounts of swallowed air can become a problem for some MS patients. The other books written for MS patients don't say that. And I've seen no data from epidemiologic studies regarding this question. Given what the introduction of this book says about the importance of epidemiologic studies for determining whether an association is valid, why should anyone believe that in the absence of such studies?

In some cases, lack of data doesn't mean lack of an association. Lack of studies could just be due to nobody ever having considered the question. Einstein said that in science, "imagination is more important than knowledge." He didn't mean imagination as used to write science fiction. He was talking instead about scientists imagining how nature works when data are unavailable or too incomplete to clarify the situation. George H.W. Bush talked about "the vision thing."

Regardless of what this is called, it seems obvious that MS patients with severe dysphagia could swallow more air than do normal healthy people. Such MS patients are well known to aspirate food, drink and saliva into the lungs, so the same neural impairment could presumably allow more air to be swallowed. Neural impairment of speech in MS patients with spastic dysarthria can reportedly affect all 10 motor components of speech: range, tone, strength, steadiness, speed, breath control, volume, pitch, vocal quality, and timing. Swallowing involves nearby anatomic parts and physiologic mechanisms and is as complex as speech, so the MS monkey wrench for swallowing may be as large as the one for speech.

The phrase "suck wind" is urban slang for performing poorly. An MS patient becoming severely disabled has increasing difficulty doing everything. This can include otherwise simple things like sitting in a chair. When weakness and spasticity make it increasingly hard to sit in a chair, struggling to stay in the chair makes it hard to concentrate on eating and drinking. Periodic limb movements with forcible spastic contractions of the arm and sometimes adjacent parts of the trunk 4 times a minute at supper make this harder still. Meanwhile, swallowing itself also becomes more difficult over time. When trying to finish a glass of juice, I sometimes struggle to do this because of spasticity and poor posture; while struggling to swallow the juice, I often inhale sharply, which may increase air swallowing.

It wouldn't surprise me if esophageal impedance studies found that MS patients with severe dysphagia swallowed more air than normal controls. But problems with too much air in the stomach and colon also could arise from normal air swallowing and decreased burping [fewer, smaller or both]. Normal adults usually swallow several liters of air per day.[Poderoux P, Gulchin EA, Shezang L, et al. Esophageal bolus transit imaged by ultrafast computerized tomography. Gastroenterology 1996;110:1422– 8.][Levitt MD, Furne J, Aeolus MR, Suarez FL (1998). "Evaluation of an extremely flatulent patient: case report and proposed diagnostic and therapeutic approach". *Am J Gastroenterol* **93** (11): 2276–81. doi: 10.1111/j.1572-0241.1998.00635.x.] But only a small portion of this air gets excreted from the rectum where it accounts for only about a quarter of the flatus in an average adult, [Tomlin J, Lowis C, Read NW. Investigation of normal flatus production in healthy volunteers. Gut 1991;32:665–9.] [Suarez F, Furne J, Springfield J, Levitt M. Insights into human colonic physiology obtained from study of flatus composition. Am J Physiol. 1997; 272 (5 Pt 1): G1028-33.]

A study of a dozen healthy adults showed an average of thirty-three burps per day, far more than usually recognized. [Bredenoord AJ, Weusten BL, Timmer R, Smout AJ. Air swallowing, belching and reflux in patients with gastroesophageal reflux disease. Am J Gastroenterol. 2006 Aug;101(8):1721-6. Epub 2006 Jun 30.] This implies that most burping may be done subconsciously as the body removes swallowed air on auto-pilot.

Why might decreased burping occur in MS patients? Impaired neural control could make it happen as could postural problems due to weakness and spasticity. Being slumped over chronically may cause decreased burping of swallowed air because the physiologic reflex that triggers transient lower esophageal sphincter relaxation and a burp is a response to a sufficiently large air bubble rising to the top of the stomach. When severely slumped over, the air bubble doesn't rise to the top of the stomach.

An MS patient might come to have too much swallowed air for other reasons as well. As disability increases, the patient becomes slower doing everything and may try to compensate by speeding up whenever possible to please others. Gobbling food is one way. If eating too fast results in excessive air swallowing, this could be one mechanism. But gobbling food could also cause more rectal gas if swallowed as larger chunks with less chewing; large chunks are more likely to flow downstream undigested and get metabolized by colonic bacteria to produce 3 gases --CO_2, H_2, and CH_4 which usually make up ~3/4 of flatus.

Another mechanism could be swallowing smaller amounts per bite by patients trying to avoid aspiration. One study suggested that each 10 ml swallow of water in normal control patients was accompanied by 17 ml of air. [Poderoux P, Gulchin EA, Shezang L, et al. Esophageal bolus transit imaged by ultrafast computerized tomography. Gastroenterology 1996;110:1422– 8.] If a smaller swallow is associated with swallowing a similar amount of air or if there is an obligatory minimum amount of air per swallow, taking smaller bites could result in more air being swallowed.

What made me think that MS patients might be so afflicted? I seemed to develop the problem myself during my 23rd year of MS. I suspect that MS was likely the cause. As mentioned in Chapter 1, there are "truths that are neither for all men nor for all times," and this is one of many examples that I could list of MS-related problems that are absent early in the disease but can appear later.

What problems did I develop suggestive of aerophagia? In the 23rd year, I started having increased regurgitation and aspiration of stomach contents. At the time, I assumed that those changes were simply due to progression of MS. But I also started having increased rectal gas in the afternoon despite eating and drinking exactly the same amounts of exactly the same foods and drinks for breakfast and lunch. I had had problems due to increased rectal gas from eating foods associated with increased gas production (e.g., soybean products) during the five years before that, but this time I had added no such food. Moreover, taking 12 tablets of Beano with breakfast, lunch and supper had no effect on this increased rectal gas in the afternoon; this made inadvertent daily ingestion of beans an unlikely explanation for the increased gas. But again, I did not initially suspect excessive swallowed air to be the cause.

The increased rectal gas had several effects : 1) it could cause rectal urgency when little to no stool was present in the rectum [this, in turn, could cause tenesmus and prolonged sitting on the toilet for no reason or rushing to the toilet to have a bowel movement that was a very small bit of stool and a large gush of gas]; 2) it could cause an unstable patient like me to fall and break a bone [I did that]; and 3) it could cause urinary urgency by inflating the colon and causing pressure on the bladder.

In the 24th year, the regurgitation got still worse - becoming more frequent and causing aspiration of larger volumes of stomach contents. My last regurgitation and aspiration was followed by immediate dyspnea and nonstop coughing, both of which lasted for an hour. For the next three days, I woke sensing something in my throat that led me to try to clear my throat multiple times and then swallow. This was not the same sensation of thick saliva clogging my epiglottis that I got when sleeping in the recliner, which was associated with vigorous coughing on waking. These developments were sufficiently ominous that I began thinking more about the problem. After doing so, I began to recognize a pattern - my regurgitations tended to happen when I felt the need to burp. Until then, I had always ignored this feeling because burping is usually considered trivial. But large, symptomatic aspiration is not trivial, so I decided to try to brace myself for a burp by grabbing hold of walker handles, grab bars, or chair armrests and trying to pull myself more erect in order to try to burp prophylactically and prevent regurgitation and aspiration of liquid gastric contents. When I did that, the burp was only air (i.e., no regurgitated liquid stomach contents came up to my throat, though sometimes I could feel liquid stomach contents start to come up with the burp but immediately stop, as if unable to rise the full height of the esophagus against gravity). That seemed to do the trick. I stopped having regurgitation of stomach contents. After 14 months of doing that with no regurgitation or aspiration of stomach contents, I felt sure that burping of swallowed air when bent over (the way spastic, paretic MS patients often are) might be an important contributing cause of regurgitation and aspiration of stomach contents in MS patients.

During that time, I also started burping at times that I never had before. For example, when I sat up in bed for nocturia, I burped several times, and some nights did this each time I woke. Does audible burping when sitting up in bed mean that I had swallowed too much air? Not necessarily, and it doesn't mean that I was burping more per day than in the past. I could have been burping less per day but more at night—perhaps because of increasing accumulated air.

My new nocturnal burping suggested that there might be more air in my stomach, supporting the idea that my increased rectal gas and increased regurgitation might be due to excess swallowed air as well.

After my intentional burping worked to prevent regurgitation of stomach contents when I felt a burp coming on, I started trying to raise myself up more erect more frequently after eating a meal when I did not feel the need to burp and found that air was often present in the stomach at those times as well, which could lead to several burps in a row. Doing this and trying to swallow less air with food (e.g., stirring breakfast cereal until all air bubbles popped before starting to eat) were associated with fewer problems of fecal and urinary urgency due to rectal gas. I also found that I could burp two or three times after eating grapes before my breakfast cereal (i.e., air swallowing was occurring with swallowing solid food like it did when I swallowed liquids). And it did not have to be ingestion of a full meal; I could burp two or three times after eating grapes before my breakfast cereal or after swallowing tomato juice with pills at night. I should mention that trying to burp during other parts of the day (e.g., an hour before supper) usually produced no burps at all, implying that the swallowed air was occurring mainly with food and drink.

So, multiple features of my illness suggested that excessive air could be a problem for at least one MS patient (me). Are there data showing that excessive swallowed air can cause such problems for other types of patients? There are. Not all studies by even the same group of authors agree on this point, but the largest and most recent by Breedenoord and colleagues reported that patients swallowing more air at mealtime were more likely to regurgitate both liquid and air from the stomach after the meal. [Bravi I, Woodland P, Gill RS, Al-zinaty M, Breedenoord AJ, Sifrim D. Increased prandial air swallowing and postprandial gas-liquid reflux among patients refractory to proton pump inhibitor therapy. *"Clinical Gastroenterol Hepatol.* 2013; Jul;11(7):784-9. doi: 10.1016/j.cgh.2012.12.041. Epub 2013 Jan 30.] A study by the same group of investigators of patients found to have aerophagia because of plain abdominal radiographs showing their bowels distended by air reported increased air swallowing, increased burping and problems from increased rectal gas. [Hemminck GJM, Weuston BLAM., Bredenoord AJ, Timmer R, Smout AJPM. Aerophagia: excessive air swallowing demonstrated by esophageal impedance monitoring. *Clin Gastro Hepatol.* 2009; 7:1127-29.]

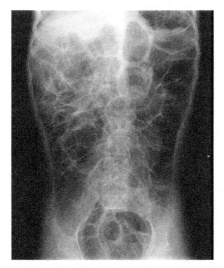

Figure 46-1 An abdominal x-ray shows air overfilling the entire bowel from stomach to rectum in a patient with aerophagia (excessive air swallowing). Swollen bowels can cause bloating and discomfort and cramp an MS patient's spastic bladder, resulting in urinary urgency and incontinence. A normal bowel filled with normal secretions and excretions would be thinner and light gray in an x-ray (by contrast, gases like air look much darker, as shown).

Two recent reviews of this topic concluded that regurgitation of stomach contents was usually related to transient relaxation of the lower esophageal sphincter (the physiologic reflex that triggers a burp). [Blackshaw LA. New insights in the neural regulation of the lower esophageal sphincter. *Eur Rev Med Pharmacol Sci.* 2008;12 Suppl 1:33-9.] [Kessing BF, Conchillo JM, Bredenoord AJ, Smout AJ, Masclee AA. Review article: the clinical relevance of transient lower esophageal sphincter relaxations in gastroesophageal reflux disease. Aliment Pharmacol Ther. 2011 Mar;33(6):650-61. doi: 10.1111/j.1365-2036.2010.04565.x. Epub 2011 Jan 10. Review.]

Chapter 47
Would a Power Recliner Be Useful to MS Patients Too Weak to Use a Manual Recliner?

I t helped me.

Sleeping in such a recliner allowed me to 1) walk less, allowing fourth metatarsal and femoral fractures to heal, 2) take the weight off of and straighten my back for an hour or two during the day when I was having back pain due to vertebral compression fractures or spasms (providing more pain relief than acetaminophen), and 3) take weight off of my butt for an hour or two when I was having trouble healing a buttock furuncle with heat alone, allowing the furuncle to heal.

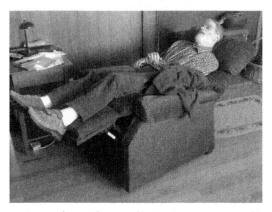

Figure 47-1 The author reclining in a power recliner.

The semi recumbent position (10°-20°) puts less pressure on the vertebral column and the buttocks than sitting upright. Doing this for as little as a half hour in the morning and a half hour in the afternoon was sufficient to help relieve the pain of vertebral compression fractures and associated back muscle spasms made worse by staying upright all day long (without requiring the longer time required for me to remove clothes and get in bed); the pain relief persisted to some degree for hours afterwards. Using the semi recumbent position for a similar amount of time per day also helped me heal buttock furuncles made worse by sitting upright all day long.

A power recliner has been available to physically disabled Medicare patients with sufficient paralysis to meet Medicare criteria.

But sleeping in the recliner also had several downsides. MS patients often have impaired glottic reflexes, making aspiration of saliva more likely and predisposing to aspiration pneumonia. Every time I started sleeping in the recliner, I woke multiple times with gobs of saliva clogging my airway at the epiglottis, causing me to cough to clear the airway; this didn't happen when I slept in bed. In bed, the body is lying flat. In my recliner, the back of the recliner doesn't recline to a fully horizontal position, leaving the section from one's buttock to head up about 10°-20° from horizontal. That small amount of incline appears to allow gravity to favor more aspiration of saliva. I also had a greatly increased frequency of periodic limb movements in my more spastic left leg; this was a problem in multiple ways – the movements sometimes woke me or made it hard to go back to sleep and twice removed my left shoe, which is a tricky problem for an MS patient waking up for urgent nocturia. A weak spastic MS patient like me has trouble standing on the slick surface of an oak floor wearing socks without shoes. Another downside of sleeping in the recliner was that this put more pressure on my bottom than did sleeping flat in bed. This small increase in pressure applied all night every night might cause pressure related problems in the buttocks or sacrum of weaker, less mobile MS patients.

Chapter 48
How Best to Counter the Yucky Taste of Methylprednisolone?

B efore I discovered a method for doing this, I used to gasp and gag (almost retching) with disgust every time I had to swallow methylprednisolone tablets for an MS flare. The method I developed involved chewing up a bite of banana, and then immediately using the glob of chewed banana to coat as many methylprednisolone tablets as I could conveniently swallow (either on a plate using a spoon or in my mouth using my tongue).

When mixed with the gooey banana properly, the methylpred- nisolone tablets were mostly cloaked and the entire mass could be swallowed with a gulp of tomato juice sort of like a raw oyster. It was easier for me to swallow than a raw oyster and much easier to swallow than plain methylprednisolone tablets without a banana coating. If any unpleasant methylprednisolone taste lingered, I would chase the banana mass with a few more gulps of tomato juice, which effectively cut any small bits of taste that my tongue managed to detect despite the banana coating. Taking the tablets this way, I never had to gasp in disgust.

Chapter 49
Fractures

Fractures (broken bones) are more common among MS patients because MS is associated with frequent falls (see Chapter 26) and osteoporosis (thinning of bones [Chapter 43]). The other books written for MS patients mentioned above don't say much about this, but it probably deserves its own chapter. The problem has loomed large for me.

Most of my really bad MS related pain has been due to fractures. Not all such fractures are severely painful. For example, I have had rib fractures with minimal pain (1 of 10 on an ordinal scale in which 10 is maximal pain) and a group of simultaneous posterior rib and vertebral fractures so painful (10 of 10 on the same ordinal scale) that the pain caused me to pass out, fall on the floor, and break more ribs.

After more than 200 falls, I have suffered 35 or more fractured bones: nine compression fractures of one or more vertebrae, 12 fractures of one or more ribs, a coccyx fracture, a fracture of the tip of the left elbow, a fracture of the left iliac crest, 2 fractures of the left clavicle (collarbone), 5 minor skull fractures, one fracture of my left fourth metatarsal, and four hip fractures.

In addition to causing intense pain, the pain of a fracture

generally lasts for months unless the fractured bone can be immobilized and weight bearing can be avoided. For MS patients, this usually results in chronic suffering because analgesics capable of relieving such intense pain are usually contraindicated for MS patients. Narcotic analgesics can cause increased constipation and also cause the patient to feel tipsy, increasing the risk of falling. Aspirin can cause increased bleeding, a serious hazard in patients prone to falling. Nonsteroidal anti-inflammatory drugs can cause peptic ulcers and have to be avoided in patients who have already suffered this complication. Such contraindications often leave an MS patient using acetaminophen (Tylenol), which only lowered one of my severe fracture pains from 8 (on a 10 point ordinal scale) to 7. Any lessening at all is desperately needed in this circumstance, but constant pain of 7 is still terrible.

When I had three vertebral compression fractures at the age of 15, my surgeon prescribed bed rest for six weeks followed by several months in a body cast. Lying flat on my back in bed kept the bone from moving and from bearing weight most of every day (the only exceptions were getting up to use the bathroom or eat). It worked well. Unfortunately, an MS patient with severe weakness and spasticity could not tolerate six weeks of bed rest or being in a cast, without severe difficulty.

In addition to chronic suffering due to moderate to severe pain, fractures have often caused increased disability for me – both temporary and chronic. For example, in the 17th year of my MS, I fell and fractured my clavicle (collarbone). For that reason, I had to stop washing my spastic, paretic left leg the way I had been doing it in the shower for years (i.e., I would lift that leg with my stronger right arm and grab hold of it with the paretic arm; while holding it that way I could use the stronger arm to wash the entire leg with soap and water). After I stopped doing that because of the fracture, I was never able to restart doing that again. The same was true of tying ties, putting on coats, etc. Use it or lose it.

MS patients have all sorts of questions and probably wonder

whether every bad pain after a fall indicates the need for an x-ray. I started falling three years before I retired and most of my early falls resulted in very little pain. My first seriously unpleasant fall happened shortly after I retired. I fell out the back door and down two steps, landing on my head on a wooden deck. I was stunned by the heavy blow and had a bad headache for a week. Given that I had not been prone to headaches, I wondered whether my physicians would want imaging of my head after such an unpleasant fall. I called and was told that we should "watch and wait" to see if anything bad developed. Because that fall was much worse than all of my other falls, I got the message that radiology usually was not necessary and that watching and waiting was often sufficient for an MS patient.

The first time I went to get x-rays after a fall, I was already certain that I had fractured my left clavicle. After doing that and seeing what role the radiographs played in management of my clavicular fracture, I didn't go back for more x-rays when I broke the same clavicle a second time or when I fell and broke ribs a dozen times.

After breaking vertebrae and anterior and posterior ribs, I developed a kidney stone in my left kidney and got colicky stone pain in addition to pain from all the surrounding fractures. Physicians evaluating the new stone pain ordered x-rays, which documented rib and vertebral compression fractures but didn't alter management. Such experiences led me to usually skip going in for x-rays because I can usually tell the difference between a bruise and a fracture. One way to tell is severity of the pain: the worse the pain, the more likely it represents a fracture. Several times after an especially bad fall with especially bad pain, I have developed nausea, dizziness, and malaise so bad I have to sit for 10-20 minutes until it passes. Each time I've felt that and gotten an x-ray, there was a fracture. Another sign of a fracture is longevity of the pain. Bruises usually start getting better within days without limiting mobility. Fractures often hurt just as bad or worse over the first few days unless mobility is limited (e.g., when a fractured bone can be immobilized in a cast, the pain can immediately begin disappearing).

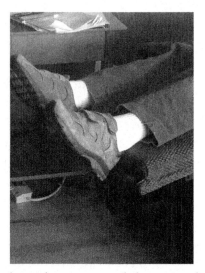

Figure 49-1 The author wore a tightly strapped Velcro shoe as a makeshift cast as shown after breaking a fourth left metatarsal bone. This required him to sleep in the recliner since he couldn't get into bed wearing a shoe.

By contrast, pain from a fractured bone that cannot be immobilized often can get worse if the fractured bone continues to be moved and especially if it is used for weight bearing. If hip pain is increasing with weight bearing 19 days after a fall, a bruise is unlikely; if that pain then subsides with reduced weight bearing, this also suggests that the pain was due to a fracture, not a bruise. After a period of immobility, the patient may be able to start moving that extremity to a certain degree and bearing weight to a certain degree without worsening. How can the patient know where to draw this line? It's hard to give an exact answer because fractures can vary from minor (e.g., hairline fractures that can get better quickly) to major (large fractures that can get much worse with moving and especially with weight bearing). The patient's weight also contributes, since being heavy puts more stress on a fractured bone in the foot or leg.

For a wheelchair patient, it's important to know that putting the foot of a leg with a broken hip on the foot rest first is a mistake.

Doing this causes increased pressure on that hip and considerable pain when lifting the other foot onto the foot rest. That can be avoided by changing the order - lifting the foot of the other leg onto the foot rest first.

Preventing fractures in patients with frequent falls and osteoporosis is difficult. Falls can be prevented by staying in a chair or bed, but doing that makes the patient weaker and more spastic. Every patient has to evaluate and choose which options to employ, understanding that there are risks as well as benefits for each approach. My approach has always been to keep walking as far as my weak spastic legs will take me but to be as careful as possible. Having a lot of fracture pain can provide powerful motivation for being careful.

Bisphosphonates such as alendronate are usually recommended to patients with osteoporosis to increase bone density. I took alendronate for years until I developed a peptic ulcer due to a nonsteroidal anti-inflammatory drug prescribed by the orthopedist caring for my first clavicular fracture. The peptic ulcer made further use of alendronate impossible.

Calcium and vitamin D supplements are often prescribed for patients with osteoporosis hoping to improve bone mineral density. There are fewer supportive data with this approach than with bisphosphonates, but one recent meta-analysis (study pooling the results of multiple other studies) reported that higher doses of vitamin D than previously recommended were more likely to prevent fractures. [Bischoff-Ferrari HA, et al. A pooled analysis of vitamin D dose requirements for fracture prevention. N Engl J Med. 2012 Jul 5;367(1):40-9. doi: 10.1056/NEJMoa1109617. Erratum in: N Engl J Med. 2012 Aug 2;367(5):481] Using this approach would require the guidance of one's physician because the optimal doses of calcium and vitamin D are not yet certain and some studies have reported harm from calcium and vitamin D supplementation.

I had more frequent fractures after stopping alendronate; it got so bad that every fall seemed to fracture bone. Feeling desperate, I agreed to increase my vitamin D dose from 1500 international units

(IU) to 2500 IU (more because of desperation than data). The 1500 IU daily dose was the result of taking a multivitamin tablet with breakfast and a Citracal (calcium citrate plus vitamin D) tablet before lunch and dinner. My vitamin D dose had been stable for years before increasing it by 1000 IU. I had less frequent fractures after the increase, but cannot cite data showing that it was responsible. For now, I'll keep taking the higher dose, hoping that it yields more benefit than harm.

Chapter 50
Bathing

Chapter 1 said that every therapy has pluses and minuses, so an MS patient must balance risks and benefits. Bathing is a good example of this. It promotes general hygiene and provides a convenient time for routine application of an antiseptic like chlorhexidine gluconate to prevent infection of abrasions and help heal minor skin infections.

But bathing also causes problems. Because of Uhthoff's phenomenon (heat related weakening), a hot bath is not a good idea, and stepping over the side of a bath tub quickly becomes an insurmountable problem for an MS patient with leg weakness.

A normal healthy person can sit in a bathtub full of water with little risk because of a normal urinary tract. A patient with an abnormal urinary tract, such as an MS patient, has potential problems. If the water is contaminated with microbes, as can happen, there is a greater risk that the contaminated water could enter the urethra and start toward the bladder.

So, showering became my primary way of bathing. How does an increasingly hemiparetic patient with increasing spasticity manage to bathe himself in the shower? I did this by leaning against a wall and making frequent use of handrails. I also turned the water off intermittently after getting wet to apply soap and shampoo. This served a dual purpose: it kept me from getting too warm and made it easier to apply soap and shampoo without the water washing it away before that soap could be well applied. For the first 15 years of my MS, taking a shower was invigorating. I would predictably be stronger after the shower than before, even though I always used warm water, not cool or cold. I could tell that I was stronger because it was easier dressing after the shower than it was removing clothes before the shower.

But after 15 years, the invigoration was probably more psychological than physical, and I began to have more problems with increased weakness and spasticity during and immediately after showering; these effects would subside over 20 to 30 minutes. If a patient tries to avoid the increased spasticity associated with a warm shower by taking a cool shower, increased spasticity occurs as a complication of that as well.

After 20 ½ years of MS, I fell coming out of the shower and decided that using a shower chair was safer for preventing falls. Sitting in a shower chair had other problems. It was cold and clammy, so I started using towels warmed in the dryer to dry off. And I had to carefully point my penis down between my legs before the shower or spastic adduction caused it to sit in my lap, which filled with water, soap suds and shampoo, irritating the urethra (and implying access to the urethra for microbes in the water).

Chapter 51
Getting Dressed (while skirting MS impairments)

When I lost the ability to dress standing up because of imbalance, I started sitting on the bed to do it. A decade later, I'm still doing that. As spasticity increased, it got harder to sit on the bed and, to make this easier, we removed the boxspring underneath the mattress; this allowed me to keep sitting on the bed and being able to reach my feet on the floor for additional years.

As my left arm became more paretic, doing all sorts of things became more difficult. It got harder to tie my shoes, but I found that substituting round laces made by Penguin allowed me to keep tying my shoes for a couple more years after regular flat shoelaces were no longer usable. When I lost the ability to tie my shoes using the round laces, I switched to using shoes with Velcro straps (Propet Hook and Loop Shoes). I later found that shoes with heel loops were easier to get on with one hand (e.g., Merrell Jungle Moccasins slip on shoes); before that I was never able to get my edematous paretic foot into a slip-on shoe even with a shoehorn. [I found that a 24 inch handled shoehorn made by Shacke and available through Amazon for $15 was easier for me to use with advancing MS related debility, which makes it hard to bend down to struggle with a shoe without falling off the bed.] A shoehorn was sometimes necessary to get my edematous paretic foot into the slip-on shoe after a midday bath, but never when getting dressed in the morning because the edema was reabsorbed while lying in bed at night.

For some reason, when I was losing the ability to tie my shoes or put on socks because of increasing weakness and apraxia of the left hand, closing my eyes made it easier for the dysfunctional left hand to participate and succeed. When I lost the ability to put on cotton socks, I switched to using cotton polyester blend socks and was able to keep putting socks on for 6 more years.

After I retired due to disability, I began wearing jeans because they were comfortable and easy for a paretic person to pull up and down in trips to the bathroom. They seemed to provide good protection for my legs when I fell. The denim also provided good friction with the floor when I needed traction for getting back up. When my paretic arm became too weak for me to be able to fasten jeans, I stopped wearing jeans and switched to slacks, which I found easier to button. I used Dockers slacks because I already had some in a closet; they had a substantial amount of cotton for protecting my legs during falls, and they were easy to fasten with one hand. Their main problem was lack of friction with the floor, making it harder to get back up after falling.

When I started having trouble fastening the button on my slacks, I kept wearing them but just pulled the zipper all the way up and stopped bothering with the button. When I started having trouble pulling the zipper up on the slacks, I switched to using polyester slacks with a partially elastic waist (an extra 3 inches of stretch). The Haggar polyester slacks were easier to put on, take off, slide up and down for toileting, and less likely to slide down to my ankles during a public moment. But, being silky, they tended to flop down around the ankles like a hobble when lowered for toileting. Moreover, if they slid under the sole of a shoe, they were very slippery and could cause a fall.

Chapter 52
Wearing Comfortable Clothes That Fit

Wearing clothes that fit is important for an MS patient – more important than for a normal healthy person. When getting into clothes that fit is already a struggle, getting into clothes that don't fit adds an extra dimension of difficulty.

A shirt too bulky is more difficult to tuck in. It can also make finding the genitalia difficult during toileting. Pants too large are more likely to fall off; this could cause embarrassment for anyone, but could also make an MS patient fall.

Having clothes too tight makes it hard to get underwear and pants back on after using the toilet repeatedly throughout the day and night. When there is an episode of urinary distress, having clothes too tight augments the urgency and makes incontinence in clothes more likely.

Wearing clothes that fit became more complicated for me when old reliable companies such as J.C. Penney that marketed very good Stafford underwear for decades recently started marketing products that might be viewed askance by their customers of prior decades. For many years, my waist size was 30 inches, and I wore Stafford underwear of that size. Perhaps because of the enlarging American waistline, Penney stopped having 30 inch waist underwear routinely available, so I tried the closest size available – 32 inches – and found that I could wear those without a problem. After doing that for a decade, I bought lots of packages as I retired due to disability, figuring that shopping was about to get more difficult. After using up all but a few of those packages, I tried to get more of the same but discovered that Stafford underwear had undergone an inexplicable change: their newly marketed 32 inch underwear had become too small for me to wear and their 34 inch underwear was too large. I spoke to their Customer Service division who were unable to explain the recent change. Other customers commented about this change in online critiques of the products. I then began searching through other brands, which took months and eventually found that none of 10 brands would fit. I had just about given up before trying Dockers 36 inch waist underwear, which fit perfectly. This was a wonderful discovery, because I needed underwear, but it was as inexplicable as the change in size of the Stafford underwear. Making it seem very strange, I could still wear Dockers slacks with a 30 inch waist but had to use the new "36 inch" Docker underwear (34 inch Docker underwear were too small)!

Elastic waistbands are important for hemiparetic patients who have difficulty with fastening buttons and tying drawstrings, but can cause problems as well. A patient with an enlarging belly can experience increased pressure over the bladder, creating problems with urinary urgency. A spastic patient with hyperactive deep tendon reflexes can fall due to an elastic waistband tugging at the popliteal fossa (the hollow behind the knee) when pants are being raised because this can cause a spastic leg to buckle.

Chapter 53
How Does a Homebound Person Go Shopping?

The Internet is a wonderful tool, but, like any other tool, it has advantages and disadvantages. Being able to shop online has become a blessing for the disabled who can't run out to a neighborhood store and need an alternate way of shopping. Amazon is a very reliable online store that protects customers' private information (e.g., credit card info), ships products promptly, and allows items that won't work (e.g. clothes that don't fit) to be shipped back free of charge for a full refund.

A disadvantage is that not all online shopping goes this smoothly. Crooks often send out emails trying to scam the gullible and steal money or private information in phishing expeditions.

When I find something I like, I'm tempted to order multiple, because products I like and order online keep disappearing: 1) Stafford underwear briefs with a 30 inch waist at JC Penney, 2) Dockers underwear briefs with a 36 inch waist, 3) Propet Hook and Loop Shoes, 4) Carex device for attaching a flashlight to a walker, 5) Sebulex shampoo, etc.

Chapter 54
If You're Going to Be Paralyzed, Does Weight Matter?

Yes. It's good to maintain an optimal weight in order to have clothes that fit. Having clothes too tight makes it hard to get underwear and pants back on after using the toilet repeatedly throughout the day and night, as mentioned above.

As a patient becomes more debilitated, getting up from the toilet and pulling one's underwear back up without falling over can be a challenge. If underwear are too tight because of a changing waistline, this is a problem for a weak arm. This makes getting it done harder and falling more likely, both of which are important problems to avoid. When there is an episode of urinary distress, having clothes too tight increases urinary urgency and makes incontinence more likely. Changing size would also require purchasing a new wardrobe, which is both inconvenient and expensive for an MS patient with dwindling amounts of time to do anything.

It's important to maintain a stable weight for multiple other reasons. Getting too heavy makes it harder for the MS patient's weakened muscles to rise out of a chair, off the bed, etc. Making ambulation more difficult for a patient already suffering fatigue is not a good idea. Extra weight also adds to the problem of pressure on the buttock of an increasingly paralyzed leg, which can result in pressure sores or pressure related infections. Obesity can predispose the patient to diabetes mellitus, which causes lots of problems and would make an MS patient still more susceptible to infection.

Chapter 55
How Does an Increasingly Hemiparetic Patient Stand up, Pull up His Pants and Fasten Them?

For me, the exact way things got done has varied over time as my hemiparesis got worse. At present, it depends on the time of day. Being stronger and less spastic in the morning, I can usually stand up and do this with one hand in the morning. As the day progresses and I get weaker and more spastic, this becomes more difficult, and I generally end up leaning against the bathroom counter to get it done or get it partially started standing beside the toilet and then sit down in my wheelchair and button my pants while sitting down.

Elastic waistbands can be important for hemiparetic patients who have difficulty fastening buttons and tying drawstrings, but can cause problems as well. New pants that are too small or an enlarging belly can cause increased pressure over the bladder, creating problems with urinary urgency. A spastic patient with hyperactive deep tendon reflexes can fall due to an elastic waistband pulling

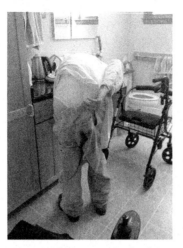

Figure 55-1 The author propped against the bathroom counter to prevent falling and using his only functional arm to raise and fasten his pants.

at the popliteal fossa (the hollow behind the knee) when pants are being raised, because this can cause a spastic leg to buckle.

Polyester pants have advantages and disadvantages. advantages include being easier to put the pants on and take them off, pull them down and up for toileting, and being less likely to have the paretic leg trap the other leg by sitting on the other pants leg when trying to get into the wheelchair. Disadvantages of polyester pants include less friction, which means that the patient is more likely to slide out of a chair when falling awkwardly onto an edge of the chair seat, which has happened to me multiple times. Less friction also means that a hemiparetic patient is unable to hold a flashlight between legs while trying to screw on the front of the light after a battery change, and that fecal incontinence is more likely because it's harder to pinch the butt closed.

As mentioned, in Chapter 23, partially flexing one knee made my spastic left hand less spastic and more helpful for raising pants (as compared with standing with both knees fully extended). I only had to resort to this device in certain evenings when my cumulative spasticity got bad enough to require this.

Chapter 56

How Does a Person with Hemiparesis Get up off the Toilet without Leaking Urine All over Everything?

With difficulty. The simplest tasks can seem challenging with hemiparesis.

My earliest approach to this problem was briefly described in Chapter 6. 24 years later, staying dry has become more complicated. My current approach requires multiple steps as itemized below.

1) mold the incontinence pad (iPad) so that it will be correctly configured (i.e. invaginated) and optimally cover the male genitalia. 2) take a stack of toilet paper as thick as necessary to blot up the usual amount of post void dribbling for that particular stage of MS and position it over the urethral meatus with my stronger right hand, 3) wedge my weaker, paretic left hand over the stack of toilet paper to hold it in place between adducted thighs as I rise, 4) position my underwear so that the just remolded iPad won't get unmolded in the process of getting up, 5) position the pants so that when I stand up, my bare leg won't be pressing against the cold porcelain

of the toilet (because the cold could cause a myoclonic jerk and consequent fall), 6) position the foot of my stronger right leg against the toilet so that I can brace that leg against the toilet as I stand up for stability, 7) grab the grab bar with my stronger right arm and use that to leverage myself up off the toilet into a standing position braced against the toilet, 8) use my right hand to pin the stack of toilet paper against the urethral meatus and release the weaker left hand from that responsibility, 9) reposition the stack of toilet paper so that it is centered over the urethral meatus, if necessary, 10) using the palm of my stronger right hand to hold that stack of toilet paper in place, I stretch out that hand to go over and under the male genitalia to reach the perineum (the space between the male genitalia and the rectum) so that I can massage that area with my second or third fingertip, which always releases additional urine (currently for me, 2-10 mL).

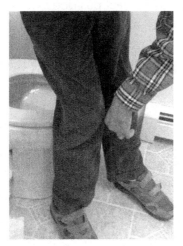

Figure 56-1 The author's stronger right leg is propped firmly against the toilet to allow him to rise from the toilet without falling and blot the urethral meatus to prevent urine leakage.

Male genitalia dangling in the way makes this a difficult process, like having a hot dog and two large raw oysters in the way of a single hand trying to do this. This may sound like a small obstacle course, but I think of it as being more like a minefield, because a hand pressed the wrong way against testicles can cause considerable pain. On a warm day and sometimes even on a winter day when wearing corduroy pants, this can become still more difficult because the warmed genitalia enlarge and the scrotum can cling to the hand trying to do all of this multitasking.

11) use the stronger right hand to grasp the glans penis and stretch the penis a bit so that my weaker left hand can try to grab the stretched penis (operating sort of like a lobster's pinchers), 12) try to wring out what's left in the urethra into the stack of toilet paper using both hands, 13) take a single sheet of toilet paper (because it's more bibulous than the stack) and touch it to the urethral meatus several times. This usually completes the drying process.

14) pull up the underwear and iPad, 15) reconfigure the iPad over the genitalia (pulling up the underwear almost never results in the iPad settling into perfect position over the genitalia), 16) raise the pants, tuck in T shirt and shirt, and fasten pants. The process of tucking my undershirt into my underwear, tucking my shirt into my pants and raising my pants and buttoning them is a very difficult process with one hand, which often causes the careful configuration of the iPad to become displaced and have to be reconfigured.

Some might ask why bother with all of the blotting if wearing an iPad, but urine can spill onto underwear, pants, shoes, shirt, toilet seat, and the floor as well as the iPad. If someone can figure out how to avoid such spillage and direct all spillage to the iPad, she would have to decide whether feeling and smelling urine was acceptable. I have felt more comfortable avoiding that.

Chapter 57

How Does a Paralyzed Person Answer the Telephone When It Starts Seeming Impossible?

One option is to switch to using a cell phone which can accompany the patient wherever he goes except into the shower. Unfortunately, even if the patient has a cell phone in a holster or a pocket, holding and answering a cell phone is often difficult with hemiparesis.

To answer the landline telephone, I use a headset with DECT technology which allows the patient to answer the phone from 400 feet away through any walls of the house. I can answer the phone when sitting in the backyard in a wheelchair.

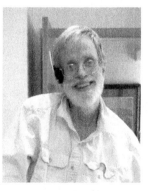

Figure 57-1 The author wearing an Office Runner headset, which is useful for dictating into the Dragon NaturallySpeaking computer software program and for answering a landline telephone when within 400 feet of the phone.

Chapter 58
What Is the Best Way for a Paralyzed Person to Read a Heavy Book or Turn on Music?

This is obviously an opinion not based on data. I believe that the optimal way for paralyzed people to read books, especially heavy ones, is with an electronic tablet like the Kindle, Nook or I-Pad. I find it much easier even if the book is only a paperback, which I frequently drop, losing my place. Being bent over by poor posture also often results in poor illumination of a conventional book.

I can buy a textbook of medicine that would conventionally weigh about 10 pounds, but, in the Kindle, the book is much easier to access, turn pages, etc. with all of the color illustrations. A tablet can also be used for watching a movie. I find all this very convenient.

Readers may be concerned about electronic tablets causing insomnia if used during the evening before bed, but the studies reported much milder effects on sleep than those caused by my MS (e.g., one study found a delay in getting to sleep of about 10 minutes after iPad reading for four hours). I don't generally read for such long durations in the evening and have perceived no additional problem from using my Kindle Fire or computer or television to watch a movie in the evening.

The Amazon Echo is even more user-friendly for a paralyzed patient wishing to play music or listen to an audiobook; it is paired with an Amazon Kindle, so all of the music and all of the audiobooks in the Kindle can be easily played through the Echo's speaker. The patient can just say, "read *The Christmas Carol* by Charles Dickens" or "play Beethoven's Moonlight Sonata," without having to pick anything up, press a button, etc. This device can also facilitate communication with the nurse's aide because an Echo remote control can be attached to a motorized wheelchair and go everywhere the patient goes. This means that a patient in the bathroom can say "Jane, I need help in the bathroom" through the Echo's speaker. This is much easier than shouting for help.

Chapter 59
How Does a Hemiparetic Patient Get into Bed?

The way I did it was by sitting down on the bed, pulling back the cover, grabbing my weak, spastic left leg with my stronger right arm and lifting it up onto the bed as I fell onto my left weak side. Then I used my stronger right leg to push my right foot under the cover (this is an important step because having the cover over a leg helps to anchor the leg and keep it from sliding off the bed). After the right leg was under the cover, I would then grab my weak left leg with my stronger right arm and pull it further over onto the bed. Next, I would use the stronger right arm to pull the cover completely up over my body, providing further anchorage. Then I would again use my stronger right arm to pull the weak left leg further onto the bed and use the stronger right leg to help push the weak left leg down under the cover as I rolled onto my back. Because the left leg was very weak, this could take 5 to 10 times before the left leg was maneuvered sufficiently far from the edge of the bed that I could sleep comfortably without risk of sliding off the edge. This process was also facilitated by wearing socks to bed. In winter, I started wearing wool socks to bed just for warmth, but they gave considerably better traction for anchoring the right foot while trying to move the left leg further into the bed. For that reason, I started wearing socks to bed year-round.

Getting into bed is even harder for an MS patient on the night after the sheets have been washed, because clean sheets have less friction. This makes it harder for the stronger leg's foot to serve as an anchor. I struggle to do that wearing socks, which is necessary for my weaker leg to slide further into the bed. These things have to be done iteratively every time. Whether it's a good night or a bad night, it has to be done more when first getting into bed and especially after the sheets have been washed.

It's always easier after I've been asleep for a couple of hours and sleep makes me stronger.

As mentioned in Chapter 23, I had to remove the boxspring in order to keep being able to sit on the bed for dressing as my spasticity increased. Removing the boxspring was equally important for continuing to get into the bed without assistance.

Chapter 60
Incontinence Pads (I-Pads)

Some books about MS imply that everything will be fine if you use a high absorbency incontinence pad, but that's not so. I'd never had urinary incontinence resulting in wet clothes that had to be changed until after I started using such pads for a different reason and then had to change clothes four times in one day despite having a pad in each time that the incontinence occurred.

The books leave out exactly how these things work. For this reason, an MS patient can be using something that might work but doesn't do so optimally because some information has been omitted. For example, the incontinence pad comes folded in a package and has to be unfolded and molded into an optimal shape before being stuck with its adhesive surface to the inside of one's briefs. The package (and the books) didn't say anything about this, so the patient could be using these things incorrectly for months before figuring out how they should be used optimally.

What I do is take a pad out of the package and then mold it into roughly the shape of a hollowed out canoe (to work optimally for the male anatomy). I do this by putting the absorptive surface down on my right thigh and rubbing the kinks out of the pad, moving it back-and-forth over my knee. The skin needs to be normal so that the pad stays clean; a skin lesion (e.g., abrasion, psoriasis plaque, etc.) can contaminate the pad, so that should be avoided.

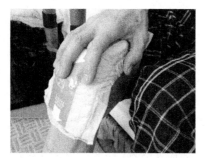

Figure 60-1 An incontinence pad being molded by rubbing it over a clean, healthy knee.

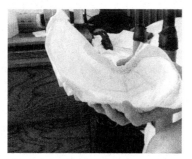

Figure 60-2 An incontinence pad demonstrating the desired canoe shape for application over the male genitalia.

After the pad is first molded and successfully adheres to the inside of one's briefs, there may be a temptation to think that this is all that is needed for optimal pad function. That would be incorrect. For best results, this has to be done repeatedly every time one's pants are lowered (i.e., a very frequent occurrence for an MS patient). If this isn't done, my pad develops lumps in inappropriate places, which make optimal positioning of the penis inside the pad impossible. Sometimes, if remolding of the pad is not done, it gets sufficiently disarrayed that the sticky side that adheres to the underwear can get turned around and stick uncomfortably to my genitalia (ouch!). You don't have to have that happen more than once to become convinced about the need for remolding the pad each time pants are lowered. In addition to discomfort, disarray of the pad makes leakage from incontinence more likely.

The first brand of incontinence pads purchased for me didn't work well, because it was not designed for the male anatomy (i.e., there was no invagination and, as a result, the penis would drift out from behind the pad and wet the underwear).

The second pad that I tried (Depends brand) was designed for the male anatomy, but there was no invagination as it came out of the package; the patient had to try to fashion a cup. This was not always easy to do for a physically disabled person with one functional hand.

The third pad that I tried (Assurance brand sold by Walmart) was also not invaginated as it came out of the package, but it was easier to invaginate than the second pad I tried. It also held more water than the second brand that I tried. I opened a pad, placed it on a plate, filled a measuring cup with water and poured 500 mL onto the pad. It absorbed all of the water; none spilled onto the plate. When I tried the same experiment with the second brand of pads, it held about 400 mL before water started spilling onto the plate. I didn't continue experimenting with additional pads. Because the third brand was easier to invaginate and held more water during the brief experiment, I switched and started using it. It certainly was not perfect, but I had fewer problems with it than with the first two brands that I tried. At the time of the comparison, the third brand (Assurance) also cost $3 less per package (of 52 pads) than the second brand.

After switching over to regular use of iPads, I didn't develop a urinary tract infection for the next year and three months. When I did develop a UTI, I don't believe that it had anything to do with the pad (the UTI began seven hours after a new nursing aide gave me a sponge bath during which she grabbed hold of the glans penis with a washcloth she had used cleaning my buttocks).

Chapter 61
Postural Problems

"Bowed by the weight of centuries he leans
Upon his hoe and gazes on the ground,
The emptiness of ages in his face,
And on his back, the burden of the world."— Edwin Markham,
"The Man with a Hoe" (a poem about Jean-François Millet's 1863 paint-
ing with the same name)

During 24 years with MS, weakness and spasticity progressively
impaired my posture until my back was so bent over that my
silhouette began to resemble a question mark, if not the famous
painting of "The Man with a Hoe."

But poor posture is more than an aesthetic concern. Some of
my postural problems have included worsening pain in the back
and ribs throughout the day, acute worsening of this pain when
trying to walk with a walker, and an intense right upper quadrant
pain from flopping forward (presumably gouging my liver with ribs).
Slumping over also puts more stress, wear and tear on the joints of
my sole functional arm, causing worse pain and disability. Slouching
forward makes imbalance worse and makes it harder to stand up

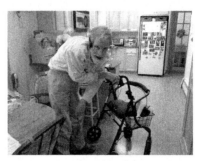

Figure 61-1 The author's posture is slumped by MS weakness and spasticity as he maneuvers with his walker.

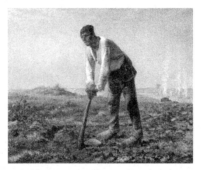

Figure 61-2 *The Man with a Hoe*, an 1863 painting by Jean-François Millet, shows a similarly slouched posture.

and get dressed, to maneuver with a walker, or to use a handheld urinal. It's harder to look forward when walking, to look in a mirror, to watch a movie, to search for infections, to apply heat to a furuncle, to check the success of a heat application, to shave a beard, etc. Slouched posture can make a Skype session difficult because the other person sees only the top of your head.

I also have had more frequent trigeminal neuralgia when bent forward, and regurgitation and aspiration of stomach contents increased as my posture got worse.

Chapter 62
How Does an MS Patient with Hemiparesis Keep Walking?

"It brings on many changes."—M*A*S*H theme song
"Come on baby, do the locomotion." "The Locomotion," - Grand
Funk Railroad

With difficulty. My hemiparesis started with my first attack and remained present for 24 years, but the extent of the problem changed over time, requiring me to change many times. First I walked without a visible limp. Next I walked with a limp. Then I had to use a cane to walk outdoors but still did okay indoors. The next stage was holding onto and leaning against walls. After that, I started using a rollator walker and grab bars.

When a patient with hemiparesis has such bad weakness and spasticity of the paretic arm that it becomes difficult to use a rollator walker with two hands, should the patient stop trying to walk with the walker? My answer to this question is both yes and no, depending upon the situation. When I first started having problems with my paretic hand losing the grip on the walker, this caused me to fall several times. If falling and fracturing bones is a predictable

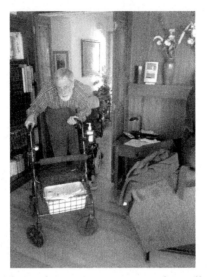

Figure 62-1 The author maneuvering with a rollator walker
from a motorized wheelchair to a power recliner.

outcome, then walking with the walker may be too hazardous for
that patient. But my weakness and spasticity fluctuated hour to
hour and day to day and I kept trying to use the walker. By doing
that, I learned that I could keep going using only the stronger arm
if I would push the walker forward about one step, set the brake and
then take a step with each foot before pushing the walker forward
another step. In doing this, I have to be careful to lock the hip of my
paretic leg before I shift my weight with each step. Such progress
may appear tedious, but it has worked for me.

Chapter 63
Time

"Time is different here." – Thomas Mann, *The Magic Mountain*

In his novel, Slaughterhouse Five, Kurt Vonnegut talks about his protagonist Billy Pilgrim getting stuck in a "chronosynclastic infundibulum"– a fictional time warp.

MS patients have significant problems with time. They begin to move so slowly that they feel like tortoises trying to keep up with rabbits.

A physical therapist watching me walk in my 21st year of MS said my gait was "incompatible with life." It's worse now.

In a jungle – real or urban – a slow moving MS patient can be "easy pickin's." In my town, a paralyzed patient was assaulted and robbed in his apartment by an acquaintance who admitted to police that he did it because "it was so easy."

Chapter 64
Wheelchair Issues

"Pride goeth before destruction, and an haughty spirit before a fall." –Proverbs 16:19

When to Get One

The optimal time is whenever walking becomes difficult, which most patients don't want to admit. A physical therapist recommended that I get a motorized wheelchair before I absolutely needed it so that I could practice using it before I became so disabled that practicing would be difficult. Since then, I have heard about patients doing the latter and crashing their motorized chairs into a wall. As recommended, I started learning how to use it while I was still able to do that. I used it increasingly over the years, with one of the first heavy uses being whenever company was in the house, because company and the distractions that socializing entails often resulted in falls. Being in a motorized wheelchair made falling less likely when interacting with people. And when I got to the point that I just could not keep walking around the house with the walker, I was already adept at driving it around, which facilitated conversion.

Should the Patient Have Difficulty Walking throughout the Day before Getting a Wheelchair?

No, if the patient has difficulty walking any time during the day, the wheelchair is necessary for safety during that time.

Are all wheelchairs pretty much the same?

I don't have as much experience with wheelchairs as some, but I have owned one manual wheelchair (Breezy made by Sunrise Medical) and two motorized wheelchairs (Quantum 600 made by Pride Mobility and Quickie QM -710 made by Sunrise Medical). The manual wheelchair was very handy for maneuvering while traveling by airplane or car provided someone was present who could fold it up and prepare it for being carried in the trunk or in the hold of the airplane and able to push the chair at our final destination. It has also been useful for going outside because it is light and goes over the threshold more easily. If I am suddenly stricken with urinary or fecal urgency on finishing a meal, it is safer to proceed to the bathroom in the manual wheelchair than to try to maneuver with my walker to the motorized wheelchair.

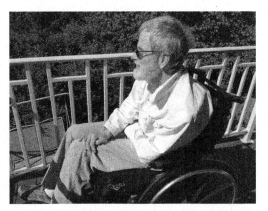

Figure 64-1 The author enjoying some sunshine in a manual wheelchair while sitting on an alternating air cushion.

I have used the motorized wheelchairs for getting around inside my house after hemiparesis made it hard to walk. The general design of the two wheelchairs was similar with a control panel located on the armrest of my sole functional arm. A toggle switch is used by both for going backwards and forwards, steering, and turning. The two chairs seemed to have comparable maneuverability and precision of guidance with the toggle stick. A problem that I have encountered with both chairs was that the control panel will occasionally do things I don't want when accidentally bumped. This problem is at least 100 fold more frequent with the Sunrise Medical chair than with the Pride Mobility chair (e.g., turning the chair on when off, changing the speed, causing the chair to move, etc.). One reason for this is that the former has raised buttons that are easier to bump. Another reason is that the control panel sits up at a 45° angle above the armrest while the control panel for the Pride Mobility chair sticks straight out.

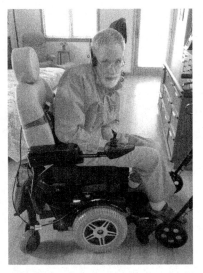

Figure 64-2 The author in a motorized wheelchair, again sitting on an alternating air cushion.

My feet also slide off of the Sunrise Medical foot rest more easily than they do off of the Pride Mobility foot rest.

Such motorized chair difficulties are not merely a nuisance. They pose significant safety hazards.

Both motorized wheelchairs occasionally locked up and would not move or respond when I pressed buttons or toggled the joystick. When I asked my neurologist and the company that provided the motorized wheelchairs, I got no clue as to what might be the reason this happened. Because motorized wheelchairs contain computer chips (like most every other modern day appliance), it seemed possible that the reason could be similar to the reason that a computer locks up with the power on and won't respond to tapping keys or moving the mouse. So, I tried the same remedy that I applied to the computer when it locked up that way: I pressed the power button and held it. The same thing happened. After some seconds of holding it, the power turned off. When I pressed power again, the wheelchairs would turn back on and operate normally. So the answer was that this was a computer problem. And being used to computers running amok, I found that doing the same thing worked the same way.

When I got my first motorized wheelchair, I was told that I would have to be measured before it could be ordered because the wheelchair should be the optimal size for the patient. When I started having trouble with my first motorized wheelchair (i.e., locking up while the power was on and becoming unresponsive to pressing buttons or moving the toggle switch), I was told that motorized wheelchairs were usually replaced after five years and that I would need a new one. Once again I was told that I would have to be measured before it could be ordered because the wheelchair should be the optimal size for the patient. After I was measured by a physical therapist who specialized in wheelchair seating, a demonstration model was brought to my house for trial. After trying the demonstration model, I told the physical therapist and salesmen accompanying her that the two wheelchairs were not the same size. The demonstration model was much larger than my first motorized wheelchair – so large that when I tried to sit down my butt did not come near the back of the seat. This meant that there was no back support until the foot rest was moved down and I climbed up into the more spacious demonstration model. I said that the demonstration model was too big for me and I preferred the smaller size of my first motorized chair, which had very good back support (after I added a lumbar cushion). The new wheelchair was ordered and delivered and was the same size as the overly large demonstration model. I was in shock. I couldn't believe that three people listening to me say that the demonstration model was too large would ignore me. I also couldn't believe that I was told that I had to be measured so that the optimal size would be ordered because the sizes of the two chairs were very different. After a couple of months of trying to get used to the new motorized wheelchair, I decided that that was hopeless and requested a modification of the chair. The supplying company moved the seatback forward about 6 inches so that when I sat down my butt rested against the seatback, providing support for my back. This change made the new chair much more comfortable, and I started using it more. The new chair had several advantages over the old chair. Its battery seemed to last longer between charges. It also had a tilt feature that allowed me to tilt the chair backwards, taking the weight off my buttocks and my back. A third advantage was a seat elevation feature, which allowed me to raise the seat when I needed to see out of a window, open the microwave above the stove, reach into a cabinet for a dish, etc. A fourth advantage was that the foot rest when closed was tucked further under the chair making it easier to stand up as my hemiparesis worsened. A fifth advantage was that the foot rest hinge could be tightened with one hand with a 6 mm allen wrench (the Pride foot rest is also tightened with a 6 mm allen wrench but requires two hands [one hand keeping the nut still at the other end of the hinge].).

Tightening the foot rest hinge is mandatory (not optional), because a foot rest that flops down and cannot be positioned out of the way traps a wheelchair user in the chair. This means that transferring to the toilet can be impossible. This could cause a desperate situation if a wheelchair user gets left home alone. The foot rest hinge on each of my motorized wheelchairs gets loose and has to be tightened regularly.

The government believes that an MS patient should be allowed to have only one device for assisting with locomotion (i.e., a cane, a walker, a manual wheelchair, or a motorized wheelchair, depending upon the degree of disability). There are a number of problems with this position on the part of the government, most important being that this is bad medical care. The reason that is bad is that a patient being paralyzed should be practicing using the motorized wheelchair before complete paralysis, at which point getting used to operating the chair is more difficult. Moreover, there are times when a motorized chair is needed before the patient becomes fully paralyzed (worse times of the day, some days worse than others, times when friends or family are visiting making distraction and falling more likely if the MS patient is trying to socialize without the safety of the motorized chair, etc.). It's also important to note that problems develop with anything and when the motorized chair stops working and has to be repaired, there has to be a fallback way of moving around, which requires the availability of other devices such as a manual wheelchair. When the patient needs to be using the motorized wheelchair most of the day, there is still a need to be using a walker if the patient is able to get up and walk with a walker because that is an important form of exercise and stretching of the arms and legs that helps counteract the accumulating spasticity. If the patient is not doing that, the spasticity can get so bad that it becomes an irreversible process making contractured extremities more likely.

Other wheelchair issues: 1) Ball bearings started spilling from the casters (these look like tiny BBs that I have noticed dropping onto the floor or just lying near where the wheelchair has been). Each time this happened I just had casters replaced (the first time all four and the next time just the front two casters). 2) Battery charging and replacements: when I bought my first motorized wheelchair (mostly paid for by health insurance for patients with paralysis due to MS), I was told to optimally recharge the battery daily and that the usual lifespan of such a battery was one year. I followed directions, recharging it frequently and the battery was clearly failing at nine months but I got it to limp along for the rest of the year before calling for a replacement battery. With the second battery, I decided to try letting it discharge almost fully each time before being recharged (the Pride Quantum wheelchair has a battery indicator that lets you know when it's getting very low). This approach seemed safe to try since I had no intention of taking the wheelchair outside and motoring across the countryside. After 9.7 years, the second battery was still working like new. 3) As discussed above, I used alternating air cushions to prevent pressure related problems on the buttock of my paretic leg. One of those problems was discomfort. The alternating air cushion has worked well in this way, except when placed on the hard seat pan of a motorized wheelchair, where it was less comfortable than when placed on the seat cushion of a regular chair. I was surprised at this discomfort, which I called the Princess and the Pea phenomenon since I seemed to be sensing the hard seat pan through the alternating air cushion. This applied to both motorized wheelchairs but was worse with the Sunrise Medical chair—presumably something about the design because the hard seat pans were equally hard. To see whether interposing another cushion between the seat pan and the alternating air cushion would fix this problem, I ordered a Sammons Preston Gel Right checkerboard wheelchair seat cushion (three-quarter inch depth) and fixed it to the hard seat pan with Velcro. (One has to be careful to avoid using anything so thick it makes the cushion fall off the chair.) I then placed an alternating cushion on top of the Gel Right cushion and was surprised to find that a new cushion so thin could solve the problem (because most medical hypotheses turn out to be false). It worked. I was able to sit on the wheelchair for hours without discomfort (i.e., very different).

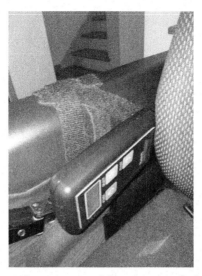

Figure 64-3 The armrest of the motorized wheelchair with the remote control device of the alternating air cushion fixed to it with Velcro straps.

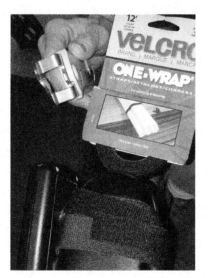

Figure 64-4 The shears and type of Velcro used by the author to fix the remote control device of the alternating air cushion to the armrest of the motorized wheelchair using only one hand.

Chapter 65
Walker Related Issues

O ccasionally it's important to tighten the brakes. But it's important to understand that tightening the brakes won't solve the problem if the wheels are slipping because of dirt or MiraLAX powder. Tightening the brakes in that situation would be counterproductive because tightening the brakes too much can cause problems for the walker and wheels slipping due to dirt or powder won't stop slipping until they are cleaned. The way I have cleaned them is with a paper towel damp with water, followed by a dry paper towel. This approach was more labor-intensive than the next approach that I found to be helpful. If my nurse helper sprays Swiffer wet jet mop liquid on the floor, I can, while in a wheelchair, maneuver my walker over the wet area enough to mostly clean the four wheels.

After figuring that out, I began using this much quicker way of cleaning wheelchair tires as well.

After four years of using an Evolution brand walker (Sprite Grande model), I decided to buy a second one just in case the company was considering canceling the model and so it would be available immediately if the first one became irreparably damaged in one of my falls.

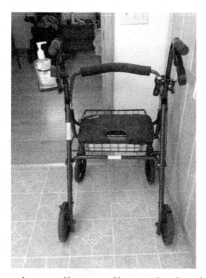

Figure 65-1 The author's rollator walker with a bottle of Purell hand sanitizer mounted near the left hand grip for hand sanitizing when needed, an LED flashlight mounted near the right hand grip for navigating at night when needed, and a cell phone mounted just below the seat on the right side for emergency communications.

Shopping by telephone, I was told that the model was still identical to the one I had purchased four years earlier. When the new walker arrived, I was disconcerted to find that the handles had been changed from foam grips to hard rubber grips. This change made it harder for my spastic paretic left hand to grasp the grip and the hard rubber also got chilly in the winter and summer (the latter from air conditioning). The problem with chilly handles is that they increase my spasticity and urinary urgency if I am proceeding toward the bathroom with a full bladder. After contemplating this problem for a while, I inquired about the availability of foam walker handles at Evolution. They were available, but with shipping costs were 10 times more expensive than foam bicycle handles the same size. I tried the latter and they worked great.

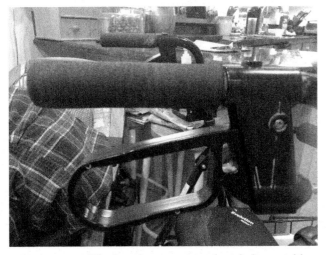

Figure 65-2 Walker handgrips covered with foam rubber, easier for my paretic, spastic hand to grip.

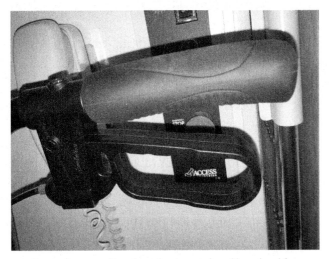

Figure 65-3 Walker handgrip made of hard rubber, harder for my paretic, spastic hand to grip.

Chapter 66

Why Is Shearing Skin on the Buttock a Problem for Hemiparetic MS Patients? Can It Be Prevented?

Intact skin provides protection against infection from microbes in the environment. Shear injury leaves a hole in the skin, which is important whenever and wherever it occurs.

This complication happens more frequently in patients with advancing paresis for multiple reasons. Flesh of the paretic leg becomes flaccid and less able to withstand the ordinary pressures of sitting on the butt. Skin on the paretic leg also becomes more friable and easily torn. How does shear injury differ from the pressure-related problems discussed in Chapter 28? Pressure sores and pressure-related furuncles usually occur from increased pressure and sitting too long without moving. Shear injury usually occurs from increased pressure while moving. This can reportedly occur when sitting on a variety of surfaces, but after 24 years of MS, I have only experienced shear injury when trying to get up off the toilet.

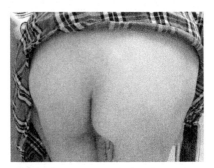

Figure 66-1 The atrophic, sagging flesh of the left
buttock in a leg being paralyzed by MS is obviously
less robust than the flesh of the right buttock.

I should probably acknowledge that the average MS patient
might not be able to distinguish a furuncle from a pressure sore
from a shear injury. In my case, this was easy (partly because I was
a physician) because a furuncle never looks like the other two; it
starts as a small, red, painful "pus bump," defined by Webster's
Dictionary as "a painful circumscribed inflammation of the skin
or a hair follicle usually caused by a staphylococcal infection." I
have only had two pressure sores, one on a knee and the other on a
shoulder (after being left lying on the floor all night); both looked
like impressive, large blood blisters the following day and remained
intensely red as superficial layers of skin died over the next few
days, leaving shallow ulcers. By contrast, my shear injuries always
occurred on the buttock of my paretic leg and looked and felt like
2- to 3-cm diameter blebs of torn skin without the discoloration or
pain associated with my pressure sores. Having said that, the two
conditions could overlap (e.g., with shear contributing to a pressure
sore). A physician (especially a dermatologist) might be helpful in
the differential diagnosis of skin lesions (i.e., telling them apart).

Why might rising from the toilet cause shear injury? Possible
contributors include the following: 1) The toilet seat is harder than
most chair cushions and the bed mattress. 2) The butt can also
become plastered to the surface of the toilet seat (this becomes

more frequent with duration of sitting, heat, humidity, etc.), making friction during the movement of getting up more likely; when temperature and humidity are right, it doesn't take long for fragile skin to become stuck to the toilet seat (e.g., about five minutes seems sufficient). 3) When a normal healthy person rises from the toilet, she stands straight up (like a helicopter taking off). By contrast, when a person with hemiparesis tries to get up from the toilet, she can't rise straight up and has to try to get up by grabbing something like a grab bar with the stronger arm and pulling. This makes the body's first motion horizontal, not vertical. Think of this as being more like an airplane trying to take off, or more precisely like a glider taking off, which has no motor of its own and is being pulled by something else. To make the analogy more exact, think of the glider being pulled despite having no wheels so that the fuselage is being severely scraped along the runway.

When jerked horizontally across a toilet seat, fragile skin stuck to the toilet seat can be torn. I did this 3 times before figuring out how this worked (the tears getting larger each time). These injuries occurred after 16 years of MS, which had made my paretic left leg weak enough that this could happen. But I was still in sufficiently good shape that I was able to find the tear using a mirror and apply polymixin, neomycin and bacitracin ointment and a Band-Aid to get the tear to heal. A little bit further into the disease and I would not have been able to do that without assistance.

After I understood how the shear was occurring, I was able to stop it from happening by adjusting my position on the toilet seat before trying to get up. For the next seven years, it didn't happen.

The probability that this sequence happened by chance (i.e., three months [25%] with new shear injury to the buttock during 12 months of not routinely adjusting my position as compared with none [0%] in the next 84 months while routinely adjusting my position before trying to get up from the toilet) was 0.0019, Fisher's exact test, 2 tailed. This means that this change was unlikely to have been due to chance (i.e., the change probably prevented new shear injuries).

Chapter 67
Is MS Stigmatizing?

My first inclination is to say that I don't know. But I was told this by another MS patient right after I was diagnosed, and I have since heard others say that. For example, I was listening to a national MS Society telecast and heard a speaker say that an MS patient told someone at work about his diagnosis and word started spreading, which began "hurting business." That sounds like stigma.

My only real experience with this phenomenon probably occurred only in reverse (i.e., something good happened because I didn't make my diagnosis public knowledge). Why did I avoid making it public knowledge? Because of what the other MS patient told me.

In the seventh year after being diagnosed, I was nominated to be president of a national scientific society for a third year in a row (The Society for Healthcare Epidemiology of America). I was elected.

If I had announced the diagnosis, I doubt that I would have been nominated once, much less three times and doubt still more that I would have been elected. Even if the reasons were innocent (e.g., some might think that a person with such a serious illness shouldn't be bothered with the mundane trivia of governing a scientific society), they would likely prevent nomination and election.

But MS patients have a disease that can impair the brain and one's ability to function in a variety of ways. Concern about these things could certainly prompt someone to vote for a different candidate. And then there's stigma, something more invidious, which also would tend to prevent nomination and election.

All I can advise is that patients should be aware of this possibility and think about how much they should reveal when and to whom.

Appendix 1
Two final notes about the MS
Patient's Sluggish Colon

First

Chapter 7 stated that the MS patient's sluggish colon usually produces smaller bowel movements, I should note that my paretic colon
still seems capable of more work than it usually performs. How do I
know? Is this just imagination and poetic license (e.g., as in Wallace
Stevens' famous line, "Let be be finale of seem")? No, under a couple
of circumstances, my colon definitely performed more vigorously
than it had for years.

While my colonic function declined over 13 years, I got treated
with high-dose methylprednisolone (500 mg per day) for MS relapses,
and during this treatment my colon always became more vigorous
and produced larger bowel movements (not looser, just larger).

After a particularly bad fracture that occurred with a fall as
I was maneuvering toward the bathroom, I sat on the toilet for
about 20 minutes trying to recover from nausea and dizziness
that followed the fall. I then had the largest bowel movement my
colon had produced in more than a decade (easily twofold larger
than the usual largest bowel movement I had had during the last
year – far larger than the mild [10%-20%] increase that occurred
with high-dose steroid treatment). It was amazing to see that my
colon remained capable of producing such a large bowel movement.
Even more unexpected, I had to have a second bowel movement
(about half the size of the first one) before I could finish wiping my
bottom after the first. Taken together, these observations imply that
the paretic spastic colon is capable of producing more under certain

conditions (e.g., high-dose steroid therapy and perhaps the effects of the autonomic nervous system on the colon following a large fracture with a lot of pain).

I mentioned that the paretic colon may be capable of more than it usually displays not because there is something obvious an MS patient can do about this but because understanding the biology can help with figuring out a new approach. Someone else may someday look at this appendix and use it to figure out a new approach.

I should probably also add that it's not surprising that weak, spastic colonic muscles can achieve more than their usual output because my weak, spastic leg muscles also can achieve more than their usual output (i.e., long after volitional ability to raise my left leg was gone, spasticity could cause the same leg muscles to raise my left leg straight out like a ballet dancer and hold the leg straight out for a full minute [until my spastic bladder finished voiding, ending a crisis of urinary urgency]).

Second

When an MS patient suffers hours of tenesmus, increased urinary urgency, and urinary incontinence because of a "bowel movement" parked in the rectum, there may be multiple reasons for this misery. One could be the precise location of the parking space – close enough to the anus to cause bladder problems, but too far from the anus to allow the bowel movement to proceed to completion. Are there medical studies showing this? Not that I have seen. Then how do I know? Whenever I have felt desperate enough to resort to digital stimulation to stimulate defecation and end the misery, that's usually where the stalled bowel movement seemed to be located.

Appendix 2
Where Does MS Come from?

"Nothing comes from nothing, nothing ever could..."
– The Sound of Music

This is usually true of disease causation (e.g., smoking causes lung cancer, human immunodeficiency virus (HIV) causes AIDS, *Mycobacterium tuberculosis* causes tuberculosis, etc.). But before medical science determines the cause of a disease, it is said to have unknown cause. And after the cause is discovered, it often turns out that multiple factors contribute to causation as discussed in Chapter 1. For example, HIV causes AIDS, but multiple risk factors make acquiring HIV significantly more likely.

Diseases can be caused by something in a patient's genes or environment. For MS, the etiology is multifactorial, and both genes and environmental factors contribute. The general rate of MS in the U.S. population is about one per thousand. The rate of MS in children of a parent with MS is about 2% (a 20-fold increase). The concordance rate of MS in identical twins is 30%. The concordance rate in dizygotic (fraternal) twins is 5%. The rate of MS in children of parents who both have MS is almost as high as the concordance rate of identical twins. These data show that one's genes play an important role in risk for developing MS, but also that genes are not the only cause (i.e., if genes were the only cause, the concordance rate in identical twins would be 100%).

Patients with ancestors from northern Europe, especially Scotland, are more likely to develop MS than those with ancestors from southerly climes. An MS patient's spouse and adopted child develop MS at the rate of the general population, showing that the illness is not contagious from one person to another and that the reason an MS patient's children are at increased risk is their genes, not their residence in the house with an MS patient.

Most patients diagnosed with MS have never had anyone else in the family that had the disease (this is called "sporadic" MS, to be distinguished from familial MS [i.e., those patients with somebody in the family that had MS before them]). Sporadic and familial MS don't seem to differ in any important way. [Tipimeni A, et al. MRI characteristics of familial and sporadic multiple sclerosis patients. *Multiple Sclerosis.* 2012.]. In a couple of large studies, the proportion of MS patients with a positive family history ranged from 20% to 26%.

Migration studies show that those moving before puberty develop MS at the rate generally observed in the area to which they are moving, whereas those moving after puberty develop MS at the rate generally observed in the area from which they moved. Such studies suggest that the environment may play an important role in the risk for developing MS.

What are some environmental factors that make MS more likely? Most but not all ecological studies have found that the rate is higher in those living in latitudes further from the equator, which have less solar intensity. Why is that? It was proposed in 1974 that this could be due to less solar intensity resulting in less vitamin D. Since that time, multiple studies have reported increased risk of MS with less sunlight exposure and with lower vitamin D levels.

A recent American study confirmed the association with latitude, but found that the association weakened in recent decades as MS risk increased in the American South. Why might that be? Don't know, but if southerners were more worried about getting melanoma and avoiding sun exposure, something like that could possibly contribute. There are other exceptions – Lapps in Scandinavia and Inuits in Alaska have low rates of MS. The Inuits get little sun exposure but get plenty of vitamin D from their subsistence on marine fish and mammals.

In a very large cohort study of nurses, those who took vitamin D supplements larger than 400 IU per day had a 41% reduction in risk of developing MS vs nonusers. [Ascherio A, Munger KL. Environmental risk factors for multiple sclerosis. Part II: noninfectious factors. *Ann Neurol* 2007; **61:** 504–13.] In a very large study of American military personnel, soldiers with serum vitamin D levels greater than 99.1 nmol/L had a 62% reduction in risk of developing MS as compared with those in the lowest quintile of serum vitamin D levels. [Munger KL, Levin LI, Hollis BW, Howard NS, Ascherio A. Serum 25-hydroxyvitamin D levels and risk of multiple sclerosis. *JAMA* 2006; **296:** 2832–38.]

Month of birth has also been suggested as a factor that affects MS risk. In a pooled analysis of data from Canada, the UK, Denmark, and Sweden including more than 40 000 individuals with MS, significantly fewer (8·5%) people with MS were born in November and significantly more (9·1%) were born in May.[Willer CJ, Dyment DA, Sadovnick AD, Rothwell PM, Murray TJ, Ebers GC. Timing of birth and risk of multiple sclerosis: population based study. *BMJ* 2005; **330:** 120.] The proposed reason that month of birth might be a risk factor is different sun exposure during different seasons, implying that risk for MS may begin in utero before birth. This association has been confirmed by multiple but not by all studies of this question.

Obesity has been linked to lower serum vitamin D levels and two cohort studies found that obesity at the end of adolescence (i.e., 18 to 20 years of age) was associated with a twofold higher risk of developing MS. [Munger KL, Chitnis T, Ascherio A. Body size and risk of MS in two cohorts of US women. Neurology. 2009; 73:1543-50.]

In a study of 129 patients with presumed early MS, smokers were 80% more likely to progress to definite MS than were non-smokers. [Di Pauli F, Reindl M, Ehling R, Schautzer F, Gneiss C, Lutterotti A, O'Reilly E, Munger K, Deisenhammer F, Ascherio A, Berger T. Smoking is a risk factor for early conversion to clinically definite multiple sclerosis. Mult Scler. 2008 Sep;14(8):1026-30. doi: 10.1177/1352458508093679. Epub 2008 Jul 16.]

In another study, patients with high Epstein-Barr virus titers were 40% more likely to develop MS. [Simon KC, et al. Epstein-Barr virus neutralizing antibody levels and risk of multiple sclerosis. Multiple sclerosis. 2012; 18:1185-7.]

Knowing that genes, latitude, sun exposure, vitamin D levels, smoking, and viral infections all may influence development of multiple sclerosis, it seems unlikely that dietary saturated fat could be the primary cause. If increased dietary salt is another risk factor for autoimmune diseases such as multiple sclerosis, [Kleinewietfeld M, et al. Sodium chloride drives autoimmune disease by the induction of pathogenic TH 17 cells. *Nature*. 2013; 496:518-22.] as some recent studies suggest, then it seems even less likely that dietary saturated fat could be the primary cause.

The reader may wish to know whether the author was an obese smoker born in May who never went out in the sun. I was born in November, never smoked, didn't have infectious mononucleosis, never took vitamin D supplements until after developing MS, and up until the age of 18, had lots of sun exposure and was not overweight. But at the age that the two cohort studies suggested was more important than one's entire adult life, I went off to college and joined a fraternity where dessert was routinely served and eaten by all. My family had not routinely eaten dessert, so this was a new norm for me. Over the next two years, I routinely ate dessert and got much less sun exposure, spending lots of time in the library (I had a 4.0 GPA in college, partly from spending so much time in the library). I gained 10 to 15 pounds during that time of dietary excess, "the freshman 15." From college, I went to medical school, where I continued to get little sun exposure and my weight slowly returned to baseline. After medical school I became a resident physician at the University of Virginia and continued to get very little sun exposure (e.g., during the first year of medical residency, we were on call every third night and got one day off every third week). After medical residency, I did a fellowship in infectious diseases, which again was very busy, allowing little time for sun exposure. After the ID fellowship, we moved to London for a couple of years, where I was a graduate student and researcher in epidemiology, which allowed little time to be outside, and the outside in England had little solar intensity. It has been said that physicians make it through the years of medical education and training through deferred gratification.

Exposure to sunlight was one of the things I deferred. And even after training was completed, life remained hectic as an assistant professor and associate professor climbing an academic ladder with clinical, teaching and research responsibilities, leaving little time for the great outdoors.

Appendix 3
When Does MS Start?

Mean age at the first attack of MS in women is 24 years and in men is 29 years, but the disease usually begins well before the first clinically evident attack. This isn't unusual, since most diseases begin before the patient is aware that anything is happening. For infectious diseases, the period from the time a microbe infects the patient until symptoms begin is called the incubation period. For cancer, the disease usually begins well before symptoms start. For atherosclerotic cardiovascular disease, the initial deposition of fat in arterial walls can begin as early as adolescence. The mean age of a first heart attack is 66 for men and 70 for women.

When did my MS begin? My first recognized attack occurred 6 weeks after I turned 40 years of age. At the time an MS patient is diagnosed with a first attack, there is often considerable evidence of old MS lesions detectable by MRI. That was true for me.

So, when did the disease actually start? Some data suggest that timing of a mother's pregnancy affects risk for her fetus later developing MS (perhaps because of sun exposure and vitamin D levels). In some patients, the first attack of MS begins in childhood, implying that the disease can begin very early in life. A number of studies suggest that environmental exposures before the midteens can be critical in determining risk for developing MS, also suggesting that disease pathogenesis could begin that early. It's thus possible that MS may begin years to decades before the first attack makes MS obvious.

Before 40, I was not aware of having any MS symptoms. But some things happened earlier that, in retrospect, now seem suspicious. When I was 20, I was doing push-ups and, for no apparent reason, my left arm buckled. I fell on the floor. I wondered why that happened, but no physician thought it was anything but a fluke. Knowing that my first clinically evident attack prominently involved my left arm and that lots of old, non-enhancing MS plaque was already present in my cervical spinal cord at that time, I now wonder whether early bits of disease caused the fall.

When I was 21, I was playing basketball and the toe of my left foot turned under as I took a step causing a fourth left metatarsal fracture. At the time, neither I nor any of the physicians helping me thought the fracture was due to due to anything but accidental trauma. 22 years after onset of MS, I was walking toward the bathroom with my walker and the toe of my left foot turned under as I took a step causing a fourth left metatarsal fracture.

When that happened, I couldn't help noticing the similarity of the two incidents. Because the second incident was obviously related to foot drop in my left leg caused by MS, I began to wonder whether the first incident could have been related to the cryptic, subclinical phase of MS affecting the left side of my cervical spinal cord.

Six months before onset of my first attack, I was walking through a mile of hallways from the parking garage to my office and the toe of my left foot dragged the floor a single time (i.e., foot drop), almost tripping me. It was extremely rare for me to have headaches, but I had one over the next few days. I called a neurologist and told him what happened. He advised me to go jogging and if everything seemed normal while jogging to forget the single misstep and the headache as mere flukes. I felt fine jogging and followed his advice, but now wonder in retrospect whether early bits of disease were already operating and somehow causing the single misstep and the headache (my left leg was compromised by my first attack and is very weak and spastic 24 years later).

I asked multiple neurologists whether a single incident such as foot drop in the months to years before recognized onset of the disease could have been due to MS. Each time, I was told, "no." They said neurologic symptoms of MS always lasted for more than 24 hours. What they were telling me is definitely the party line.

But with MS, a single incident of foot drop after weeks to months of no foot drop has caused me to fall lots of times. The fact that foot drop happened intermittently always made the fall unexpected. If this happens after the first recognized, full-fledged attack, why not before? Especially since an MS patient (like me) can have a large number of MS plaques visible on MRI at the time the first recognized, full-fledged attack occurs. Those plaques presumably were causing damage to the central nervous system – recognized or unrecognized. It seems possible that such damage could potentially cause an occasional incident of foot drop.

And it wasn't just my observations of unexplained occurrences that I later regarded as suspicious. Several people also said things implying that they may have observed abnormalities before I was aware of them when I considered myself completely well.

For example, when I was 16, a swimming team coach working with several team members on the butterfly stroke commented privately that my trunk seemed unusually stiff. I had spent four months in a body cast because of three vertebral compression fractures several months before and assumed that that might be the explanation.

When I was 23 years old, I was a freshman in medical school and ran in a race against one of our professors who challenged our class to have four of us each run 2 miles as part of a relay team running a total of 8 miles and he would run the entire 8 miles. I had the fastest qualifying time on the team and ran first. I lapped the professor. But after running 2 miles, I felt an unusual tightness in my legs. Not long after that several of my classmates and I met with a cardiology professor for a clinical correlation session. As part of the session, he asked for one of us to get on his treadmill and walk. I volunteered. When I started walking on the treadmill, the professor said, "he's spastic." My classmates dismissed what the professor said, assuring him that I was the fastest runner in the class, assuming that that meant I couldn't be ill.

After getting married at 25, I spent more time with my wife than with anybody else, and she had many opportunities to observe possible abnormalities in motion. When I was about 27, we took a walk holding hands, and she said that my hand kept coming up rather than just hanging down in a relaxed fashion. With spasticity, an arm often flexes at the elbow, which would cause the hand to rise. In retrospect, decades later, I have to wonder whether this reflected an early manifestation of MS.

At about the same age, we signed up for a dance class and danced together during each of the sessions. When we were dancing, she said something about stiffness that reminded me of what the swim coach had said 11 years earlier. I felt completely well at the time and didn't know what to think about the comment.

A year later, I was doing something that required very little strength, but my wife noted that I was grimacing as I did it as if it required great strength. Again, I didn't know what to make of the comment. I told her that I hadn't intended to make a face – that any face made was non-volitional. In retrospect, once again, I have to wonder whether this was an early manifestation of the disease because spastics often grimace when doing all sorts of trivial things.

Index

86, 176, 276, 283, 284, 286, 289, 291, 292, 321, 322, 326

digital stimulation 86, 88, 89, 91, 92, 113, 398

direct sustained pressure 114, 129

dressing 40, 75, 124, 227, 300, 301, 354, 371

dysarthria xxiii, 179, 334, 336

dysphagia xxiii, 40, 157, 248, 252, 255, 256, 336

dyssynergic defecation 90, 130

E

edema 104, 142, 155, 209, 264, 269, 306, 356

electronic tablets 368

epidemiologist xxvii, 23, 26, 137

epidemiology xv, 1, 2, 21, 27, 233, 256, 261, 394, 402

exercise xxv, 5, 8, 13, 27, 38, 40, 57, 59, 138, 145, 146, 147, 171, 172, 173, 174, 175, 176, 177, 193, 194, 214, 217, 219, 251, 252, 307, 308, 311, 312, 318, 328, 385

F

falling vii, 32, 41, 54, 58, 69, 79, 84, 111, 112, 134, 146, 147, 149, 156, 182, 183, 204, 218, 219, 220, 221, 222, 223, 224, 225, 227, 228, 230, 240, 243, 247, 267, 268, 271, 275, 281, 306, 307, 308, 309, 310, 314, 348, 349, 356, 360, 363, 365, 378, 380, 385

falls xvii, 6, 27, 54, 69, 71, 85, 119, 134, 135, 139, 143, 149, 150, 152, 155, 156, 158, 162, 163, 171, 180, 183, 191, 196, 198, 199, 201, 204, 207, 211, 218, 219, 220, 221, 222,

223, 224, 225, 226, 227, 247, 261, 263, 265, 266, 268, 269, 274, 277, 282, 306, 307, 308, 309, 331, 332, 339, 347, 349, 350, 351, 354, 356, 357, 358, 363, 365, 378, 380, 386, 389, 397, 406, 407

fatigue xxviii, xxx, 19, 27, 28, 34, 37, 38, 42, 43, 59, 61, 145, 146, 188, 305, 308, 310, 361

fecal incontinence 6, 83, 84, 86, 89, 93, 96, 98, 121, 122, 123, 124, 125, 168, 228, 237, 238, 260, 261, 263, 271, 272, 309, 363

feculent odor xvii, 251, 281, 283, 284, 285, 287, 288, 289, 290, 293, 294, 295, 297, 302

fiber xxiv, 33, 36, 69, 72, 73, 75, 76, 77, 78, 81, 85, 86, 104, 113, 282, 326

flannel patch 202

flatus xvii, xxv, 113, 129, 281, 282, 283, 284, 286, 288, 289, 290, 291, 293, 294, 295, 297, 302, 303, 337, 338

food poisoning 98, 121, 163, 240, 243, 273, 274

fracture xvii, 30, 31, 32, 46, 47, 58, 64, 90, 92, 93, 135, 136, 138, 139, 140, 143, 144, 149, 150, 151, 156, 163, 166, 171, 185, 194, 196, 197, 198, 199, 200, 201, 204, 211, 212, 221, 223, 224, 227, 240, 247, 261, 305, 306, 307, 308, 309, 310, 318, 319, 327, 343, 344, 347, 348, 349, 350, 351, 352, 397, 398, 406, 407

fractures xvii, 30, 31, 32, 46, 47, 58, 64, 90, 92, 93, 135, 136, 138, 139, 140, 143, 144, 149, 150, 151, 156, 163, 166, 171, 185, 194, 196, 197, 198, 199, 200, 201, 204, 211, 212,

120, 135, 208, 243, 247, 256, 259,
348, 361
suicide 61, 62, 63
swallowed air xxi, 249, 335, 337, 338,
339, 340

T

tenesmus 79, 86, 97, 123, 124,
339, 398
testimonial xviii, 4, 24, 234
tomato juice 32, 40, 152, 156, 157,
158, 159, 243, 259, 340, 346
torn rotator cuff xxv, 5, 140, 161,
166, 167, 314, 315, 316, 328
transient relaxation of the lower
esophageal sphincter 342

U

Uhthoff's phenomenon xviii, 147,
160, 161, 167, 176, 227, 353
urinal 68, 101, 115, 119, 153, 154,
324, 376
urinary incontinence 33, 37, 64, 80,
83, 91, 101, 102, 104, 116, 119, 121,
122, 135, 228, 291, 304, 306, 310,
372, 398
urinary tract infection xviii, 6, 19,
31, 32, 34, 35, 37, 107, 125, 126,
241, 242, 245, 258, 259, 260, 261,
262, 263, 264, 277, 279, 324, 325,
326, 374
urinary urgency xviii, xxx, 6, 8, 11,
33, 74, 77, 80, 82, 83, 84, 86, 87,
91, 95, 96, 102, 103, 104, 105, 106,
109, 110, 111, 112, 113, 114, 115,
116, 117, 118, 119, 120, 122, 124,
135, 158, 167, 179, 180, 185, 189,
190, 197, 198, 206, 222, 231, 259,
277, 304, 306, 307, 308, 309, 310,

325, 339, 340, 341, 358, 360, 362,
389, 398
urine dipstick 279, 280, 325

V

vaccine 2, 25, 26, 27, 246, 252,
332, 333
Valsalva maneuver 88, 111, 114,
129, 308

W

walker 5, 6, 46, 47, 57, 58, 64, 110,
115, 119, 122, 123, 135, 136, 141,
153, 154, 162, 177, 183, 196, 200,
201, 212, 221, 222, 223, 224,
227, 229, 230, 231, 243, 287, 307,
308, 309, 312, 339, 360, 375, 376,
377, 378, 381, 385, 388, 389, 390,
391, 406
warm moist compress xvii, 90,
136, 168, 237, 238, 270, 271, 272,
277, 278
weakness xviii, xxiv, xxx, 29, 38, 46,
58, 63, 67, 68, 82, 89, 139, 147, 148,
149, 156, 161, 164, 170, 171, 172,
174, 175, 176, 177, 179, 181, 183,
185, 186, 188, 219, 220, 221, 223,
229, 238, 241, 243, 244, 253, 274,
305, 307, 308, 310, 311, 328, 336,
337, 348, 353, 354, 356, 375, 376,
377, 378
wheelchair xxiv, 5, 42, 47, 52, 58, 114,
115, 116, 122, 138, 190, 204, 229,
269, 278, 350, 362, 363, 368, 369,
378, 380, 381, 382, 383, 384, 385,
386, 387, 388

Z

About the Author

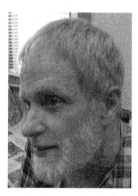

Dr. Barry Farr was Professor of Medicine and Hospital Epidemiologist at the University of Virginia as well as President of The Society for Hospital Epidemiology of America before retiring due to MS. After 24 years of battling MS, he wrote *Multiple Sclerosis: Coping with Complications* to help other patients cope, sharing strategies he developed that helped him.

CPSIA information can be obtained
at www.ICGtesting.com
Printed in the USA
LVOW04s1743070616

491605LV00010B/247/P